Handbook of
Kidney
Transplantation

Handbook of Kidney Transplantation

Third Edition

Edited by

GABRIEL M. DANOVITCH, M.D.

Medical Director, Kidney Transplant Program,
UCLA Medical Center; Professor, Department
of Medicine, UCLA School of Medicine,
Los Angeles, California

LIPPINCOTT WILLIAMS & WILKINS
A **Wolters Kluwer** Company
Philadelphia · Baltimore · New York · London
Buenos Aires · Hong Kong · Sydney · Tokyo

Acquisitions Editor: Timothy Y. Hiscock
Production Editor: Melanie Bennitt
Manufacturing Manager: Colin J. Warnock
Cover Illustration: Patricia Gast
Compositor: Circle Graphics
Printer: R.R. Donnelley—Crawfordsville

Library of Congress Cataloging-in-Publication Data

Handbook of kidney transplantation / edited by Gabriel M. Danovitch.—3rd ed.
    p. ; cm.—(LWW handbook series)
  Includes bibliographical references and index.
  ISBN 0-7817-2066-4
  1. Kidneys—Transplantation—Handbooks, manuals, etc. I. Danovitch, Gabriel M. II. Series.
  [DNLM: 1. Kidney Transplantation. WJ 368 H236 2000]
  RD575 .H236 2000
  617.4'610592—dc21

                         00-032255

Care has been taken to confirm the accuracy of the information presented and to describe generally accepted practices. However, the authors, editor, and publisher are not responsible for errors or omissions or for any consequences from application of the information in this book and make no warranty, expressed or implied, with respect to the currency, completeness, or accuracy of the contents of the publication. Application of this information in a particular situation remains the professional responsibility of the practitioner.

The authors, editor, and publisher have exerted every effort to ensure that drug selection and dosage set forth in this text are in accordance with current recommendations and practice at the time of publication. However, in view of ongoing research, changes in government regulations, and the constant flow of information relating to drug therapy and drug reactions, the reader is urged to check the package insert for each drug for any change in indications and dosage and for added warnings and precautions. This is particularly important when the recommended agent is a new or infrequently employed drug.

Some drugs and medical devices presented in this publication have Food and Drug Administration (FDA) clearance for limited use in restricted research settings. It is the responsibility of the health care provider to ascertain the FDA status of each drug or device planned for use in their clinical practice.

10 9 8 7 6 5 4 3

Cover: Schematic diagram of the structure of a representative class I MHC molecule (HLA-A2). The α_1 and α_2 domains form a peptide-binding site with the binding groove, which faces the T-cell receptor at the top (see Chaps. 2 and 3). (This remarkable structure is described in detail by PJ Bjorkman, MA Saper, B Samraoni, et al. Structure of the human class I histocompatibility antigen, HLA-A2. *Nature* 1987; 329:506. Reprinted with permission.)

For Nava, my "emotionally-related" spouse,
And for our "1-haplotype–matched" children,
Itai, Roy, and Yaël

Contents

Contributing Authors ix

Preface xiii

1. Options for Patients with End-Stage Renal Disease 1
   William G. Goodman and Gabriel M. Danovitch

2. Transplantation Immunobiology 17
   J. Harold Helderman and Simin Goral

3. Histocompatibility Testing, Crossmatching, and
   Allocation of Cadaveric Kidney Transplants 39
   Steven Katznelson, Steven K. Takemoto, and J. Michael Cecka

4. Immunosuppressive Medications and Protocols
   for Kidney Transplantation 62
   Gabriel M. Danovitch
   Part I: Immunosuppressive Agents in Current Clinical Use
   Part II: Biologic Immunosuppressive Agents
   Part III: Clinical Trials and New Immunosuppressive Agents
   Part IV: Immunosuppressive Protocols

5. Living and Cadaveric Kidney Donation 111
   H. Albin Gritsch, J. Thomas Rosenthal,
   and Gabriel M. Danovitch

6. Evaluation of the Transplant Recipient 130
   Elizabeth Kendrick

7. The Transplant Operation and
   Its Surgical Complications 146
   H. Albin Gritsch and J. Thomas Rosenthal

8. The First Two Posttransplantation Months 163
   William J. C. Amend, Jr., Flavio Vincenti, and
   Stephen J. Tomlanovich

9. Long-Term Posttransplantation Management
   and Complications 182
   Bertram L. Kasiske
   Part I: Causes of Late Allograft Failure
   Part II: Management of Recipients in the Late
           Posttransplantation Period

10. Infectious Complications of Kidney Transplantation
    and Their Management 221
    Bernard M. Kubak, David A. Pegues, and Curtis D. Holt

11. Hepatitis in Kidney Transplantation 263
    Fabrizio Fabrizi and Paul Martin

12. Diagnostic Imaging in Kidney Transplantation 272
    Peter Zimmerman, Nagesh Ragavendra, Carl K. Hoh,
    and Zoran L. Barbaric

13. Pathology of Kidney Transplantation 290
    Cynthia C. Nast and Arthur H. Cohen

14. Kidney and Kidney–Pancreas Transplantation in
    Diabetic Patients 313
    John D. Pirsch and Hans W. Sollinger

15. Kidney Transplantation in Children 332
    Samhar I. Al-Akash and Robert B. Ettenger

16. Psychiatric Aspects of Kidney Transplantation 365
    Kirk Murphy

17. Ethical and Legal Issues in Kidney Transplantation .. 380
    Leslie Steven Rothenberg

18. Nutrition in the Kidney Transplant Recipient 394
    Susan Weil Guichard

19. Psychosocial and Financial Issues in Kidney
    Transplantation 411
    Marcy H. Gitlin, Terri H. Sayama, and Robert S. Gaston

Subject Index 421

Contributing Authors

Samhar I. Al-Akash, M.D. *Associate Director, Department of Pediatric Renal Transplantation, UCLA–Mattel Children's Hospital; Clinical Instructor, Department of Pediatrics, UCLA School of Medicine, Los Angeles, California 90095*

William J. C. Amend, Jr., M.D. *Professor of Clinical Medicine, Department of Medicine, Kidney Transplant Program, University of California at San Francisco, San Francisco, California 94143*

Zoran L. Barbaric, M.D. *Chief, Department of Abdominal Imaging, UCLA Medical Center; Professor, Department of Radiological Sciences, UCLA School of Medicine, Los Angeles, California 90095*

J. Michael Cecka, Ph.D. *Professor, Department of Pathology, UCLA School of Medicine, Los Angeles, California 90095*

Arthur H. Cohen, M.D. *Attending Pathologist, Cedars Sinai Medical Center; Professor, Departments of Pathology and Medicine, UCLA School of Medicine, Los Angeles, California 90095*

Gabriel M. Danovitch, M.D. *Medical Director, Kidney Transplant Program, UCLA Medical Center; Professor, Department of Medicine, UCLA School of Medicine, Los Angeles, California 90095*

Robert B. Ettenger, M.D. *Professor, Department of Pediatrics, Head, Department of Pediatric Nephrology, and Vice Chairman, Clinical Affairs, UCLA School of Medicine, Los Angeles, California 90092*

Fabrizio Fabrizi, M.D. *Staff Nephrologist, Department of Nephrology, Maggiore Policlinico Hospital, Milano, Italy 20122*

Robert S. Gaston, M.D. *Professor of Medicine and Surgery, Department of Transplantation, University of Alabama at Birmingham, Birmingham, Alabama 35214*

Marcy H. Gitlin, M.S.W., L.C.S.W. *Lecturer, Department of Psychiatry and Biobehavioral Sciences, UCLA / NPI; Clinical Social Worker, Department of Social Services and Kidney Transplant Program, UCLA Medical Center, Los Angeles, California 90095*

William G. Goodman, M.D. *Associate Director, General Clinical Research Center, UCLA Medical Center; Professor, Department of Medicine, UCLA School of Medicine, Los Angeles, California 90095*

Simin Goral, M.D. *Staff Physician, Department of Nephrology, Vanderbilt University Medical Center; Assistant Professor, Department of Nephrology, Vanderbilt University School of Medicine, Nashville, Tennessee 37232*

H. Albin Gritsch, M.D. *Surgical Director, Department of Urology, Renal Transplant Program, UCLA Medical Center; Associate Professor, Department of Urology, UCLA School of Medicine, Los Angeles, California 90095*

J. Harold Helderman, M.D. *Medical Director, Department of Medicine, Vanderbilt Transplant Center; Professor, Departments of Medicine, Microbiology, and Immunology, Vanderbilt University School of Medicine, Nashville, Tennessee 37240*

Carl K. Hoh, M.D. *Assistant Professor, Departments of Molecular and Medical Pharmacology and Radiological Sciences, UCLA School of Medicine, Los Angeles, California 90095*

Curtis D. Holt, Pharm.D. *Assistant Clinical Professor, Department of Surgery, Liver and Pancreas Transplant Program, UCLA Medical Center, Los Angeles, California 90095*

Bertram L. Kasiske, M.D. *Chief, Department of Nephrology, Hennepin County Medical Center; Professor, Department of Medicine, University of Minnesota College of Medicine, Minneapolis, Minnesota 55455*

Steven Katznelson, M.D. *Transplant Nephrologist, Department of Transplantation, California Pacific Medical Center, San Francisco, California 94115; Associate Professor, Department of Medicine, University of California at Davis, Sacramento, California 95619*

Elizabeth Kendrick, M.D. *Transplant Nephrologist, Kidney Transplant Program, UCLA Medical Center; Clinical Instructor, Department of Medicine, UCLA School of Medicine, Los Angeles, California 90095*

Bernard M. Kubak, M.D., Ph.D. *Associate Professor, Department of Medicine–Infectious Diseases, UCLA School of Medicine, Los Angeles, California 90095*

Paul Martin, M.D. *Director, Department of Hepatology, Dumont–UCLA Transplant Program, UCLA Medical Center; Associate Professor, Department of Digestive Diseases, UCLA School of Medicine, Los Angeles, California 90095*

Kirk Murphy, M.D. *Attending Psychiatrist, Department of Psychiatry, UCLA Medical Center; Assistant Clinical Professor, Department of Psychiatry, Neuropsychiatric Institute, UCLA School of Medicine, Los Angeles, California 90095*

Cynthia C. Nast, M.D.   *Attending Pathologist, Department of Pathology, Cedars Sinai Medical Center; Professor, Department of Pathology, UCLA School of Medicine, Los Angeles, California 90095*

David A. Pegues, M.D.   *Epidemiologist, Department of Infectious Diseases, UCLA Medical Center; Associate Clinical Professor, Department of Infectious Diseases, UCLA School of Medicine, Los Angeles, California 90095*

John D. Pirsch, M.D.   *Director, Medical Transplantation Service, Departments of Medicine and Surgery, University of Wisconsin Hospital and Clinics; Professor, Departments of Medicine and Surgery, University of Wisconsin Medical School, Madison, Wisconsin 53792*

Nagesh Ragavendra, M.D.   *Chief, Ultrasound Section, UCLA Medical Center; Professor, Department of Radiological Sciences, UCLA School of Medicine, Los Angeles, California 90095*

J. Thomas Rosenthal, M.D.   *Transplant Surgeon, Renal Transplant Program, UCLA Medical Center; Professor of Surgery, Department of Urology, UCLA School of Medicine, Los Angeles, California 90095*

Leslie Steven Rothenberg, J.D.   *Director, Program in Medical Ethics, UCLA Medical Center; Associate Professor, Department of Clinical Medicine, UCLA School of Medicine, Los Angeles, California 90095*

Terri H. Sayama, L.C.S.W.   *Clinical Social Worker, Department of Social Services and Kidney Transplant Program, UCLA Medical Center, Los Angeles, California 90095*

Hans W. Sollinger, M.D., Ph.D.   *Chairman, Department of Surgery and Organ Transplantation, University of Wisconsin Hospital and Clinics; Folkert O. Belzer Professor, Department of Surgery, University of Wisconsin Medical School, Madison, Wisconsin 53792*

Steven K. Takemoto, Ph.D.   *Associate Adjunct Professor, Department of Pathology, UCLA School of Medicine and UCLA Immunogenetics Center, Los Angeles, California 90095*

Stephen J. Tomlanovich, M.D.   *Clinical Professor, Department of Medicine, Kidney Transplant Program, University of California at San Francisco Medical Center, San Francisco, California 94143*

Flavio Vincenti, M.D.   *Professor, Department of Medicine, Kidney Transplant Program, University of California at San Francisco Medical Center, San Francisco, California 94143*

Susan Weil Guichard, M.D.   *Department of Medicine, Dialysis Unit, UCLA School of Medicine, Los Angeles, California 90024*

Peter Zimmerman, M.D.   *Staff Radiologist, Department of Radiology, West Los Angeles Veterans Affairs Medical Center; Assistant Professor, Department of Radiology, UCLA School of Medicine, Los Angeles, California 90095*

Preface

Four years elapsed between the publication of each of the three editions of the *Handbook of Kidney Transplantation*. This rapid pace reflects the dizzying rate of change in the world of organ transplantation. Exciting discoveries continue to advance our understanding of the immunobiology of the alloimmune response. Donor-specific tolerance and xenotransplantation, once topics of a transplantation fantasy-world, now appear to be attainable goals. New and potent immunosuppressive agents are being tested in clinical trials and introduced into clinical practice. Innovative surgical techniques have helped expand the donor pool. The success rate of kidney transplantation continues to improve.

Yet all the news is not good. The demand for cadaveric organs grows inexorably while the supply remains essentially stagnant. The last decade has seen the waiting time for cadaveric organs lengthen from months to years and many dialysis patients wait with frustrated anticipation, and their condition often deteriorates before a kidney becomes available for them. Attempts to expand the donor supply by the use of "marginal" kidneys may lead to the acceptance of organs for transplantation whose long-term function is intrinsically limited.

Transplant immunosuppression, always a potentially dangerous but once a relatively uncomplicated undertaking, has become more complex. New, effective, and potent agents have been introduced based on their short-term impact before their long-term benefits or optimal use has become firmly established. The transplant practitioner is faced with a varied array of protocol options, yet remains limited in his or her capacity to individualize therapy. Chronic allograft failure remains largely beyond therapeutic bounds and cardiovascular disease, cancer, and infection are constant threats to long-term survival.

The third edition of the *Handbook of Kidney Transplantation* reflects these changes. Each chapter has been thoroughly updated and new chapters on viral hepatitis and the social and financial implications of transplantation have been added. Like its predecessors, this edition is designed to make the rapidly changing world of kidney transplantation fully accessible to those who are entrusted with the care of our long-suffering patients with end-stage kidney disease.

Gabriel M. Danovitch

Handbook of
Kidney
Transplantation

1

Options for Patients with End-Stage Renal Disease

William G. Goodman and Gabriel M. Danovitch

Before 1970, therapeutic options for patients with end-stage renal disease (ESRD) were limited. Only a small number of patients were receiving regular dialysis because few dialysis centers had been established. Patients underwent extensive medical screening to determine their eligibility for ongoing therapy, and treatment was offered only to patients with renal failure as the predominant clinical management issue. Those with other systemic illnesses in addition to ESRD were not considered for chronic dialysis therapy. Kidney transplantation were in their early stages of development as a viable therapeutic option. Transplant immunology and immunosuppressive therapy were in their infancy, and for most patients, a diagnosis of chronic renal failure was a death sentence.

In the decade that followed, the availability of care for patients with ESRD grew rapidly throughout the medically developed world. In the United States, the passage of Medicare entitlement legislation to pay for maintenance dialysis and for renal transplantation provided the major stimulus for this expansion.

Despite advances in knowledge and skill in treating chronic renal disease, patients with ESRD often remain unwell even when maintained by regular dialysis. Constitutional symptoms of fatigue and malaise persist despite the dramatic improvement that followed the introduction of erythropoietin for the management of the anemia of chronic renal disease. Progressive cardiovascular disease (CVD), peripheral and autonomic neuropathy, bone disease, and sexual dysfunction are common even in patients who receive adequate amounts of dialysis as judged by established objective criteria. Patients may become dependent on family members or others for physical, emotional, and financial assistance. Rehabilitation, particularly vocational rehabilitation, remains poor. Such findings are not unexpected, however, because the most efficient hemodialysis regimens currently provide only 10% to 12% of the small-solute removal achieved by two normally functioning kidneys. Removal of higher-molecular-weight solutes is even less efficient.

For most patients with ESRD, kidney transplantation offers the greatest potential for restoring a healthy, productive life. Renal transplantation, however, does not occur in a clinical vacuum. All transplant recipients have been exposed, at least to some degree, to the consequences of ESRD. Practitioners of kidney transplantation must consider the clinical effects of ESRD on the overall health of renal transplantation candidates when this therapeutic option is first considered. They must also remain aware of the potential long-term consequences of previous ESRD (see Chapter 6) throughout what may be decades of successful posttransplant clinical follow-up (see Chapter 9).

DEMOGRAPHICS OF THE ESRD POPULATION

United States

Each year, the United States Renal Data System provides updated information about the demographics of the ESRD population in the United States. The 1999 report is based on data updated through September 1998 that are complete only through December 1997. At that time, about 222,000 patients were receiving maintenance dialysis in the United States (Table 1.1). This number increased at an annual rate of 6% from 1992 to 1997, and it is expected to rise by at least another 4% in subsequent years. The average age of the dialysis population continues to increase each year. Nearly half of patients undergoing regular dialysis are older than 65 years of age, and the mean age of those beginning dialysis is 62 years. This phenomenon has been described as the "gerontologizing" of nephrology, and it is reflected in the increasing age of patients being evaluated for renal transplantation (see Chapters 3 and 6).

In the ESRD population, men slightly outnumber women, and about one third of patients are black. Despite improvements in the clinical management of both diabetes mellitus and hypertension, these two diagnostic categories remain the most common causes of ESRD. Indeed, the percentage of diabetic patients in the United States ESRD population is rapidly approaching 50%.

Table 1.1.   Demographics of the dialysis population in the United States (percentage of new patients in 1997)

Demographic	Percentage
Age (yr)	
<20	<1
20–44	18
45–64	37
65–74	26
>75	19
Sex	
Male	53
Female	47
Race	
Black	37
White	56
Asian	3
Native American	2
Cause of end-stage renal disease	
Diabetic nephropathy	38
Hypertension	28
Glomerulonephritis	13
Cystic kidney disease	3
Other[a]	18

[a] Nearly 10% of patients with end-stage renal disease have a failed transplant.
From: United States Renal Data System. Excerpts from the 1999 Annual Data Report. *Am J Kidney Dis* 1999;34 (Suppl 1), with permission.

Older patients and those with diabetes are more likely to be accepted for dialysis in the United States than in other countries. In addition, patients beginning dialysis in the United States have more comorbid medical conditions than those accepted for treatment in the 1980s. Congestive heart failure is present in 35% of the incident dialysis population, whereas coronary artery disease can be found in up to 40% in some series.

In contrast to the steady rise in the number of patients receiving regular dialysis, the number of cadaveric kidney transplantations performed each year has grown only marginally to about 9,000 in 1999. The number of living donor transplantations has increased to about 4,000 per year, largely as a result of transplants from donors who are not biologically related (see Chapter 5). As a result, the number of patients receiving dialysis who are awaiting cadaveric renal transplantation is progressively rising, and exceeded 45,000 at the beginning of 2000. The gap between the supply of and the demand for cadaveric donor kidneys is illustrated graphically in Fig. 1.1. Consequently, the average waiting time for a cadaveric renal transplant has increased substantially, and it is now measured in years (see Chapter 3).

Worldwide

Compared with the United States, most countries have a lower incidence of treated ESRD (Fig. 1.2). This difference reflects, in part, the high incidence of ESRD in blacks in the United States. Other factors, such as limitations on the availability of dialysis for elderly patients in some countries, also play a role. There is no age restriction for providing dialysis in the United States, and this helps explain the steady rise in the average age of the U.S. dialysis population.

Modalities for the management of ESRD vary among countries. In the United Kingdom, Australia, and Canada, home dialysis is used extensively, whereas this therapeutic approach is uncommon in Japan. Age is an important factor for patient selection in many countries. Renal transplantation rates from both cadaveric and living donors vary considerably among industrialized countries (Fig. 1.3). Certain legal constraints and cultural barriers to the acceptance of brain-death criteria or living donation (see Chapters 5 and 16) are important determinants of national transplantation rates.

TREATMENT OPTIONS FOR ESRD: DIALYSIS

Hemodialysis

Hemodialysis is the predominant technique for treating ESRD throughout the world. The procedure can be done either in medical facilities specifically designed for this purpose or in the patient's home. When performed in a dialysis facility, hemodialysis treatments typically range in length from 2.5 to 5 hours, and they are usually done three times a week. For highly motivated patients with a suitable living environment and a willing assistant, usually a spouse, hemodialysis can be done at home, freeing the patient from the need to visit a dialysis center and to adhere to a rigid treatment schedule.

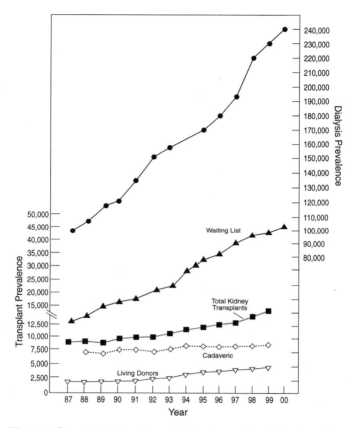

Fig. 1.1.   Comparative numbers of patients receiving dialysis and awaiting and receiving transplants in the United States between 1987 and 2000. (From United States Renal Data System 1999 and United Network for Organ Sharing.)

During dialysis, solutes are removed by diffusion across a semipermeable membrane within a dialyzer, or artificial kidney, from blood circulated through an extracorporeal circuit. Fluid retained during the interval between treatments is removed by regulating the hydrostatic pressure across the membrane of the dialyzer. Most hemodialysis machines now control fluid removal, or ultrafiltration, using volumetric systems controlled by electronic microcircuits to ensure accurate and predictable results. Hemodialysis is generally well tolerated, although ultrafiltration can cause hypotension, nausea, and muscle cramps. Older patients and those with established CVD may tolerate the procedure less well. Vascular access failure from repeated cannulation procedures and the need for intermittent heparinization to prevent clotting in the extra-

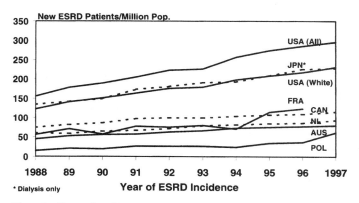

Fig. 1.2. Treated end-stage renal disease incidence rates per million population for Australia, Canada, selected European countries, Japan, and the United States for 1988 through 1997. (From United States Renal Data System 1999.)

corporeal blood circuit are additional concerns, particularly in diabetic patients. The intermittent nature of hemodialysis treatment, which results in rapid changes in extracellular fluid volume, blood solute concentrations, and plasma osmolality, may contribute to postdialysis fatigue and malaise.

Most dialysis membranes are cellulosic, and they provide reasonably efficient removal of low-molecular-weight solutes. Urea clearances of 180 to 240 mL/min are readily achieved during hemodialysis. The efficiency of solute removal declines markedly, however, as molecular weight increases. Thus, the clearance of vitamin B_{12}, which has a molecular weight of about 1,350 daltons, rarely exceeds 40 to 60 mL/min, a value far less than that provided by two normal kidneys.

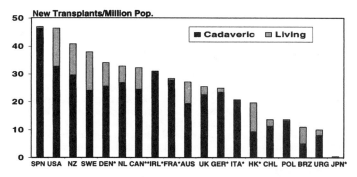

Fig. 1.3. New renal transplants per million total population for selected countries as of 1997. (From United States Renal Data System 1999.)

Although the minute-by-minute removal of low-molecular-weight solutes during hemodialysis may exceed that provided by normal endogenous renal function, the intermittent nature of hemodialysis as used in clinical practice substantially undermines the overall efficiency of this form of renal replacement therapy. Even for patients receiving 12 to 15 hours of hemodialysis per week, adequate solute clearance is provided for less than 10% of a 168-hour week. During the remaining 153 to 156 hours of each week, no additional solute removal is achieved unless there is some residual endogenous renal function. This residual function needs to be considered when recommending native kidney nephrectomy before transplantation (see Chapter 6).

Concerns regarding dialysis efficiency and adequacy have received considerable attention in the nephrology literature in recent years, particularly with respect to their effects on patient morbidity and mortality. Annual mortality rates in the United States are higher than in Europe, where the average weekly duration of hemodialysis is considerably longer. The decline in annual mortality in the United States ESRD population in recent years corresponds temporally with educational efforts to raise clinician awareness about the need for more efficient weekly dialysis prescriptions and with the more widespread use of objective measures of dialysis efficiency to monitor ongoing therapy. Whether these developments will continue to affect favorably the annual mortality rate for ESRD patients in the United States remains to be determined.

Hemodialysis requires access to the patient's circulation to provide continuous blood flow to the extracorporeal dialysis circuit. For ongoing hemodialysis therapy, an autologous arteriovenous (A-V) fistula is the most reliable type of vascular access. Long-term patency is greatest with A-V fistulas, and the incidence rates of thrombosis and infection are low. A-V grafts that use synthetic materials are often placed in elderly patients and in diabetic patients whose native blood vessels may not be adequate for the creation of a functional A-V fistula. Complication rates are considerably higher, however, with grafts than with fistulas. Thrombosis is a recurrent problem, and it frequently occurs because of stenosis at the venous end of the graft, where it forms an anastomosis with the native vein. Infections and the formation of pseudoaneurysms are more common with grafts than with fistulas.

Temporary venous dialysis catheters are used to establish vascular access when hemodialysis must be started urgently. Other venous catheters, designed to be used over longer intervals, have been increasingly used as a method for providing vascular access in patients undergoing regular hemodialysis, particularly when treatment is first begun or when permanent access sites require surgical revision. Reliance on these approaches should be limited, and permanent access should be established using A-V fistulas or A-V grafts as soon as ESRD is deemed to be inevitable. Stenotic lesions in large proximal veins in the thorax are an increasingly recognized complication of indwelling venous dialysis access catheters. These may involve the subclavian and innominate veins and the superior vena cava. Their presence can interfere with successful placement of permanent vascular access by producing venous hypertension that interferes with venous blood return from A-V fistulas or grafts. The sustained use of venous dialysis access catheters should be avoided.

Peritoneal Dialysis

Peritoneal dialysis is a widely practiced alternative to hemodialysis that exploits the fluid and solute transport characteristics of the peritoneum as an endogenous dialysis membrane. It can be done either as *continuous ambulatory peritoneal dialysis* (CAPD) or as *continuous cycling peritoneal dialysis* (CCPD). Access to the peritoneal cavity is achieved by surgically placing a Silastic catheter (often called 'Tenckhoff' catheter) of varying design through the abdominal wall. Surgery is done several weeks before starting treatment, and patients are subsequently trained to perform their own dialysis procedures.

Peritoneal dialysis is accomplished by instilling a specified volume of peritoneal dialysis fluid, typically between 1,500 and 3,000 mL, into the abdominal cavity by gravity-induced flow, allowing the fluid to remain in the abdomen for a defined period, then draining and discarding it. During each dwell period, both solute removal and ultrafiltration are achieved. Solute removal occurs by diffusion down a concentration gradient from the extracellular fluid into peritoneal dialysate, with the peritoneal membrane acting as a functional semipermeable dialysis membrane. The efficiency of removal of small solutes is relatively low compared with hemodialysis, whereas the clearance of higher-molecular-weight solutes is somewhat greater. Ultrafiltration is accomplished by osmotic water movement from the extracellular fluid compartment into hypertonic peritoneal dialysate that contains a high concentration of dextrose, ranging from 1.50 to 4.25 gram percent. The lower rates of solute removal that characterize peritoneal dialysis are offset by prolonged treatment times.

For CCPD, an automated cycling device is used to regulate and monitor the dialysate flow into and out of the abdominal cavity. Four to 10 dialysis exchanges, ranging from 1 to 3 L each, are done nightly over 8 to 10 hours. A variable amount of dialysate is left in the abdomen during the day to provide additional solute and fluid removal. For CAPD, dialysis is done 24 hours a day, 7 days a week, using manual exchanges of peritoneal dialysate four or five times per day.

Peritoneal dialysis has certain advantages over hemodialysis, including the maintenance of relatively constant blood or serum levels of urea nitrogen, creatinine, sodium, and potassium. Hematocrit levels are often higher than for patients receiving hemodialysis, and gradual and continuous ultrafiltration may provide better blood pressure control. Because it is a form of self-care, peritoneal dialysis promotes patient independence.

The major complication of peritoneal dialysis is bacterial peritonitis. Its frequency varies considerably among patients and among treatment facilities, but it occurs with an average frequency of one episode per patient per year. When bacterial peritonitis is diagnosed promptly and treatment is immediately begun, infections are generally not severe, and they resolve within a few days with appropriate antibiotic therapy. Episodes of peritonitis are an ongoing threat, however, to the long-term success of peritoneal dialysis, and they can lead to scarring of the peritoneal cavity and to the loss of the peritoneum as an effective dialysis membrane. In the past, gram-positive organisms, such as *Staphylococcus epidermidis* or *Staphylococcus aureus,* accounted for most cases of peritonitis, but almost half of episodes are now due to gram-negative bacteria. Fungal peritonitis typically causes extensive intra-abdominal scarring and fibrosis, and it often leads to the failure of peritoneal dialysis as an effective mode of treatment.

With few exceptions, there are no particular medical advantages of hemodialysis over peritoneal dialysis. Both effectively manage the consequence of uremia (Table 1.2). Matters of individual lifestyle and other psychosocial issues should be considered when selecting a particular mode of dialysis. Home hemodialysis provides an opportunity for independence and rehabilitation, but it can be a cause of substantial emotional stress for the dialysis assistant and other family members. In some home settings, neither hemodialysis nor peritoneal dialysis is advisable. In-center hemodialysis can provide ongoing social interaction for older, single patients with few friends or family members available for support.

Table 1.2.   Comparison of hemodialysis and peritoneal dialysis

	Hemodialysis	Peritoneal Dialysis
Advantages	Short treatment time Highly efficient for small solute removal Socialization occurs in the dialysis center	Steady-state chemistries Higher hematocrit Better blood pressure control Dialysate source of nutrition Intraperitoneal insulin administration Self-care form of therapy Highly efficient for large solute removal Liberalization of diet
Disadvantages	Need for heparin Need for vascular access Hypotension with fluid removal Poor blood pressure control Need to follow diet and treatment schedule	Peritonitis Obesity Hypertriglyceridemia Malnutrition Hernia formation Back pain

Technical Advances in Dialysis

Numerous technical and procedural advances have significantly improved the quality of life for patients who require renal replacement therapy by dialysis.

Hemodialysis

The development of synthetic dialysis membranes with higher hydraulic conductance and increased permeability for higher-molecular-weight solutes has made it possible to increase the overall efficiency of hemodialysis. Many of the newer hemodialysis membranes are considered to be biologically more compatible than previously used materials. Cytokine release and complement activation during dialysis are less, and these differences may have long-term benefits. The use of advanced microcircuits and automated controls in modern dialysis equipment permits precise control of the rate of fluid removal, and the capacity to vary dialysate sodium concentrations can improve tolerance of the dialysis procedure in some patients. With better mass transport characteristics, some dialyzers can achieve equivalent amounts of solute removal with shorter treatment times than older, less efficient models.

The use of high-efficiency hemodialysis has grown in popularity, particularly among patients for whom the shortened treatment time is appealing. The long-term consequences of this approach are not known, however, and there are concerns that manifestations of uremia or inadequate dialysis may develop after months or years. Indeed, guidelines for implementing and monitoring dialysis prescriptions in the United States have increasingly recognized the critical role of cumulative weekly procedure length as a key element for maintaining hemodialysis adequacy. Reports on the use of daily hemodialysis suggest that blood pressure and extracellular volume are better controlled and that overall metabolic control improves. *Such findings suggest that more dialysis is better than less dialysis.* More dialysis reduces the substantial disparity between the amount of solute removal provided by the standard thrice-weekly hemodialysis schedule and that achieved by normal endogenous renal function.

Peritoneal Dialysis

Efforts continue to lower the risk for bacterial contamination and peritonitis in patients undergoing peritoneal dialysis. The devices that establish the connections among peritoneal dialysis catheters, fluid transfer sets, and plastic bags containing peritoneal dialysate are continually being refined for both CAPD and CCPD.

Long-Term Complications of Dialysis

As survival for patients on regular dialysis improves, a number of debilitating complications of either long-term renal failure or protracted dialysis may develop, even in well-rehabilitated and medically adherent patients. As the waiting time for cadaveric renal transplants inexorably increases (see Chapter 3 and Fig. 1.1), these complications are more likely to manifest clinically. Their presence may influence the medical indications for transplantation, and they may affect the choice of renal transplantation as a therapeutic option (see Chapter 6). The longer patients receive dialysis, the greater the risk for posttransplantation morbidity and mortality. The following discussion concentrates on those long-term complications that are most relevant to the posttransplantation course.

Cardiovascular Disease

The incidence of CVD in the ESRD population has been described as reaching epidemic proportions. Factors that contribute to the excess risk for CVD can be identified even in the early stages of progressive chronic renal disease. Nearly all patients at some time during their clinical course develop hypertension, and many require multiple antihypertensive medications. The incidence of hypertension and diabetes as primary causes of ESRD is increasing more rapidly than that of other diagnoses. Proteinuria and the associated hyperlipidemia, increases in extracellular fluid volume, anemia, high plasma levels of thrombogenic factors, and homocysteine all represent additional cardiovascular risk factors. Uremia may contribute to atherogenesis and to the development of cardiomyopathy.

Patients with renal disease are at greater risk for left ventricular hypertrophy (LVH) than the general population even before ESRD becomes established. The prevalence of LVH varies directly with the degree of renal dysfunction. At the time that regular dialysis is begun, 50% to 80% of patients have LVH, and the prevalence of coronary artery disease may reach 40%.

Patients receiving regular dialysis have an adjusted death rate from all causes that is estimated to be 3.5 times higher than that of the general population. CVD accounts for 50% of this mortality, occurring at a rate of 9% per year, which is 10 to 20 times greater than in the general population. Hypertensive patients have worse outcomes after dialysis, and patients with LVH have a two- to three-fold higher death rate from cardiac causes. Progressive calcification of the coronary arteries occurs over the years spent on dialysis and can be recognized even in young adult dialysis patients. Mortality rates after myocardial infarction in dialysis patients are substantially higher than in the general population, a finding that probably reflects the severity of underlying CVD in patients with ESRD. The passage of time receiving regular dialysis represents ongoing exposure to multiple cardiovascular risk factors, and worsening myocardial function has been described, particularly during the first year of treatment. These observations may explain the finding that the longer patients spend on dialysis the worse is their long-term posttransplant prognosis (see Chapter 3.)

Renal Osteodystrophy

Secondary hyperparathyroidism and high-turnover bone disease often develop in patients with ESRD. Several factors contribute to excess parathyroid hormone (PTH) secretion in patients with renal failure. These include hypocalcemia, diminished renal calcitriol production, skeletal resistance to the calcemic actions of PTH, alterations in the regulation of pre-pro-PTH gene transcription, reduced expression of receptors for both vitamin D and calcium in the parathyroid glands, and hyperphosphatemia due to diminished renal phosphorus excretion. Progressive parathyroid gland hyperplasia often occurs. Severely affected patients experience bone pain, fractures, and hypercalcemia, and soft tissue and vascular calcifications may develop.

Low-turnover lesions of renal osteodystrophy include osteomalacia and adynamic bone. In the past, osteomalacia was found in patients with tissue aluminum accumulation, but aluminum-related bone disease is now uncommon. Most ESRD patients with osteomalacia have evidence of vitamin D deficiency, mineral deficiency, or both.

The adynamic lesion of renal osteodystrophy occurs in patients with normal or only modestly elevated serum PTH levels. It can be a manifestation of aluminum toxicity, and affected patients have bone pain, muscle weakness, and fractures. When aluminum is not the cause, patients have few symptoms, but episodes of hypercalcemia occur more often than in patients with high-turnover skeletal lesions. Adults with adynamic bone are at increased risk for vertebral fracture. Adynamic renal osteodystrophy is somewhat more common in patients undergoing peritoneal dialysis than in those treated with hemodialysis, and it often develops after the treatment of secondary hyperparathyroidism with large intermittent doses of calcitriol, or 1,25-dihydroxy-vitamin D. The effects of transplantation on uremic bone disease are discussed in Chapter 9.

Uremic Neuropathy

Peripheral neuropathy is a feature of chronic renal failure, and progressive encephalopathy will develop if appropriate renal replacement therapy is not instigated. A mild stable sensory neuropathy is common in nondiabetic dialysis patients; it is usually largely sensory and detected clinically by impaired vibration and position sense. It may be a source of pain and "restless legs." Occasionally, a devastating polyneuropathy develops that may be reminiscent of Guillain-Barré syndrome. Neuropathy may recover dramatically after successful transplantation.

Severe encephalopathy is rare in appropriately dialysed patients. Impaired concentration and memory loss may represent discrete manifestations of cognitive impairment in dialysis patients, and improvement after transplantation is gratifying. Autonomic neuropathy in nondiabetic patients receiving dialysis can be recognized by impaired heart rate variability and is also reversible after transplantation.

Neuropathy may contribute to sexual dysfunction in dialysis patients. About half of men suffer from erectile dysfunction, and menstrual disturbance and infertility are common in women. Improvement after transplantation is variable and is discussed in Chapter 9.

Amyloidosis

Patients undergoing long-term dialysis may develop a unique form of amyloidosis in which the amyloid deposits are composed of beta$_2$-microglobulin, a protein that is present normally on the surface of all cells. Beta$_2$-microglobulin is released into the circulation, freely filtered at the glomerulus, and subsequently degraded by cells of the proximal tubule. In renal failure, beta$_2$-microglobulin accumulates in the plasma, and it eventually forms amyloid deposits in various tissues.

Tendons and articular cartilage are the most common sites of beta$_2$-microglobulin deposition, and the amyloid deposits at the wrist may cause carpal tunnel syndrome. Cystic lesions at the proximal ends of long bone are frequently seen. Patients have typically been treated with dialysis for at least 5 years, and amyloid deposits can be documented in most patients after 8 years. Severe disease with joint deformity can lead to marked disability, and the clinical course is progressive. Renal transplantation may result in symptomatic improvement, but there is little evidence that amyloid deposits disappear after successful transplantation.

Interactions between blood constituents and hemodialysis membranes, particularly cellulosic membranes, are thought to promote the development of dialysis-related amyloidosis by stimulating beta$_2$-microglobulin production. Amyloid deposition can occur, however, in patients receiving peritoneal dialysis; therefore, blood–membrane contact may not be essential for its development. Lower disease prevalence has been reported with improved water purification methods during dialysate production, with certain high-permeability dialysis membranes, and with bicarbonate-containing dialysate. Only symptomatic relief is available for patients with dialysis-related amyloidosis.

Acquired Cystic Disease

Patients with chronic renal failure of any cause may develop acquired cystic disease involving the kidneys after several years of treatment by dialysis. The condition is characterized by multiple, usually bilateral, renal cysts in small, contracted kidneys and is, therefore, easily distinguishable from adult polycystic kidney disease. Cysts may become infected, bleed, or cause localized pain, and they can undergo malignant transformation. "Suspicious" cysts should be imaged at intervals, and concern about malignant transformation may be an indication for pretransplantation nephrectomy. Acquired cystic disease can occur in patients treated by either hemodialysis or peritoneal dialysis. The capacity for malignant transformation should not be forgotten in the posttransplantation period.

Dialysis Access Failure

Early referral before starting regular hemodialysis is essential for establishing optimal long-term vascular access. For patients managed with hemodialysis, reliable vascular access is a life-sustaining aspect of medical care. Vascular access failure not only threatens the near-term well-being of patients but also has long-term implications with regard to the success of ongoing renal replacement therapy. Access-related morbidity accounts for almost 25% of all hospital stays for ESRD patients and for close to 20% of the cost of ESRD care.

As discussed previously, A-V fistulas are the gold standard for long-term vascular access for hemodialysis. A-V grafts almost invariably undergo thrombosis; their 3-year cumulative patency rate has been estimated to be about 50%. Because the number of sites that are suitable for permanent vascular access placement is limited, the choice of A-V grafts for long-term vascular access conveys the risk of ultimately losing all remaining vascular access sites, rendering further hemodialysis technically impossible.

TREATMENT OPTIONS FOR ESRD: TRANSPLANTATION

The relative prevalence of the major ESRD treatment options between 1987 and 2000 in the United States is shown in Figure 1-1. Cadaveric transplantation accounts for two thirds of kidney transplantations in the United States, the remainder being from living donors. A critical shortage of donor organs is the major limitation to expanding the use of this therapeutic modality (see Chapter 3). The rate of renal transplantation varies considerably among patient groups. Transplantation rates are lower in older patients, who represent a relative high-risk group (see Chapter 6). Transplantation rates tend to be lower in black ESRD patients, partly because of biologic reasons that tend to restrict access to cadaveric organs (see Chapter 3). A tendency to restrict access to transplantation based on race, gender, insurance status, and type of dialysis center has also been described.

Patient and graft survival rates in the United States are shown graphically in Chapter 3 (see Figs. 3.4 and 3.5). Mean 1-year graft survival for all types of live donor transplants is about 95%, and in many centers, it is 90% or greater for all match grades of cadaveric transplants.

Patient Survival

Difficulties With Data Analysis

To help select the most appropriate therapeutic option for patients with ESRD, clinicians and patients are understandably interested in comparative survival rates for various treatment modalities. Such comparisons are difficult, however, because data in the literature often do not reflect the fact that patients change treatment modalities frequently and that the characteristics of patients selected for each modality may differ substantially when therapy is begun. For dialysis patients, a number of comorbid factors can adversely affect survival; these include increased age, diabetes, coronary artery disease, chronic obstructive pulmonary disease, and cancer. Overall, blacks have a better survival rate with ESRD than nonblacks, whereas certain renal diagnoses, such as amyloidosis, multiple myeloma, and renal cell cancer, are associated with poorer prognoses. Nutritional status, as measured by serum albumin and prealbumin levels, has been increasingly recognized as an important predictor of survival during long-term dialysis (see Chapter 18). If these factors are not considered, accurate comparisons among therapeutic modalities cannot be made.

Comparison of Treatment Modalities

Most of the data comparing survival rates for patients treated with hemodialysis, CAPD, and cadaveric kidney transplantation suggest that the patient's state of health before treatment, rather than the treatment modality itself, is the most important factor that determines survival. Healthier dialysis patients are more likely to be placed on the waiting list for transplantation, and these patients enjoy a reduction in the relative risk for death if they subsequently receive a transplant rather than continuing to receive dialysis. This phenomenon is illustrated graphically in Fig. 1.4, which records the relative risk for death of more than 46,000 dialysis patients who were placed on a cadaveric transplant waiting list.

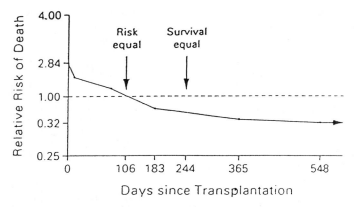

Fig. 1.4.   Adjusted relative risk for death among 23,275 recipients of a first cadaveric transplant. The reference group was 46,164 patients receiving dialysis who were on the waiting list (relative risk, 1.0). (From Wolfe RA, Ashby VB, Milford EL, et al. Comparison of mortality in all patients on dialysis, patients on dialysis awaiting transplantation, and recipients of a first cadaveric transplant. *N Engl J Med* **1999; 341:1725, with permission.)**

About half of these patients underwent transplantation, and their long-term survival rates were better. This survival benefit was detected within the first posttransplantation year despite the higher mortality rates associated with the surgical procedure and with immunosuppressive therapy. The magnitude of the survival benefit varies according to patient characteristics at the time of initial placement on the waiting list (Fig. 1.5) and is most marked in young diabetic patients.

Cost of Therapy

The annual cost of medical care for patients undergoing chronic hemodialysis in the United States is about $50,000. Medical costs during the first year after renal transplantation are considerably higher and are estimated to be nearly $100,000. The cost of care is less, however, after the first posttransplantation year compared with the cost of dialysis despite the approximately $10,000 annual cost of immunosuppressive therapy (see Chapter 19). The mean cumulative costs of dialysis and transplantation are about the same for the first 4 years of therapy. Thereafter, overall costs are lower after successful renal transplantation.

Survival by Diagnosis

When the most common causes of kidney disease are assessed using the Cox proportional hazards model, only diabetes mellitus has an adverse effect on patient survival. Other common causes of renal failure do not significantly affect survival. The survival rate of patients with ESRD due to other less common renal diseases, such as collagen vascular disease and vasculitis, is generally similar to that of nondiabetic patients with common causes of ESRD.

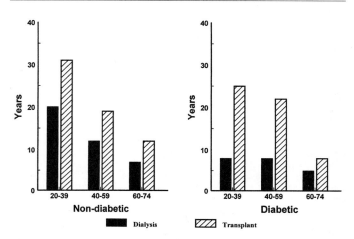

Fig. 1.5. Projected years of life for patients receiving dialysis awaiting a transplant and patients who receive a cadaveric transplant. (Modified from Wolfe RA, Ashby VB, Milford EL, et al. Comparison of mortality in all patients on dialysis, patients on dialysis awaiting transplantation, and recipients of a first cadaveric transplant. *N Engl J Med* 1999;341:1725, with permission.)

Not surprisingly, systemic and renal malignancies confer a poorer prognosis.

Quality of Life

Most studies demonstrate that the quality of life of patients receiving peritoneal dialysis exceeds that of patients receiving hemodialysis in a dialysis center. Home hemodialysis patients reportedly have a high quality of life, although selection factors, such as the level of patient motivation and the patient's overall health status at the beginning of treatment, make it difficult to attribute this higher quality of life to the modality alone.

Most dialysis patients select renal transplantation in the hope of improving their quality of life, and recipients of successful transplants consistently report a better quality of life than patients receiving regular dialysis; this includes both peritoneal dialysis and home hemodialysis. Life satisfaction, physical and emotional well-being, and the ability to return to work are all significantly better in transplant recipients than in dialysis patients. Transplantation may correct or improve some complications of uremia that are typically not fully reversed by dialysis; these include anemia, peripheral neuropathy, autonomic neuropathy, and sexual dysfunction (see Chapter 9). The quality of life after live donor transplantation compares favorably to that seen in the general population.

Initiation of End-Stage Renal Disease Therapy

An in-depth discussion of the indications for commencement of dialysis is beyond the scope of this text. Most patients with progressive renal failure develop symptoms and require treatment for ESRD when the glomerular filtration rate (GFR) falls to below 10 mL/min or the serum creatinine level increases to more than 10 mg/dL. Many patients, particularly those with diabetes, develop symptoms at lower serum creatinine levels and at higher GFR values. Hemodialysis or peritoneal dialysis access should be arranged sufficiently far in advance that treatment can be started when needed on an elective basis; patients can then be spared the suffering and risk that are inevitably associated with advanced renal failure. Because permanent vascular access for hemodialysis requires 4 to 8 weeks to mature, placement should be undertaken early so that urgent placement of temporary venous catheters can be avoided. For peritoneal dialysis, peritoneal catheter placement can be delayed until dialysis is more imminent because only 2 to 4 weeks is required before the access can be used. The decision to start dialysis is a clinical one, and it should be based not only on the plasma levels of creatinine, urea nitrogen, and electrolytes but also on a careful assessment of uremic symptoms. Outcome after dialysis is better for patients who start early rather than late.

Predialysis transplantation is discussed in Chapter 6. Predialysis patients who are placed on the cadaveric transplant waiting list and those prepared for live donor transplantation should be warned explicitly not to delay access placement and dialysis if it becomes necessary before a donor organ is available. This avoids an unduly hurried pretransplantation evaluation that can be dangerous and emotionally stressful both for patients and caregivers.

SELECTED READINGS

Ayanian JZ, Cleary PD, Weissman JS, et al. The effect of patients' preferences on racial differences in access to renal transplantation. *N Engl J Med* 1999;341:661.

Chugh KS, Jha V. Differences in the care of ESRD patients worldwide: required resources and future outlook. *Kidney Int* 1995;48:S7.

Goodman WG, Goldin J, Kuizon BD, et al. Coronary artery calcifications in young adults with end-stage renal disease who are undergoing dialysis. *N Engl J Med* 2000;342:1478.

Hakim RM, Lazarus JM. Initiation of dialysis. *J Am Soc Nephrol* 1995;6:1319.

Hariharan S, Johnson CP, Bresnahan BA. Improved graft survival after renal transplantation in the United States, 1988 to 1996. *N Engl J Med* 2000;342:605.

Holley JL, McCauley C, Doherty B, et al. Patients' views in the choice of renal transplant. *Kidney Int* 1996;49:494.

Ifudu O. Care of patients undergoing hemodialysis. *N Engl J Med* 1998;339:1054.

Luke RG, Beck LH. Gerontologizing nephrology. *J Am Soc Nephrol* 1999;10:1824.

Parfrey PS, Foley RN. The clinical epidemiology of cardiac disease in chronic renal failure. *J Am Soc Nephrol* 1999;10:1606.

Pereira BJ. Optimization of pre-ESRD care: The key to improved dialysis outcomes. *Kidney Int* 2000;57:351.

Schwab SJ. Vascular access for hemodialysis. *Kidney Int* 1999;55:2078.

Tilney NL. A crisis in transplantation: too much demand for too few organs. *Transplant Rev* 1998;12:112.

United States Renal Data System. Excerpts from the 1999 Annual Data Report. *Am J Kidney Dis* 1999;34(Suppl 1).

2

Transplantation Immunobiology

J. Harold Helderman and Simin Goral

Renal transplantation is the preferred mode of renal replacement therapy for virtually all patients with end-stage renal disease. Despite the increasing success of renal transplantation, acute and chronic transplant rejection remain major problems. New discoveries have led to a better understanding of transplant immunobiology, out of which have come a number of novel immunosuppressive regimens.

The following is a brief glossary of the terminology used by transplant immunologists to describe the cells and tissues encountered in the transplant setting. Transplantation of one's own tissue to another site is called an *autologous graft* (or *autograft*). A graft transplanted between two genetically identical individuals is called an *isogeneic* or *syngeneic graft* (or *syngraft*). A graft transplanted between two genetically different individuals of the same species is called an *allogeneic graft* (or *allograft*). A graft transplanted between members of different species is called a *xenogeneic* graft (or *xenograft*). The antigens that are recognized as foreign on allografts are called *alloantigens,* whereas those recognized as foreign on xenografts are called *xenoantigens.* The lymphocytes that recognize and respond to the alloantigens or xenoantigens are called *alloreactive* or *xenoreactive lymphocytes,* respectively.

MAJOR HISTOCOMPATIBILITY COMPLEX

Human Leukocyte Antigen

After several unique discoveries in organ transplantation, it has become clear that rejection and acceptance of a transplant are inherited characteristics. An array of inherited proteins on cell surfaces contribute to transplant rejection. The genes that encode for these proteins, termed *histocompatibility genes,* are located on different chromosomes in each species. The histocompatibility genes are responsible for the recognition of the graft as similar to one's own tissues or as foreign. Because of its central role in antigen recognition and transplant immunobiology, this group of genes has been defined as the *major histocompatibility complex* (MHC). The incompatibility of the MHC antigens between a donor and a recipient of an allograft leads to graft rejection.

Although discovered and named for the capacity to induce graft rejection, the principal immunologic function of the MHC gene product is to present antigens as fragments of foreign proteins, forming complexes that can be recognized by T lymphocytes through specific antigen receptors. In individuals, these antigen receptors are specific for foreign antigens recognized in the context of MHC molecules. Because MHC molecules are membrane associated, antigen-specific T lymphocytes can recognize fragments of the antigens only when they are bound to the surface of other cells that bear the MHC molecule. These cells that bear MHC molecules present the antigen to T cells. Mature T cells recognize and react to foreign antigens but do not react to self proteins because, during the ontogeny of the immune system, self reactive T lymphocytes are removed in the thymus by a variety of processes, including *clonal deletion,* which permits *self tolerance* (see the section on tolerance).

The MHC is a complex of genes found in all vertebrates; in humans, it has been located on the short arm of chromosome 6. The MHC genes in humans encode polymorphic cell-surface molecules, alloantigens known as *human leukocyte antigens* (HLAs). The polymorphism of HLAs involves specific hypervariable regions of the molecule and contributes both to recognition of self and to antigen binding. HLA gene products are inherited in a mendelian codominant fashion. At least six separate genes are involved in the HLA system; phenotypically, each one is represented by two codominant alleles, one from the paternal gamete and one from the maternal gamete. Developed in the gamete during meiosis and located on a single strand of parental chromosome, alleles of the HLA system constitute a *haplotype* unless a crossover has occurred (see Chapter 3). HLAs have been divided into two general types—class I and class II—according to their cellular distribution, chemical and crystallographic structure (Fig. 2.1), and immunologic function.

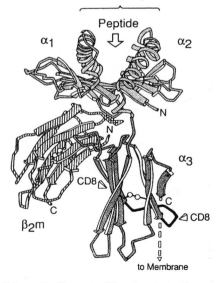

Figure 2.1.   **Schematic diagram of the structure of a representative class I major histocompatibility molecule (HLA-A2). The alpha$_1$ and alpha$_2$ domains form a peptide-binding site, with the binding groove that faces the T-cell receptor at the top. (From Bjorkman PJ, Saper MA, Samraoni B, et al. Structure of the human class I histocompatibility antigen, HLA-A2. *Nature* 1987;329:506, with permission.)**

Class I Antigens

HLA class I antigens (HLA-A, -B, and -C) are found on virtually all cell surfaces, although the concentration of these molecules varies widely. These molecules are composed of one highly polymorphic MHC-encoded polypeptide chain designated alpha (heavy) and a monomorphic chain, beta$_2$-microglobulin, encoded by genes on chromosome 15 (Figs. 2.1 and 2.2). Allospecifity of class I molecules resides in the alpha chain, a polypeptide with a prominent groove. The beta chain interacts noncovalently with the heavy chain and has no direct attachment to the cell. The aminoterminus portion of the heavy chain that extends into the extracellular space is composed of three domains: alpha$_1$, alpha$_2$, and alpha$_3$. The alpha$_1$ and alpha$_2$ domains interact to form the sides of a cleft (or groove), with a floor formed by strands of beta-pleated sheets. The cleft is the site where foreign proteins bind to MHC molecules for presentation to T cells. The size of the cleft is too small to bind an intact globular protein; therefore, native globular proteins need to be processed into smaller fragments that can bind to MHC molecules. The highly variable amino acid residues located in the groove determine the specificity of peptide binding and T-cell antigen recognition. Both class I and class II molecules bind foreign protein antigens and form complexes that are recognized by antigen-specific T lymphocytes. Class I molecules function as immunorecognition sites for endogenously synthesized foreign proteins, such as viral

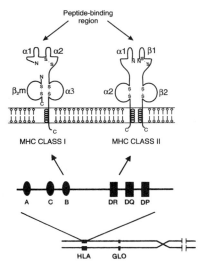

Figure 2.2. The *lower half* of the figure depicts the major histocompatibility complex class I and class II genes on the short arm of chromosome 6. The *upper half* is a schematic diagram of the class I and class II molecules, which are the transmembrane glycoprotein products of these genes. N, amino terminus of the polypeptide chains; C, carboxy terminus of the polypeptide chains; S . . S, intrachain disulfide bonds.

proteins and tumor antigens. Antigens associated with class I molecules are recognized by cytotoxic CD8+ T lymphocytes. The non-polymorphic alpha$_3$ region contains the binding sites for CD8+ T cells, which enhances the affinity of the antigen-bearing MHC with the T-cell antigen receptor (see the section on T-cell receptor [TCR]–CD3 complex).

Class II Antigens

In contrast to class I antigens, class II antigens (HLA-DR, -DP, and -DQ) have a more restricted cell distribution because they are generally expressed by *antigen-presenting cells* (APCs), such as B monocytes, macrophages, dendritic cells of lymphoid organs, renal mesangial cells, Kupffer's cells, and alveolar type 2 lining cells, and certain other elements of the immune system, such as lymphocytes and thymic epithelial cells. A subset of activated T lymphocytes may also express class II molecules. All parenchymal cells of the germline retain the genes for class II molecules. Engagement of the appropriate promoter sequences at the 5' end of the coding start site by inflammatory cytokines, such as *interferon-gamma* (IFN-gamma), can initiate coding for the synthesis of the class II protein.

Class II genes are composed of two MHC-encoded and noncovalently associated polymorphic chains (alpha and beta chains; Fig. 2.2). Each alpha and beta chain is composed of two extracellular domains (alpha$_1$ and alpha$_2$ and beta$_1$ and beta$_2$). Similar to class I molecules, x-ray crystallography reveals a spatial configuration of helices surrounding beta-pleated sheets, into which are embedded antigen-binding grooves or clefts. For class II molecules, there are two separate grooves, in contrast to the single groove for class I, formed by domains of alpha$_1$ and beta$_1$, which permit binding of peptide fragments of about 12 amino acids in length rather than the 9 for class I.

Class II molecules play a central role in the initiation of the immune response to transplantation antigens. Recognition of foreign class II molecules activates helper CD4+ T lymphocytes, which begins the process of clonal expansion and also supports cytotoxic T-cell clonal expansion by stimulating the CD4+ lymphocyte generation of regulatory cytokines (Fig. 2.3). Additionally, the class II region of the MHC contains genes, such as the *transporter in antigen processing* (TAP) *1* and *2* genes, that are necessary for the assembly of peptide fragments with the MHC and for ultimate surface expression of class I MHC molecules.

Both class I and class II antigens play essential roles in the recognition of nominal, nontransplantation antigens by the immune system. Receptors on the cells that are responsible for initial recognition of antigens recognize not only some piece of the molecular structure of the antigen but also surface proteins, which are self identifying molecules. Certain antigens are preferentially recognized in association with class I antigens, whereas other antigens are recognized in association with class II antigens. This role of self identification by the MHC is the essence of its immunoregulatory function. In rejection, allogeneic class I and class II molecules become the targets for the efferent responses of the immune system.

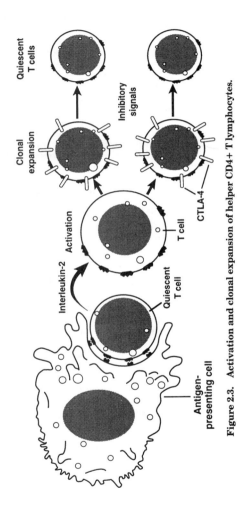

Figure 2.3.   Activation and clonal expansion of helper CD4+ T lymphocytes.

Minor Histocompatibility Antigens

The observations of rejection of skin grafts between MHC-identical mice and the development of severe graft-versus-host disease in bone marrow transplantation between MHC-identical siblings imply the existence of structures other than MHC that can be recognized by T cells to activate the immune response. As many as 20 gene regions, termed *minor loci,* encoded by a large number of chromosomes, are thought to function as *minor histocompatibility antigens* (MiHAs). There is compelling evidence that MiHAs are small endogenous peptides that occupy the antigen-binding site of self MHC molecules and can trigger T-cell responses between MHC-identical individuals. Whereas MHC antigens can be recognized by both B and T lymphocytes, responses to MiHAs appear to be strictly T-cell mediated and therefore MHC restricted. MHC restriction is the most fundamental characteristic of MiHA recognition. Most MiHAs are processed and presented to recipient T cells in association with either donor MHC or self MHC molecules. The MiHAs become important for initiating rejection in patients receiving allografts from living-related donors matched for the entire HLA. Only for transplantations between identical twins, for whom one can establish identity at both major and minor gene regions, can one dispense with the need for immunosuppression.

ALLOGENEIC RECOGNITION

The recognition of transplantation antigens by T cells is referred to as *allorecognition* or *alloresponse* and is determined by the inheritance of codominant MHC genes. Because of the resemblance of a foreign MHC molecule to an MHC molecule bound to a foreign peptide, this recognition of a foreign MHC molecule is actually a cross-reaction of a TCR that recognizes a self MHC molecule bound to a foreign peptide. As many as 2% of the host peripheral blood lymphocytes are capable of recognizing and responding to a single foreign MHC molecule. The reason for strong allograft rejection is the presence of this high frequency of T cells reactive with allogeneic MHC molecules. The principal target of the immune response to the graft is the MHC molecule itself, and T-cell allorecognition of MHC is the major event that triggers rejection.

There are at least two distinct pathways of allorecognition (Fig. 2.4). In the *direct pathway,* recipient T cells have direct allorecognition of intact MHC molecules (foreign MHC) with or without relevant antigen fragments carried in the groove of the MHC structure on the surface of donor target cells. This pathway accounts for the generation of a primary cytotoxic CD8+ T-cell response and thus plays the dominant role in early allograft rejection. The graft contains a significant number of donor-derived passenger APCs, which present intact donor MHC molecules and provide the necessary costimulatory signals to CD8+ T cells. In the *indirect pathway* of allorecognition, CD4+ helper TCRs recognize donor MHC allopeptides derived from the catabolism of donor MHC molecules after processing and presentation by self APCs. The donor MHC may be shed from the surface of parenchymal cells of the graft into the circulation to be engulfed by APCs, processed, and presented by self MHC; alternatively, phagocytic cells may encounter the donor MHC in the graft itself, where processing can be accomplished. In any case,

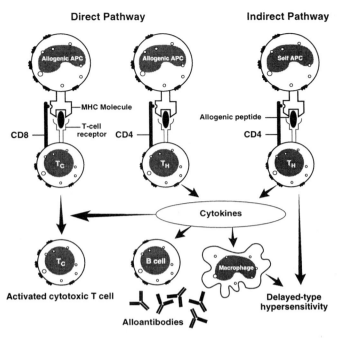

Figure 2.4. Pathways of allorecognition.

recipient APCs internalize the exogenous foreign proteins shed from the graft and process the peptides for presentation (in the context of self HLA) to T cells, thereby providing the requisite signal for lymphocyte activation. This is the usual pathway used by the immune system for the processing and presentation of nominal antigens. CD4+ helper T cells activated by the indirect pathway have been shown to initiate the effector mechanisms of rejection, which include delayed-type hypersensitivity responses, cell-mediated toxicity, and alloantibody production. Observations suggest that the indirect pathway enhances and amplifies acute rejection and is predominant for chronic rejection. Animals immunized with donor class II MHC allopeptides reject their grafts in a significantly accelerated fashion with marked vascular rejection as well as severe cellular rejection, supporting the role of indirect allorecognition in allograft rejection. After the antigen-specific TCR on the surface of the helper T cell is triggered, a series of intracellular events is initiated, culminating in the synthesis of an array of new molecules targeted to the nucleus, the cytosol, the cell membrane, and the external milieu.

T-Cell Receptor–CD3 Complex

T cells express protein receptors that specifically bind the peptide–MHC complexes. The TCR is a heterodimer that consists of two polypeptide chains, alpha and beta chains, linked to each other by disulfide bonds (Fig. 2.5). Both chains have variable (V) and constant (C) regions. The C-terminal end of the V region is encoded by a joining (J) segment gene and, in the beta chain only, a diversity (D) segment gene. The V regions of these TCR proteins are responsible for antigen binding. The structure and the genes encoding TCR molecules with V, D, J, and C regions are similar to those of immunoglobulin (Ig). Both TCR and Ig are members of a family of molecules called the *Ig superfamily.*

Although the TCR allows T cells to recognize antigen–MHC complexes, the cell-surface expression of TCR molecules and the initiation of intracellular signaling depend on a complex of additional peptides known as the *CD3 complex* (Fig. 2.5). The CD3 complex consists of at least five peptide chains—gamma, delta, epsilon, zeta, and eta chains—which noncovalently bind to each other and are closely arrayed in the membrane alongside the TCR (Fig. 2.5). This relationship is necessary for surface expression and the function of both TCR and CD3 proteins. When the TCR binds the antigen, there is a conformational change in CD3 that activates intracellular signal pathways, including tyrosine kinase, thus transferring the activating signals to the cytoplasm of the T cell. This antigen-driven signal transduced by the TCR–CD3 complex is called *signal one* and is essential *but not sufficient alone* for the activation of T cells. Full activation of T cells requires two synergistic signals. A second, antigen-independent signal (*signal two*) must be provided through additional so-called accessory molecules. The provision of signals through the TCR alone leads to clonal and antigen-specific anergy, in which the T cell does not produce cytokines and does not divide, but instead becomes unresponsive to appropriate stimulation for up to several weeks or undergoes programmed cell death (apoptosis). This process is called *clonal anergy.* T cells receiving signal one without signal two not only do not activate but also are refractory to activation

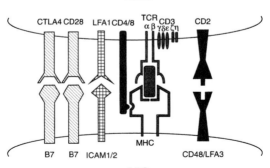

Figure 2.5.   T-cell receptor–CD3 complex with accessory molecules binding to a major histocompatibility complex containing a peptide in its groove.

even when all necessary activation elements are later presented (see later section on tolerance).

Accessory Molecules

Accessory molecules, nonpolymorphic membrane proteins that can serve as cell surface markers, are often involved in adhesion reactions and are identical on all T cells of a species. Accessory molecules play at least three roles in the alloimmune response:

1. Accessory molecules on T cells stabilize the interaction between cytotoxic T cells and the target cell by binding their specific ligands on the surfaces of target cells, an essential step in the cytotoxic effector response.
2. Accessory molecules provide the non–antigen-driven second signal for T-cell activation and play a direct role in signal transduction.
3. *Adhesion molecules* enhance antigen recognition by increasing the affinity between the TCR and the MHC-bearing antigen.

CD4 and CD8 molecules, expressed as T-cell–surface proteins, are accessory molecules that enhance the interaction between the TCR and APCs through the MHC. By binding class II MHC molecules, the CD4 molecule facilitates TCR–CD3 complex–mediated signal transduction and assists the actions of class II–restricted T cells. Similarly, the CD8 molecule binds to class I MHC molecules and stabilizes the interaction of the class I MHC–restricted T cell with a target cell–mediating signal transduction. CD4/CD8+ TCR–CD3 complex proteins function together in initiating the signals for T-cell activation. It has been shown that monoclonal antibodies against CD4 or CD8 molecules inhibit T-cell activation and thus are important potential targets for immunosuppression.

Several other T-cell membrane proteins, including CD2, CD28, lymphocyte function–associated antigen-1 (LFA-1), and very-late-activation molecules (VLA), also affect T-cell activation. These proteins belong to a family of cell adhesion molecules: the *integrin superfamily.* By binding to its ligand LFA-3, CD2 serves as an intercellular adhesion molecule. In addition, evidence suggests that the CD2–LFA-3 interaction may provide a costimulatory signal to T-cell activation and proliferation. Studies support the primacy for CD28 binding to its ligands B7-1 (CD80) and B7-2 (CD86) for transplantation allorecognition and through the provision of a strong signal two for T-cell activation. The binding of B7 to CD28 is also important for the delivery of costimulatory signals that are necessary for full activation of T cells. LFA-1 is a cell-surface protein that is expressed on all bone marrow–derived cells and that mediates a potent stimulatory signal for T-cell activation. Intercellular adhesion molecule-1 (ICAM-1) and ICAM-2 are specific ligands for LFA-1. ICAM-1 is expressed on both hematopoietic and nonhematopoietic cells, including endothelial cells, keratinocytes, and fibroblasts. It has been demonstrated that anti–LFA-1 monoclonal antibody can be used in HLA-mismatched bone marrow transplantation to prevent rejection. The VLA molecules VLA-4, VLA-5, and VLA-6 are expressed on resting T cells. These molecules interact with their extracellular matrix ligands (fibronectin and laminin) and provide additional signals to T cells.

VLA-4 also interacts with vascular cell adhesion molecule-1 (VCAM-1) and mediates the binding of lymphocytes to endothelium at inflammatory sites. T cells also express CTLA-4, a molecule structurally similar to CD28 that also binds B7-1 and B7-2. CTLA-4, however, transmits an inhibitory signal that helps to terminate the immune response. The CD40:CD40 ligand pathway has also been described as a key pathway in both B-cell and T-cell activation. CD40 is expressed on B cells, macrophages, dendritic cells, and endothelial cells, whereas its ligand is expressed on activated CD4 T cells. Several additional cell-surface proteins, such as CD44, Thy-1, and CD45, also transduce signals for T-cell activation on binding their ligands.

T-CELL ACTIVATION

T cells thus require at least two different signals to be activated. The first signal is initiated by the binding of the alloantigen or the processed antigen presented by self MHC to the TCR–CD3 complex. The second signal for T-cell activation is provided by the interaction between a number of accessory molecule–ligand pairs on APCs and on T cells, such as that between the CD28 molecule on the T lymphocyte with its ligand B7 on the surface of the APC. On specific ligand binding, a signal is delivered that acts synergistically with TCR-induced signals to produce T-cell activation. These dual signals trigger the CD4+ T cell to activate the cytokine interleukin-2 (IL-2) and IL-2 receptor gene expression, leading to induction of the expression of other cytokines. Then, cytokines engage their receptors to provide a further signal, *signal three,* which permits the entire cascade of T-cell activation to proceed, leading to cell division (Fig. 2.6). If a TCR is triggered without an accompanying second signal, the cell is driven into an anergic state in which it is not only inactivated but also becomes refractory to the full range of activating signals.

Within minutes of stimulation, T cells leave the quiescent phase of cell division (G_0). The specific events of this activated cell are described in terms of the synthesis and the cell content of RNA, DNA, and protein concentrations that culminate in the attainment of new molecules targeted for the cell surface, called *activation markers,* for the cytosol, for the nucleus, and for the external milieu. In the first phase of the cell cycle (G_{1a}), T cells begin to transcribe and express cellular protooncogenes, such as c-*myc,* c-*myb,* c-*fos,* and c-*jun,* and the genes for IL-2 and its receptor. The products of the cellular protooncogenes, c-*fos* and c-*jun,* are believed to function within the nucleus to regulate cell growth, including transcriptional regulation of the IL-2 gene, whereas c-*myc* and c-*myb* regulate DNA synthesis required for ultimate mitosis and cell division. The binding of IL-2 to its receptor propels the cell into the G_{1b} phase, in which an array of proinflammatory cytokines and additional cell-surface receptors, such as that for transferrin, are synthesized. Eventually, the cell enters the S phase of the cell cycle, doubles its DNA content, arranges its chromosomes along a spindle pattern, and undergoes mitotic division in a process called *postantigenic differentiation,* which leads to *clonal expansion* (Fig. 2.3). The net result of the clonal expansion of both helper (CD4+) and CD8+ T cells is the development of *cytotoxic T lymphocytes,* which act as effector cells capable of inducing graft rejection (see

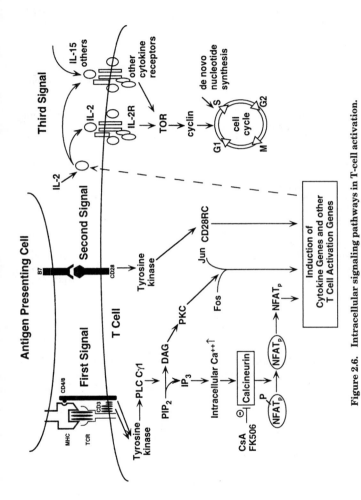

Figure 2.6.   Intracellular signaling pathways in T-cell activation.

the section on acute rejection). The vigor of S phase of the cell cycle is under tight regulatory control by *cyclins,* or *cell cycle regulators,* which are constitutively under inhibitory control. Cytokine signals release the inhibitory brake allowing cyclins to stimulate the tuning of the cell cycle, leading to clonal expansion.

The events that initiate and regulate the activation of T cells can be understood at the single-cell level as a series of events that begin with antigen recognition and lead to the synthesis of various second messengers. These second messengers activate the promoter sequences of the crucial genes involved in the synthesis of the regulatory molecules capable of driving the activated lymphocyte through the activation cascade (Fig. 2.6). After alloantigen recognition, the antigen-specific TCR permits the passage of signals into the cell. The immediate effect is the appearance of newly phosphorylated tyrosine residues on a number of proteins mediated by phosphotyrosine kinase. Phosphorylation of tyrosine residues activates an enzyme called *phosphatidylinositol phospholipase Cγ1,* which in turn catalyzes the breakdown of a plasma membrane phospholipid called *phosphatidylinositol 4,5-biphosphate,* leading to the signaling events, such as second messengers, inositol 1,4,5 triphosphate (IP3), and diacylglycerol (DAG). IP3 stimulates the release of ionized calcium from intracellular stores. DAG, in the presence of increased cytoplasmic calcium, activates protein kinase C (PKC) on binding to it. PKC activation leads to the synthesis of nuclear regulatory elements, such as the protooncogenes c-*fos* and c-*jun.* Cytoplasmic calcium forms a complex with the calcium-dependent regulatory protein called *calmodulin.* These calcium–calmodulin complexes activate other kinases and phosphatases, including *calcineurin.* Calcineurin, a calcium–calmodulin complex–dependent phosphatase, plays a key role in the activation of factors required for IL-2 gene transcription.

As a consequence of this enzyme activation, the activated form of a molecule called *nuclear factor of activated T cells* (NF-AT) is generated by dephosphorylation of a cytosolic precursor. Increased calcium promotes the dephosphorylation of NF-AT by calcineurin and allows NF-AT to migrate from the cytoplasm to the nucleus. In the nucleus, NF-AT binds cooperatively with c-*fos* and c-*jun,* products of cellular protooncogenes, to the distal NF-AT–binding sites in the promoter sequence of the IL-2 gene and enhances transcription of this gene. The c-*fos* and c-*jun* stabilize the binding of NF-AT to DNA. After synthesis, IL-2 functions as an *autacoid* by binding to its own receptor on helper T cells (Fig. 2.6), providing an internal signal for completion of the lymphocyte-activation cascade.

Mechanism of Action of Immunosuppressive Agents

The previous discussion, together with inspection of Figure 2.6, permits a useful overview of the site of action of many of the immunosuppressive agents in clinical use (see Chapter 4).

Agents that target signal one. The monoclonal antibody OKT$_3$ is targeted against the CD3 molecule, and after its administration, the TCR becomes dysfunctional. The polyclonal antibodies (e.g., the antithymocyte globerline) are targeted against the CD3 molecule and an array of cell surface markers. Cyclosporine and tacrolimus inhibit the phosphatase activity of calcineurin when they bind to their immunophilin-binding proteins in the cytosol (see Plate 1), leading to the inhibition of IL-2 gene transcription. They are, therefore, both called *calcineurin inhibitors*.

Agents that target signal two. There are currently no clinically approved agents that target signal two. CTLA-4–Ig and anti-CD154 are two promising agents in clinical development (see Chapter 4 and the later section on tolerance). They block the co-stimulatory molecules that provide signal two.

Agents targeted against signal three. Basiliximab and daclizumab are humanized monoclonal antibodies targeted against IL-2 (also called *tac* or CD25) receptor. Sirolimus acts on a target protein called *target of rapamycin* (TOR), which interrupts the signaling pathway between cytokine receptors and cell cycling. Mycophenolate mofetil and azathioprine impair *de novo* nucleotide synthesis.

Cytokines

Cytokines are soluble, antigen-nonspecific proteins that are synthesized in response to antigenic stimuli by several different cell types, including monocytes and T cells, especially CD4+ T lymphocytes. They initiate their action by binding to their specific receptors on the surface of the target cells. The same cell that secretes the cytokine may be the target cell (*autocrine* action). A nearby cell (*paracrine* action) or a distant cell may also be stimulated by cytokines (*endocrine* action). The molecular weights of cytokines vary between 15,000 and 25,000 daltons. Cytokines induce both humoral and cellular responses, including activation, proliferation, and differentiation of T cells, B cells, macrophages, and hematopoietic cells, by binding to high-affinity receptors on target cells (Table 2.1). Cytokines increase MHC expression and target cell injury and inflammation involving neutrophils and platelets. Cytokines also augment the expression of cellular adhesion molecules on endothelial and epithelial cells of the graft and facilitate natural killer (NK) and macrophage-mediated cytotoxicity. Cytokines influence the synthesis and the action of other cytokines, and can also play inhibitory roles to down-regulate the immune response. The balance between stimulatory and inhibitory cytokines sets the vigor of any given immune response to an antigen.

Because of the fact that there are a large number of cytokines with similar, often interchangeable functions, there is a degree of promiscuity and redundancy to these systems. Specific profiles of cytokine production have been correlated with distinct T-cell functions. A pattern of response emerges in which one set of cytokines is generally involved with the enhancement of antibody responses to an antigen and may down-regulate cellular response (subset 2 of the helper T [TH_2] cytokines, synthesized by the TH_2 subset of lymphocytes), and one set of cytokines is generally involved with the enhancement of cellular immune responses (TH_1 cytokines, a product of the TH_1 subset of lymphocytes) (Fig. 2.7). In the initiation of an immune response, several cytokines, such as *tumor necrosis factor* (TNF) and IFN-gamma, direct the maturation of the lymphocyte pool to favor the TH_1 subset of cells that elaborate IL-2, IFN-gamma, and IL-12. The antiinflammatory cytokines, such as *transforming growth factor-beta* (TGF-beta),

Table 2.1. Cytokines in transplant immunology

Cytokine	Cell Source	Cell Target	Primary Action
Interleukin-2	T cells	T cells	Growth, cytokine production
		NK cells	Growth, ↑ cytolytic function
		B cells	Growth, ↑ antibody synthesis
Interleukin-4	CD4+ cells, mast cells	T cells	Growth
		Macrophages	Inhibit activation
Transforming growth factor-beta	T cells, macrophages	T cells	Inhibit activation and maturation
		Macrophages	Inhibit activation
Gamma-interferon	T cells, NK cells	Macrophages	Activation
		Endothelial cells	Activation
		NK cells	Activation ↑ Class I and class II MHC expression
Interleukin-10	T cells	Macrophages	Inhibit function
		B cells	Stimulation
Interleukin-12	T cells, B cells, NK cells, monocytes	NK cells	Stimulation
		T cells	Stimulate differentiation
Interleukin-1	Macrophages, T cells, epithelial and endothelial cells	Macrophages	↑ Acute-phase reactants
		Vascular endothelium	Inflammation
		Liver and hypothalamus	Fever
Tumor necrosis factor	Macrophages, T cells, NK cells, mast cells	Vascular endothelium	↑ Expression of adhesion molecules
		Neutrophils	Inflammation
		Macrophages	Fever
		Liver and hypothalamus	↑ Acute-phase reactants
Interleukin-6	Macrophages, vascular endothelial cells, fibroblasts, T cells	Liver	↑ Acute-phase reactants (fibrogen)
		B cells	Growth, stimulation of differentiation

MHC, major histocompatibility complex; NK, natural killer.

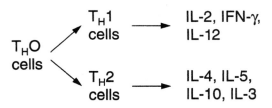

Figure 2.7.   Subsets of helper T lymphocytes.

direct the maturation process of the TH_2 cytokines IL-4 and IL-10, which dampens the cellular response to alloantigen. During rejection, all of these cytokines are found in the graft, but in states of tolerance, the TH_1 cytokines are reduced and TH_2 cytokines are enhanced, suggesting a causal relationship.

The cytokines play other roles in the alloresponse in addition to their roles in the maturation of specific T-cell subsets and in the balance between the cellular and humoral arms of immunity. As discussed in the section on lymphocyte action, IL-2 plays a pivotal role in regulating T-cell activation by providing the signals needed to complete the activation program of both helper and cytotoxic T cells and by stimulating the synthesis of the proto-oncogenes needed for DNA synthesis and clonal expansion. T-cell activation, however, can occur in the absence of IL-2. In animals with targeted deletion of the IL-2 gene (*IL-2 knockout mice*), acute rejection can still occur with the functions of IL-2 substituted by other cytokines. This is an example of the redundancy that is a frequent feature of the immune response.

IFN-gamma, in addition to its subset maturational role, regulates the quantitative expression of MHC class I and class II molecules. As with the IL-2–deficient mice, allografts transplanted into IFN-gamma–deficient recipients are also rejected, supporting the idea that IFN-gamma is not necessary for acute allograft rejection. Finally, the cytokines may play a purely inflammatory role as mediators of the constitutional responses to transplantation antigens. IL-2, TNF, and IL-6 are responsible for the fever, myalgias, arthralgias, and capillary leak syndrome that lead to edema and swelling of the graft, often perceived as graft tenderness during the rejection response. Recognition of individual cytokine gene polymorphisms may permit identification of patients at risk for episodes of rejection.

FORMS OF ALLOGRAFT REJECTION

Renal graft rejection can be defined as a series of events in which the graft is recognized as nonself. This process involves the participation of both local and systemic immune responses involving CD4+ T lymphocytes, CD8+ T lymphocytes, B cells, NK cells, macrophages, and cytokines; the establishment of a local inflammatory injury; induction of MHC expression; and eventually deterioration of renal function and necrosis of the transplanted tissue. Rejection can be classified as hyperacute, acute, or chronic on the basis of etiologic, clinical, and pathologic parameters (Table 2.2).

Table 2.2. Classification of transplant rejection

Form	Pathogenesis	Histopathology	Therapy
Hyperacute	Preformed, IgG, anti-HLA class I	Ischemic necrosis, thrombosis	No successful treatment; prevention with crossmatch
Acute	Cellular and humoral immune response	Tubulitis, vasculitis, lymphocytic infiltrates	Steroids, anti-lymphocyte antibodies
Chronic	Alloantigen dependent and alloantigen independent	Interstitial fibrosis, tubular atrophy, glomerular sclerosis	No effective treatment

HLA, human leukocyte antigen; IgG, immunoglobulin G.

Hyperacute Rejection

Hyperacute rejection occurs within minutes to hours after the vascular clamps to the transplanted organ are released. This dramatic event is caused by preformed, cytotoxic, anti-HLA class I (IgG isotype) or anti-ABO blood group antibodies (IgM isotype) in the recipient. These antibodies bind to the endothelial surfaces of the arterioles on the graft, activate complement, and lead to severe vascular injury, including thrombosis and obliteration of the graft vasculature. The endothelial cells are stimulated to secrete von Willebrand factor, which mediates platelet adhesion and aggregation. Complement activation initiates the coagulation cascade and the generation of multiple inflammatory mediators. Eventually, transplanted tissue suffers irreversible ischemic damage. The current ABO-matching policy has largely eliminated hyperacute rejection by anti-ABO antibodies (see Chapter 3). Hyperacute rejection is mediated by antibodies against alloantigens that have appeared in response to previous exposure to alloantigens through blood transfusions, prior transplantations, or multiple pregnancies. Pathologic findings show fibrinoid necrosis of the vessel walls, fibrin thrombus formation, margination of neutrophils, and ischemic necrosis. The graft may become flaccid or cyanotic and hard and may even rupture within minutes after revascularization.

Without proper precautions, hyperacute rejection often leads to graft loss. It can be largely prevented by testing recipients for the presence of the preformed, cytotoxic antibodies that react with the cells of the donor in a sensitive test called a *crossmatch* (see Chapter 3). Treatment options are discussed in Chapters 4 and 8.

Accelerated Acute Rejection

Rejection occurring within a few days after transplantation (between 24 hours and 4 days) is called *accelerated acute rejection*. It occurs when the recipient has been sensitized by prior interactions with graft antigen, generally by prior transplantations but also by transfusions, and is thought to represent an immuno-logic memory response to prior sensitization. The recipient devel-ops rejection in a rapid fashion. This event has also been seen after donor-specific transfusions in recipients of kidneys from living-related donors. This type of rejection may represent a com-bination of cellular and antibody-mediated injury. The cellular infil-tration may not be as intense as with acute rejection. This serious event may be difficult to control with current immunosuppressive regimens and may contribute to early graft loss.

Acute Rejection

Acute rejection, which generally occurs days to weeks after sur-gery, is a systemic inflammatory disorder that in its full-blown manifestation may be associated with multiple constitutional symptoms, including fever, chills, myalgias, and arthralgias. Many of these symptoms are manifestations of cytokine release (e.g., TNF, IL-1); expression of IL-2 and IFN-gamma has been shown to in-crease before the development of the typical interstitial infiltrate. Acute rejection is described in clinical and pathologic detail in Chapters 8 and 12. In this era of potent immunosuppressive agents, the constitutional inflammatory signs and symptoms are often masked, and only renal physiologic derangements may be present. Acute rejection should be diagnosed immediately to initiate the appropriate treatment and prevent irreversible damage.

About 90% of acute rejections are predominantly cell mediated and are more easily reversed with appropriate treatment than rejections in which antigraft antibodies are the predominant effec-tors. Evidence suggests that CD4+ T cells are important for the ini-tiation of rejection, and CD8+ T cells are critical at the later stages. Cytotoxic T lymphocytes and NK cells contain powerful cytolytic granules of the *effector molecules: granzymes* and *perforins.* Gran-ule exocytosis releases these molecules, which cause membrane damage and induce apoptosis. Quantification of these effector mol-ecules and cytokine genes in urinary cells may provide an innova-tive, non-invasive way of making a clinical diagnosis of rejection.

About 5% to 10% of the rejection episodes are mediated by hu-moral immune response and are more difficult to reverse. Partic-ipation of donor-specific IgG antibodies against endothelial cell alloantigens activates complement and leads to vascular injury in the graft. Perivascular infiltration with T cells, NK cells, and mononuclear cells and tubulitis, accompanied by vasculitis on biopsy, are defining features of acute rejection. Chemotactic fac-tors, such as the *beta chemokines*, may serve to facilitate environ-mental homing of T cell toxicities of inflammation. In severe forms, vascular occlusion and interstitial hemorrhage may be seen (see Chapter 12).

Chronic Rejection

Chronic rejection leading to late graft loss is characterized by glomerular sclerosis, tubular atrophy, splitting of the glomerular basement membrane, and interstitial fibrosis. It occurs slowly over months to years and leads to progressive loss of renal function. The pathogenesis of chronic rejection is not fully understood, but both immune (*alloantigen dependent*) and nonimmune (*alloantigen independent*) mechanisms are important (see Chapter 9). The healing process after repeated bouts of acute rejection, chronic graft injury by delayed-type hypersensitivity response, chronic ischemia, antibody formation, calcineurin-inhibitor toxicity, and enhanced TGF-beta production drugs have all been proposed as stimuli for the ubiquitous fibrosis.

Cytomegalovirus and Rejection

Infection with cytomegalovirus (CMV) has been implicated in the development of both acute and chronic allograft rejection in various clinical and experimental situations; late acute rejection has been ascribed to clinically covert CMV infection. CMV infection promotes a generalized immune response in a similar fashion to rejection. It has been shown that CMV up-regulates MHC molecules and the various adhesion molecules. In the kidney, ICAM-1 expression is up-regulated as a direct effect of the virus on CMV-infected proximal tubular epithelial cells or through activation of lymphocytes and the mononuclear cell release of IFN-gamma. Infection of human umbilical vein endothelial cells with CMV causes a rapid rise in ICAM-1 mRNA levels, suggesting that the viral immediate-early proteins are involved in gene activation. This finding supports a model in which CMV immediate-early gene products interact with ICAM-1 promoter elements to increase gene expression. The diagnosis, treatment and prophylaxis of CMV infection are discussed in Chapter 10.

TOLERANCE

Immunologic tolerance can be described as immunologic unresponsiveness because of an antigen-induced block in the development or differentiation of lymphocytes specific for the inducing antigen. Normal subjects have mature T lymphocytes that recognize nominal antigen in the context of self antigens. During lymphocyte ontogeny, the immune system eliminates autoreactive clones of lymphocytes and preserves the clones that can recognize foreign antigens in the context of self. In this process, the entire repertoire of response to be displayed by the mature individual is established. Self tolerance is initiated during development within the thymus and is maintained in the periphery.

The induction of human tolerance to defined foreign antigens while maintaining intact the remainder of the immune repertoire continues to be an elusive goal. In defined animal models or experiments of nature, tolerance to transplantation antigens has been induced or encountered. Tolerance can be generated by intrathymic events and can be global (central tolerance), or it can be either maintained or even developed by mature lymphocytes that have emigrated from the thymus (peripheral tolerance). The deletion of T-cell clones responding to an antigen produces tolerance through a process of activation-induced apoptosis. As an example, the cornea is a so-called immunologically privileged site where an immune response is prevented by the expression of an apoptosis-inducing ligand (*Fas ligand*), which triggers apoptosis in infiltrating Fas-positive lymphocytes.

Introduction of antigen during ontogeny into the thymus at an appropriate point of T-cell maturation leads to a similar clonal deletion for that defined antigen as for autoreactive clones. Such tolerance can be complete, or it may need to be maintained in the periphery. Introduction of antigen into the thymus after lymphocyte development may also culminate in tolerance to a defined antigen. An important contribution of an intact peripheral immune system is required because immunosuppressant therapy can either reverse or block such tolerance development.

In experimental settings, the creation of central tolerance leads to the acceptance of foreign lymphoid cells that can co-circulate unscathed in the host, a condition called *chimerism*. It has been suggested that the persistence of chimerism, even with a scant number of cells, called *microchimerism,* not only marks the tolerant state but also is mechanistically important in the maintenance of the tolerance in the periphery. Chimeric states can be introduced into the mature immune system with the provision of donor hematopoietic cells in the setting of immunosuppressant conditioning, often by forms of radiation. Total-body irradiation, a myeloablative regimen, has been used to permit allogeneic marrow or stem cell transplantation, leading to chimerism in experimental models. This technique has been limited in clinical medicine by the development of often fatal graft-versus-host disease. *Total-lymphoid irradiation* involves radiation of the immune organs and the spleen and was developed for the treatment of Hodgkin's disease. It may permit chimerism and tolerance without graft-versus-host disease in rodents and lower mammals, a promise not yet met in human biology.

Protocols have been developed to induce chimerism using polyclonal or monoclonal antilymphocyte antibody conditioning at the time of provision of donor antigen through directed donor cell transfusions or by "minimal" radiation conditioning with both donor and recipient marrow elements. In animal models, pretransplantation donor-specific transfusion of blood or bone marrow cells can lead to long-term donor-specific allograft survival when one class I or class II antigen is mismatched between donor and recipient. The fact that the immune system can be manipulated to tolerate transplanted tissues without immunosuppressive drugs encourages the continued research for the induction of transplantation tolerance. The continued presence of alloantigen either on the graft or as chimerism of cells appears to be necessary for the maintenance of tolerance.

Strategies have been described to exploit this principle, each culminating in models of antigen-specific tolerance. In one strategy, T cells of donor origin that suppress the immune response, so-called *veto cells*, have been identified as the mediators in several models when protocols employing polyclonal T-cell antibody–conditioned bone marrow have been used. Trials to induce specific T-cell tolerance are in progress using peptides derived from polymorphic regions of donor MHC molecules. CTLA-4–Ig is a recombinant fusion protein consisting of the extracellular domain of CTLA-4 linked to the constant region of IgG_1. It blocks the CD28-mediated costimulatory signal and prevents the interaction between graft B7 molecules and recipient CD28 molecules (Fig. 2.5). CTLA-4 has a much higher affinity for B7 than for CD28, and thus is a highly effective inhibitor of the B7:CD28 interaction. In mice that lack CTLA-4, a rapidly fatal lymphoproliferative disorder of activated helper T cells develops. Inhibition of the costimulatory signals at the time of TCR–MHC interaction may produce a state of T-cell anergy. It has been demonstrated that CTLA-4–Ig treatment can induce suppression of antibody production and T-cell–mediated responses to allogeneic and xenogeneic grafts *in vivo*.

Blockade of another costimulatory pair, CD40 and CD40 ligand, has also been shown to induce total tolerance in a nonhuman primate model. The importance of apoptosis of activated T cells in the generation of tolerance and the impact of concomitant immunosuppression are discussed in Chapter 4.

XENOGENEIC TRANSPLANTATION

Transplantation of organs from other mammals to humans could solve the clinical organ-donor shortage. Because of differences in the primary immune mechanisms culminating in severe graft destruction, xenografts can be separated into those between closely related species, such as human and non-human primates, called *concordant xenografts,* and those between distant species, such as swine and humans, called *discordant xenografts.* The preeminent hurdle to xenotransplantation is the immunologic reaction of the host against the graft.

The major discriminating feature of discordant xenogeneic transplantation is a form of hyperacute rejection secondary to the presence of preformed, xenoreactive "natural" antibodies and complement activation. This form of rejection can destroy an organ within minutes or hours after transplantation. Many individuals develop natural antibodies that are directed against carbohydrate determinants of other species, including anti–alpha-galactose (important in swine-to-human transplantation), antiphosphatidyl-choline antibodies, and isohemagglutinins. These antibodies bind to the endothelial cells of the xenograft and activate the complement cascade, leading to bleeding into the graft and the formation of platelet thrombi.

Complement activation depends on the combination of species. Transplantation between primates and swine triggers the antibody-dependent, classic pathway. In contrast, in transplantation between guinea pigs and rats, complement activation occurs through the alternative pathway. This type of rejection cannot be controlled with current immunosuppressive regimens. It can be inhibited by depleting xenoreactive antibodies from the xenograft recipient or by preventing activation of the complement system.

Various therapies are being developed with the goal of prevention of hyperacute rejection. Natural antibodies are rare between concordant species, and an accelerated cellular rejection response, thought to be related to either heightened indirect antigen presentation or more vigorous CD4+ delayed-type hypersensitivity response, characterizes the unique aspects of concordant xenotransplantation. After these barriers are overcome, the conventional rejection pathways will need to be addressed.

Acute or accelerated vascular rejection (sometimes called *delayed xenograft rejection*) occurs 2 to 3 days after transplantation and is a T-cell–independent phenomenon. Because xenoantibodies play an important role in initiating delayed xenograft rejection, various agents, including cyclophosphamide, mycophenolate mofetil, 15-deoxyspergualin, and leflunomide, have been used with some success to suppress their formation.

A practical way to permit xenotransplantation may be to immunoisolate the xenogeneic tissue in capsules or membranes. This technique has been attempted with pancreatic islets. A promising and potentially revolutionary approach is to use adenovirus vectors to transduce the organ graft with immunomodulatory genes and proteins. This technique has been used to prolong graft survival in experimental models using sequences encoding CTLA-4-Ig. Genetic manipulation of a xenotransplant prior to implantation could obviate the necessity for intensive immunosuppression. The danger of transmission of zoonotic diseases from animals to humans is a matter of great concern, which will need to be addressed before xenotransplantation becomes a clinical reality.

SELECTED READINGS

Burlingham WJ, O'Connell PJ, Jacobson LM, et al. Tumor necrosis factor-α and tumor growth factor-β genotype: Partial association with intragraft gene expression in two cases of long-term peripheral tolerance to a kidney transplant. *Transplantation* 2000; 69:1527.

Goral S, Helderman JH. Cytomegalovirus and rejection. *Transplant Proc* 1994;26(Suppl):5.

Helderman JH. Renal transplant rejection. In: Jacobson F, Striker G, Klahr S, eds. *The principles and practices of nephrology*, 2nd ed. St Louis: Mosby–Year Book, 1995:811–821.

Holland EJ, Schwartz GS. The new immunology: the end of immunosuppressive drug therapy? *N Engl J Med* 1999;340:1754.

Hutchinson I, Provicia V, Sinnot P. Genetic regulation of cytokine synthesis: Consequences for acute and chronic rejection. *Graft* 1998;1:186.

Lakkis FG. Role of cytokines in transplantation tolerance: lessons learned from gene-knockout mice. *J Am Soc Nephrol* 1998;9:2361.

Lambrigts D, Sachs DH, Cooper D. Discordant organ xenotransplantation in primates: world experience and current status. *Transplantation* 1998;66:547.

Matzinger P. Graft tolerance: a duel of two signals. *Nature Med* 1999; 5:616.

Pavlakis M, Lipman M, Strom TB. Intragraft expression of T-cell activation genes in human renal allograft rejection. *Kidney Int* 1996; 49:57.

Robertson H, Morley AR, Talbot D, et al. Renal allograft rejection: β-chemokine involvement in the development of tubulitis. *Transplantation* 2000;69:684.

Sayegh MH, Turka LA. The role of T-cell costimulatory activation pathways in transplant rejection. *N Engl J Med* 1998;338:1813.

Sayegh MH, Watschinger B, Carpenter CB. Mechanisms of T cell recognition of alloantigen. *Transplantation* 1994;57:1295.

Tomasoni S, Azzolini N, Casiraghi F, et al. CTLA4Ig gene transfer prolongs survival and induces donor-specific tolerance in a rat renal allograft. *J Am Soc Nephrol* 2000;11:747.

Yang L, DuTemple B, Khan Q, et al. Mechanisms of long-term donor-specific allograft survival induced by pretransplant infusion of lymphocytes. *Blood* 1998;91:324.

Waldmann H. Transplantation tolerance: where do we stand? *Nature Med* 1999;5:1245.

Woodle EW, Kulkarni S. Programmed cell death. *Transplantation* 1998; 66:681.

3

Histocompatibility Testing, Crossmatching, and Allocation of Cadaveric Kidney Transplants

Steven Katznelson, Steven K. Takemoto, and
J. Michael Cecka

The major histocompatibility complex (MHC) encodes a group of cell-surface antigens that define the "foreign" nature, or *allogeneity*, of transplanted organs and tissues. These antigens provide the major, although not sole, barrier to transplantation. This chapter deals with the structure of the MHC, its genetic determinants, techniques for its identification, its relevance to the results of clinical transplantation, and its role in public policy decisions regarding the allocation of donor organs. Other factors determining the outcome of renal transplantation are also covered.

THE HUMAN MAJOR HISTOCOMPATIBILITY COMPLEX

Nomenclature

The human MHC complex, known as the HLA (human leukocyte antigen) system, comprises a series of genes located on the short arm of chromosome 6 (see Chapter 2, Fig. 2.2). The concentration of the HLA genes in one defined area of the chromosome allows these genes to be inherited as a packet, or *haplotype*. Each person inherits one haplotype of HLA genes from each parent, and the products of the two haplotypes make up that person's HLA type, or *profile*.

The HLA antigens can be grouped into two different classes based on their structure and cellular distribution. *Class I* molecules are named HLA-A, -B, and -C, and *class II* molecules are named HLA-DP, -DQ, and -DR. In clinical kidney transplantation, it is the HLA-A, -B, and -DR antigens that are regarded as the most important. The remarkable degree of polymorphism of these antigens accounts for the great difficulty in tissue matching, as opposed to the relative ease of matching for the less polymorphic ABO blood group antigens.

The nomenclature for HLA antigens evolved as the antigens were defined based on their reactivity with antisera. When antisera were identified that indicated subsets, or *splits,* of existing specificities, new antigen numbers were assigned. Table 3.1 lists the serologically defined HLA-A, -B and -DR antigens recognized by the World Health Organization (WHO) nomenclature committee. The broad antigen groups are indicated in parenthesis next to the split antigen name. More than 81 different HLA-A, -B, and -DR antigens can be detected using serologic methods. The number of HLA alleles that can be identified using newer DNA technologies (see DNA Typing Methods) is growing rapidly. For

Table 3.1. Recognized human leukocyte antigen (HLA) specificities

No. of Alleles	Antigen	No. of Alleles	Antigen
HLA-A		3	B53
4	A1	1	B54(22)
32	A2	7	B55(22)
6	A3	5	B56(22)
5	A11	5	B57(17)
1	A23(9)	2	B58(17)
21	A24(9)	1	B59
2	A25(10)	3	B60(40)
12	A26(10)	4	B61(40)
4	A29(19)	15	B62(15)
7	A30(19)	2	B63(15)
4	A31(19)	1	B64(14)
3	A32(19)	1	B65(14)
3	A33(19)	2	B67
2	A34(10)	1	B70
1	A36	2	B71(70)
1	A43	2	B72(70)
3	A66(10)	1	B73
10	A68(28)	5	B75(15)
1	A69(28)	3	B76(15)
3	A74(19)	1	B77(15)
1	A80	4	B78
HLA-B		1	B81
14	B7	1	B82
6	B8		
4	B13	**HLA-DR**	
17	B15	6	DR1
7	B18	3	DR2
16	B27	10	DR3
28	B35	35	DR4
2	B37	2	DR6
4	B38(16)	3	DR7
19	B39(16)	26	DR8
13	B40	1	DR9
3	B41	1	DR10
2	B42	39	DR11(5)
11	B44(12)	8	DR12(5)
3	B45(12)	36	DR13(6)
1	B46	33	DR14(6)
3	B47	10	DR15(2)
5	B48	8	DR16(2)
1	B49(21)	3	DR17(3)
1	B50(21)	2	DR18(3)
17	B51(5)	14	DR51
3	B52(5)	19	DR52
		10	DR53

Note: The numbers in parentheses represent prior designations.
Data modified from Bodmer JG, Marsh SGE, Albert ED, et al. Nomenclature for factors of the HLA system, 1999. *Hum Immunol* 1999;60: 361–395, with permission.

example, 32 HLA-A2 alleles have been identified encoding 32 distinct amino acid sequences. (The number of alleles that encode different antigens for each serologically defined HLA antigen is listed in the allele column in Table 3.1.)

The additional HLA polymorphism that has been revealed through the application of DNA technologies has provided interesting insights into the role of HLA in many autoimmune diseases, but its significance in clinical transplantation remains to be seen. Allele differences between the donor and recipient of bone marrow transplants lead to graft-versus-host disease. However, an extensive analysis of HLA-DR allele mismatches among kidney transplant recipients revealed no effect on graft survival rates.

Structure of HLA

Class I antigens (A, B, and C) consist of a unique heavy chain of 45,000 daltons with three globular domains termed $alpha_1$, $alpha_2$, and $alpha_3$ (see Chapter 2, Figs. 2.1 and 2.2). The $alpha_3$ domain is associated with $beta_2$-microglobulin, which is not MHC encoded. Class I antigens are expressed on all nucleated cells. The class II antigens (DR, DP, and DQ) consist of two noncovalently associated peptides—an alpha chain (35,000 daltons) and a beta chain (31,000 daltons). Each chain has two globular domains. Class II antigens are not expressed on all cells but are found on all B lymphocytes and activated T lymphocytes, monocytes, dendritic cells, glomerular endothelium, and renal tubular cells and capillaries.

Alloantigenic sites are clustered in the $alpha_1$ and $alpha_2$ domains of the class I molecule and in the external domain of the DR beta chain. Some antigenic determinants are shared by many HLA antigens. These are called *public specificities.* Unique determinants are known as *private specificities,* or splits. Both private and public specificities are often associated with distinct amino acid sequences.

The HLA antigens play a key role in normal immunity, displaying antigen peptides that fit into a groove formed by the $alpha_1$ and $alpha_2$ domains of the class I antigens or the $alpha_1$ and beta domains of the class II antigens (see Chapter 2, Fig. 2.1). The interaction between these polymorphic domains, peptides and the T-cell receptor provides the critical first signal of the immune response (see Chapter 2, Fig. 2.6). In the transplantation setting, similarities between the donor and recipient HLA molecules allow for direct recognition of donor HLA molecules and their peptides by recipient T cells. This can occur in addition to indirect recognition of donor HLA molecules that have been processed and presented by recipient antigen-presenting cells in the groove of recipient HLA molecules (see Chapter 2, Fig. 2.4).

Inheritance of HLA

Each parental chromosome 6 provides a haplotype or linked set of MHC genes to the offspring (Fig. 3.1). Parental chromosomes also provide other minor histocompatibility antigens that are not yet identified. Haplotypes are usually inherited intact from each parent, although crossover between the A and B locus occurs in about 2% of offspring, resulting in a *recombination* (and a new haplotype). The child carries one representative antigen from each of the class I and class II loci of each parent. A child is, by definition, a one-haplotype match to each parent unless recombination has occurred.

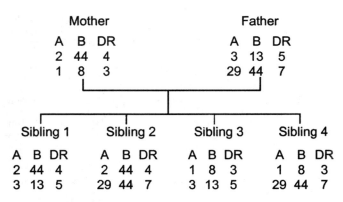

Figure 3.1.   Inheritance of haplotypes and HLA profile in four theoretical siblings. Sibling 1 is a one-haplotype match to siblings 2 and 3 and a zero-haplotype match to sibling 4. For sibling 1, A1, B8, DR3 is a noninherited maternal haplotype (NIMA) and is found in siblings 3 and 4 but not in 2.

HLA haplotypes are inherited in a mendelian fashion. Statistically, there is a 25% chance that siblings will share the same parental haplotypes (two-haplotype match), a 50% chance they will share one haplotype (one-haplotype match), and a 25% chance that neither haplotype will be the same (zero-haplotype match). In the latter case, 25% to 100% of other parental chromosomes may still be shared.

HLA Phenotypes and Genotypes

Consider an individual with the following HLA profile or phenotype:

A1, A24, B8, B44, DR4, DR15

From this phenotypic information alone it is not possible to identify haplotypes because it is not known from which parent each specificity was inherited.

Consider another individual:

A1, A3, B7, B8, DR4, DR12

If this individual is the biologic parent, offspring, or sibling of the first, it becomes possible to identify the shared haplotype of the family as A1, B8, DR4. The first individual also has an unshared haplotype A24, B44, DR15, and the second individual an unshared haplotype A3, B7, DR12. These haplotypes may appear in the other parent or siblings. A kidney transplantation between these two individuals would be a one-haplotype match, and the A1, B8, and DR4 antigens would be *genotypically identical* in the donor and recipient because they are encoded by the same genes.

If these two individuals are not related, it is not possible to identify the haplotypes. Thus, in cadaveric or living-unrelated donor transplantation, the haplotypes are unknown, and only the *phenotypic identity* of individual HLA antigens can be determined.

The two individuals whose HLA phenotypes are listed would be called a three-antigen match or a three-antigen mismatch (see HLA Matches and Mismatches). Sharing of minor histocompatibility antigens is serendipitous.

Identical and Fraternal Twins

The differentiation between identical twins and two-haplotype–matched fraternal twins is important because the recipient of a transplant from an identical twin requires no immunosuppression. The procedure is immunologically equivalent to an auto-transplantation. Two-haplotype–matched siblings, whether they are fraternal twins or not, differ in their minor histocompatibility antigens, and immunosuppression is required.

Monozygotic, or identical, twins share a single placenta and amniotic sac at birth. However, such information may be unavailable or unreliable when the patient and donor are evaluated as adults. A small skin graft can be performed from the potential twin donor to the recipient. The graft will be rejected if the twins are fraternal. For practical purposes, it may be helpful to perform extended blood typing. The genetic determinants of the Rh, MN, and other blood types are dispersed throughout the genome, and the more unlinked markers that can be identified and matched, the higher the certainty that the twins are identical. Any genetic difference that can be detected indicates that the twins are fraternal.

Linkage Disequilibrium

As noted previously, it is not possible to identify an individual's haplotypes from the phenotypic HLA typing information alone. Within racial or ethnic populations, however, there is a tendency for certain HLA determinants to be inherited together more often than would be expected by chance (e.g., HLA-A1, -B8, and HLA-A2, B44 among whites). This phenomenon is known as *linkage disequilibrium* and represents the inheritance of haplotypes within racial groups.

HLA Matches and Mismatches

It is not always possible to identify two HLA specificities of each HLA locus. Consider the HLA phenotype for the following two unrelated individuals:

1. A2, —; B27, B13; DR3, DR4
2. A2, A3; B8, B14; DR3, —

The absence of the second A-locus antigen in individual 1 and a DR specificity in individual 2 could result from a failure to identify the second antigen. More often, it reflects the inheritance of the same antigen (A2 and DR3 in these cases) from both parents (homozygous). Among whites, the latter is usually the case. A transplantation between these two individuals would be described as a 1-A, 1-DR match, a terminology that does not take into account any unidentified loci. If individual 1 were a donor for individual 2, it would be more precise to describe the combination as a 0-A, 2-B, 1-DR mismatch. If individual 2 were a donor for individual 1, the combination would be a 1-A, 2-B, 0-DR mismatch. Antigenic differences in the donor kidney are potential targets of rejection; therefore, the convention of counting the number of donor HLA antigens that are not shared by the recipient provides an estimate of the antigen dose.

TISSUE TYPING TECHNIQUES

Tissue typing has been performed using the microcytotoxicity test for more than 30 years. Using the products of an immune response (antibodies) to measure the targets of an immune response (HLA antigens) has a certain inherent logic. If an antigen had provoked an antibody response, its immunologic importance was demonstrated. Development of the polymerase chain reaction (PCR) test has made it possible to perform HLA typing using DNA techniques. These molecular genetic approaches are still evolving, but as the technology improves, the use of DNA typing will increase.

Microcytotoxicity Test

The microlymphocytotoxicity test developed by Terasaki is still the most commonly used assay for the detection of class I HLA antigens (Fig. 3.2). The great advantage of this test is that it uses the rare anti-HLA antiserum reagents sparingly. Only 1 μL of each serum per test is required. Lymphocytes are treated with carboxyfluorescein diacetate, a fluorescent dye, and then tested against a panel of antisera defining each of the HLA types. After addition of rabbit complement and further incubation, a quench solution (hemoglobin or India ink) containing ethidium bromide is added, and the test is read using a fluorescence microscope.

Anti-HLA Antisera

The serum of pregnant women and monoclonal antibodies are the primary sources for the antibodies used in tissue typing. Maternal antibodies are produced against the foreign paternal HLA antigens present in the fetus. Massive screening programs are required to identify and select reagent grade antisera that are highly specific for an HLA antigen and that have a high titer so that the cytotoxic reactivity is not lost under suboptimal conditions. Monoclonal antibodies specific for HLA antigens are produced from a single hybridoma and provide stable, high-titer reagents for typing.

Isolation of Lymphocytes

Immunomagnetic beads coated with monoclonal antibodies provide the simplest method for the selective separation of lymphocytes from whole blood or a suspension of mononuclear cells. Anti–T-cell or anti–B-cell monoclonal antibodies are used to coat the immunomagnetic beads. When mixed with a blood sample, the target cells adhere to the beads, and after placing the tube against a magnet to hold the beads in place, the remaining cells in the supernatant may be removed to another tube or discarded. The target cells may be used on the beads or may be detached from the beads.

Another simple method for cell isolation uses a monoclonal antibody–complement cocktail. The reagent contains monoclonal antibodies against the cells that are to be eliminated from the suspension, complement, and a density gradient medium. When unseparated white blood cells are added to the mixture and incubated, red blood cells, granulocytes, and platelets are lysed. After centrifugation, purified lymphocytes are deposited on the bottom

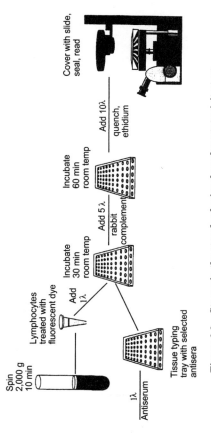

Figure 3.2. Stages in the standard microlymphocytotoxicity test.

of the tube, and the fragments of the other cells remain in the supernatant. The main advantage of this technique is that the isolation of lymphocytes takes place in one tube, thus eliminating the possibility of switching samples.

Procedure

The steps involved in standard testing for HLA are illustrated in Fig. 3.2. The standard conditions were set at a National Institutes of Health (NIH) meeting, and the test is often referred to as the *NIH test*. Lymphocytes isolated from blood are added to tissue typing trays containing typing reagents. Although any type of anticoagulated blood can be used, citrated blood has been found to be the best for long-distance transport of blood samples. Lymphocytes are purified from blood, as described previously. After incubation with the antibodies, rabbit complement is added, and the tray is incubated for another hour. Complement kills cells that have reacted with the antibody. In a two-color fluorescence assay, the viable cells appear green when read with a fluorescence microscope, and the dead cells appear red.

The reactions are scored using a rough scale to facilitate the estimation of cell killing based on the change in viability between the negative control and the test wells. A negative reaction is scored as 1; a probable negative as 2; a weak positive as 4. If most cells are killed, the score is 6, and if all the cells are killed, the score is 8. Results are analyzed and typing assigned based on the specificity of the antisera producing the positive reactions.

DNA Typing Methods

It is now possible to type individuals by DNA-based rather than conventional serologic methods. Using the extensive DNA sequence data available, it has been possible to design oligonucleotide primers and probes that specifically hybridize to sites that are unique to an HLA locus, allele, or group of alleles. Three basic methods used in conjunction with PCR employ site-specific oligonucleotide probes (SSOP), sequence-specific primers (SSP), and sequencing-based typing (SBT). SSOP is based on first amplifying genomic DNA using locus- or group-specific primers, then detecting the hybridization of allele-specific oligonucleotide probes tagged with radioactive or enzymatic markers to the amplified product. SSP depends on DNA amplification using group- or allele-specific primers and detecting an amplified product of the correct size by gel electrophoresis. Several commercial kits are available for both class I and class II typing using variations on these approaches. SBT uses group-specific primers to sequence polymorphic regions of the gene, and alleles can be assigned based on the nucleotides identified at key positions in the sequence.

DNA-based typing offers several advantages over serology. Viable lymphocytes are not required. Typing can be performed on any tissue containing nucleated cells. Buccal swabs can provide sufficient DNA for tissue typing and may be preferable to drawing blood from infants or those who are squeamish about needles. Samples can be dried on filter paper and stored without refrigeration for extended periods. The oligonucleotide reagents are more easily standardized and controlled, and they can be synthesized when needed.

The accuracy of DNA typing is better than has been achieved using serology. The more difficult HLA specificities, those for which highly specific alloantisera are rare or not widely available, can be more precise using DNA testing. For example, HLA-DR6 has been a troublesome specificity for many years because antisera could not be obtained. It is now known that HLA-DR6 is composed of at least 69 alleles of HLA-DR13 and HLA-DR14. Laboratories around the world generally have been successful in typing the DR13 and DR14 splits of DR6 using DNA typing. For the most part, the concordance of DNA and serologic typing for HLA has been high for the broad specificities, but DNA is clearly the superior method for the split specificities.

The nomenclature for HLA antigens typed using DNA technology expands on the serologic designation whenever possible. The gene is listed, followed by an asterisk to indicate a DNA typing result. The serologic designation is followed by two or more digits that represent the individual allele. The second HLA-A1 allele that was described is called HLA-A*0102. Noncoding nucleotide differences that do not alter the amino acid sequence of the antigen can be designated with a fifth digit (A*02011, A*02012), and differences in the *introns* (noncoding portions of the gene) can be indicated with 6th and 7th digits (A*2402102).

The naming of HLA class II antigens is similar but somewhat more complex than that of class I antigens because two distinct peptides combine to form the antigen. However, the DR antigens are distinguished by their DR beta$_1$ subunit; therefore, the first allele of DR1 is DRB1*0101. The naming convention for the third through seventh digits is the same as for class I antigens.

HLA Matching for Kidney Transplantations

It is difficult to find HLA-matched kidney donors outside the patient's immediate family. Even using the current convention of matching for 75 serologically defined HLA-A and -B antigens and considering only 10 broad HLA-DR specificities, fewer than 20% of cadaver kidneys are transplanted to an HLA-matched recipient. To achieve this level of matching, each cadaver donor's HLA type is compared with those of all waiting patients in the United States (more than 45,000 at the beginning of the year 2000). If all the known alleles of HLA were used for identifying a matching kidney donor, the task would be even more daunting. As seen in Table 3.1, to provide for good matches using all the known alleles, it would be necessary to match 119 A locus, 238 B locus, and 204 DR locus alleles. So far, there is no evidence that marked improvements in graft survival could be achieved by matching kidneys at the allele level. In fact, many recipients with HLA-mismatched kidney grafts continue to have good function many years after transplantation. This suggests that there may be "immunogenic" and "nonimmunogenic" HLA mismatches. If those can be identified, it may be possible to reduce the number of known specificities to a practical list relevant for organ sharing. Efforts to reduce the number of specificities still further are detailed in the next section.

Cross-reacting Group Matching

The emphasis on high resolution of the HLA alleles accentuates HLA differences that have evolved anthropologically. The result is that racial groups are more distinctly separated with regard to their HLA types. On the other hand, combining broad specificities into even broader cross-reacting groups (CREGs) tends to group individuals together, regardless of their racial background. The CREG groups are based on reactivity patterns of commonly encountered HLA antibodies. When an individual makes antibody, it usually reacts to a group of HLA antigens rather than with an individual HLA antigen. CREGs can also be defined in terms of *epitopes* (antibody-binding sites on HLA antigens) or amino acid residues shared by cross-reacting antigens. The rationale for CREG matching is that kidneys with epitopes more similar to those in the recipient are less likely to elicit a vigorous immune response. In retrospective analysis higher survival has been reported among patients receiving transplants from donors who shared these CREG groups. Decreasing the number of antigens used for matching to about a dozen HLA-A and -B locus CREGs is being attempted to determine whether more "matched" patients within smaller local pools can undergo transplantation and whether, as a result, more kidneys will be offered to minority candidates.

IMMUNOLOGIC EVALUATION
OF TRANSPLANTATION CANDIDATES

When a patient is entered to the United Network for Organ Sharing (UNOS) renal transplant waiting list, the patient's HLA-A, -B and -DR antigens are first determined using DNA or serologic typing methods. A second test that estimates the probability that the patient will have a positive donor crossmatch is also required. Evaluation of HLA antibodies in the serum of a transplant candidate is the transplantation equivalent of ABO blood group typing for a blood transfusion. The consequence of proceeding with transplantation or transfusion with the presence of reactive antibody is similar. The former produces red blood cell lysis and a transfusion reaction, and the latter results in hyperacute rejection. Assiduous attention to pretransplantation lymphocyte crossmatching has virtually eliminated hyperacute rejection as a clinical threat.

Measuring Anti-HLA Antibodies

The microlymphocytotoxicity test can be used to screen for preformed anti-HLA cytotoxic antibodies. The patient's serum is incubated separately with B cells and T cells from a panel of donors selected to represent the HLA antigens commonly found in the local population. Complement is added and cell lysis detected, as noted previously. The results are usually expressed as the percentage of panel cells that are killed by the serum. The anti-HLA antibodies that are detected are called *panel-reactive antibody* (PRA). Immunoglobulin G (IgG) antibodies reactive to HLA class I antigens (found on both T and B cells) are the most important. These antibodies react to T cells at 37°C (*T warm antibodies*). IgM antibody is characterized by reactivity at 5°C, and its activity can be removed by heating the serum to 55°C or by treatment with a reducing agent, such as dithiothreitol (DTT). IgM antibody is often autoantibody and is commonly detected in the sera of patients with systemic lupus erythematosus. Such antibodies can usually be ignored. The importance of anti-DR antibody (reactive to B cells) remains controversial.

The higher a patient's PRA, the more difficult it is to find a cross-match-negative kidney. Simplistically, the finding of 60% PRA on the T-cell panel suggests that 60% of donors will be unacceptable for the patient because there are circulating antibodies that react with one or more of the donor's HLA antigens. Patients with high levels of PRA may wait many years for their transplants.

Patients can be separated into groups based on their level of HLA antibody. An attempt should be made to determine the HLA specificity (a list of HLA antigens that react with the patient's serum) for patients with 5% to 95% PRA. These patients should be screened on a monthly basis to monitor changes in their reactivity. If an HLA specificity can be identified based on the reaction pattern, donors whose HLA profile includes that antigen can be listed as unacceptable. Patients with no HLA antibody or those with more than 95% PRA can be screened less frequently unless they receive a blood transfusion or become pregnant. Sera from patients with PRA of more than 50% (the exact level varies depending on local policy) can be placed on special trays and tested with lymphocytes from each blood group–compatible donor that becomes available to facilitate transplantation of these broadly sensitized patients.

The most potent sources of immunization to HLA antigens are prior blood transfusions, pregnancy and parturition, and a rejected prior transplant. The widespread use of erythropoietin for chronic dialysis patients and the subsequent reduction in transfusion requirements have reduced the number of patients who become sensitized while waiting for a transplant.

More Sensitive Tests for Measuring HLA Antibodies

Antihuman Globulin

Anti-HLA antibodies that do not fix complement or that are present in very small amounts may be missed using the standard NIH procedure. The cytotoxicity test can be enhanced by adding antihuman globulin (AHG) to the microcytotoxicity plate before addition of complement. AHG promotes complement fixation by cross-linking bound HLA antibody. The AHG reagent must be standardized because its titer and specificity may vary.

Enzyme-linked Immunosorbent Assay

The enzyme-linked immunosorbent assay (ELISA) uses solubilized, purified, or both types of HLA antigen pooled from a panel of many donors that has been adhered to a test plate. Patient serum is added, followed by an enzyme-labeled second antibody reactive to human IgG. The reaction is measured in an ELISA reader. Neither viable lymphocytes nor complement fixation is required. HLA specificities can be determined using a panel of HLA antigens from individual donors plated in separate wells on the test plate. Innovations of this technique have improved identification of class I and class II specificities.

Flow Cytometry Panel-reactive Antibody

Flow cytometry is the most sensitive antibody assay (its use as a crossmatch test is outlined in Fig. 3.3). To determine PRA, a pool

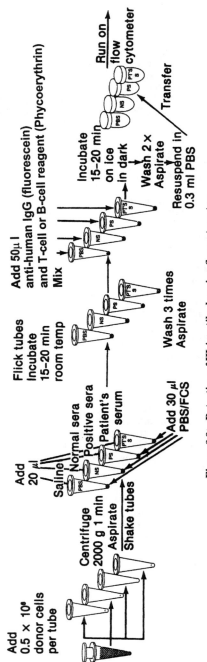

Figure 3.3. Detection of HLA antibody using flow cytometry.

of target cells composed of lymphocytes from 5 to 10 donors is used. Target cell mixtures are selected to represent CREGs and DR antigens. The patient's serum is mixed with target cells; the cells are washed and then incubated with monoclonal mouse anti-CD3 (a pan T-cell marker) antibody conjugated with phycoerythrin and an antihuman IgG antibody conjugated with fluorescein. With a flow cytometer, the T cells that stain red can be gated, making the amount of green fluorescence proportional to the concentration of anti–T-cell antibodies present in the serum. Alternatively, microparticles coated with purified HLA class I or class II antigens can be used as antibody targets. These offer the advantage of purified target antigens and may be prepared from individual donors to allow antibody specificities to be determined.

Pretransplantation Crossmatch

The crossmatch test is the final pretransplantation immunologic screening step. Using the previously described HLA antibody screening assays, the potential donor's lymphocytes serve as the target cells for the patient's serum. The presence of cytotoxic IgG antidonor HLA antibodies is a strong contraindication to transplantation. Most transplant centers use the more sensitive AHG augmentation or flow cytometry in addition to the cytotoxicity test. ELISA tests using isolating donor antigens have yet to gain widespread acceptance.

Patients with high PRA have accumulated on waiting lists because of the difficulty in finding suitable crossmatch-negative donors. To expedite the crossmatch procedure, screening tray sets with recent sera samples from sensitized patients are prepared either quarterly or monthly. Tray sets are segregated by patient ABO, and a "preliminary" crossmatch is performed by testing donor cells on the appropriate tray set at the time of donor HLA typing. Sensitized patients with a positive crossmatch are excluded, but those with a negative preliminary crossmatch and 80% or more PRA receive special consideration in the ranking of candidates (see Kidney Allocation and Distribution). When the preliminary crossmatch is negative, a final crossmatch using either AHG or flow cytometry is performed with recent or fresh sera. Some centers allow older sera to be used if the patient is unsensitized and has not received a recent blood transfusion.

IgM autoantibodies can cause false-positive lymphocytotoxic crossmatch test results (see Immunologic Evaluation of Transplantation Candidates). Sera from patients with demonstrated IgM autoantibodies should be heated or treated with DTT to eliminate IgM. Not all IgM antibodies are benign. IgM antibodies with anti-HLA specificity have been associated with hyperacute or accelerated rejections in isolated cases. Thus, the patient's antibody profile should be thoroughly evaluated before transplantation. When testing is performed by flow cytometry, the specificity of the second antibody can be used to determine the antibody class. Typically, these tests employ antihuman IgG antibody; therefore, IgM reactions are not detected.

Flow Cytometry Crossmatch

The flow cytometry crossmatch test (FCXM) is outlined in Fig. 3.3. Although a positive lymphocytotoxic crossmatch is a contraindication to kidney transplantation, the place of the flow cytometry crossmatch is still somewhat controversial. The test can detect very low levels of circulating antibodies. Positive flow cytometry crossmatches have been associated with a higher rate of early acute rejection episodes and a lower 1-year graft survival rate. Hyperacute rejection has not been reported, however, and some transplants across a positive FCXM have no early problems (if the cytotoxic crossmatch is negative). The T-cell FCXM may be particularly useful in the pretransplantation evaluation of sensitized and retransplantation candidates whose antibody levels may have fallen but who can mount a rapid memory response upon challenge. Low levels of circulating antibody may have a more profound effect when the cadaver donor is older or the kidney quality is uncertain. Although the T-cell FCXM has been used with some success, as described previously, the role of the B-cell FCXM is still being debated. Most studies have shown that a positive B-cell FCXM, when associated with a negative T-cell FCXM, does not increase the risk for early rejection or graft loss. However, B-cell FCXM results that are strongly positive may be associated with high titers of anti–HLA class II antibodies and may be predictive of poor graft outcome.

KIDNEY ALLOCATION AND DISTRIBUTION

Ideally, all patients with end-stage renal failure who are awaiting transplants would receive a well-matched high-quality kidney after a short waiting time. In the United States as of the year 2000, more than 220,000 patients were on chronic dialysis. More than 42,000 dialysis patients (a 200% increase compared with 1988) were awaiting cadaveric kidney transplants, but only about 9,000 cadaver kidneys were procured annually (see Chapter 1, Fig. 1.1). The growing discrepancy between the supply and demand for cadaveric kidneys means that the wait for a kidney transplant can vary from several months to several years.

The U.S. Congress passed the National Organ Transplant Act in 1984 to address problems of the inadequate supply of human organs and to ensure equitable distribution of those that were available. This act provided for the establishment and operation of an Organ Procurement and Transplantation Network (OPTN) and a Scientific Registry. In 1986, UNOS was awarded the contract to develop the OPTN. The mandate to UNOS includes the improvement of cadaveric organ procurement and distribution and the development of an equitable system for access to and sharing of renal and extrarenal organs.

To operate this system, the country is divided into organ procurement regions and areas, with regional Organ Procurement Organizations (OPOs) operating according to agreed distribution and sharing criteria. To be placed on the transplant waiting list, a patient must fulfill certain *listing criteria*. Renal transplant recipients must either be receiving chronic dialysis or, if they are pre-dialysis, have a glomerular filtration rate estimated at 20 mL/min or less. No priority is given for specific disease states. The distribution of kidneys by the OPOs to patients on the waiting list is discussed next.

Distribution by ABO Blood Groups

The ABO blood group antigens behave as strong transplantation antigens, and transplantation across ABO barriers usually leads to irreversible hyperacute rejection. In principle, the same criteria determine kidney distribution according to ABO as do blood transfusions with group O (the universal donor) and group AB (the universal recipient). The disproportionate percentage of type O recipients who are waiting for kidney transplants generally mandates that blood group identity rather than blood group compatibility determine the distribution of cadaver kidneys. For living-related donor transplantation, ABO compatibility is adequate.

Attempts have been made to overcome blood group barriers by removing blood group isoagglutinins with plasmapheresis or immunoabsorption, followed by intense immunosuppression. In general, ABO-incompatible transplantations have resulted in high rates of early graft loss because of isoagglutinin-mediated rejection episodes. In white populations, about 20% of blood group A individuals can be defined as A2, and these patients have reduced levels of A antigen on graft endothelium. They may permit an exception to the ABO-incompatibility barrier because A2 kidneys can be safely transplanted into O or B recipients with low preoperative titers of isoagglutinin. Transplantation of A2 kidneys into O or B recipients is routine in some centers.

The distribution of ABO groups among different ethnic groups and potential kidney transplant recipients is noted in Table 3.2. If all ethnic groups contributed equally to the donor pool and all ethnic groups suffered end-stage renal disease in direct proportion to their frequency in the general population and equally among blood groups, waiting times for the different ethnic groups and blood group categories would be the same. In fact, whites contribute disproportionately to the donor pool and blacks contribute disproportionately to the recipient pool because kidney disease is more common in blacks. As a result, patients with blood group O or B wait longer for a blood group–identical donor.

Table 3.2. Percent distribution of ABO blood groups according to ethnic groups and patients on the transplant waiting list

Blood Group	White	Black	Native American	Asian	Waiting List[a]
O	45	49	79	40	52
A	40	27	16	28	28
B	11	20	4	27	17
AB	4	4	<1	5	3
TOTAL					42,392

[a] Waiting list is compiled by the United Network for Organ Sharing research department as of June 2000.

Data modified from RH Walker, ed. *Technical manual of the American Association of Blood Banks*, 11th ed. Bethesda, MD: American Association of Blood Banks, 1993:204, with permission.

Distribution by HLA Matching and Waiting Time

The importance of matching in determining graft outcome is well established. The extent to which matching should determine kidney distribution remains controversial. Were matching to be given absolute priority in kidney distribution, the whole country would represent a single donor and recipient pool. Such a policy has been accepted for fully HLA-matched kidneys. Less well-matched kidneys are not shared nationally, but the quality of the HLA match is reflected in the UNOS point allocation within the regional OPO's.

To ensure that kidneys are allocated equitably, a point system has been established for use in the United States (Table 3.3). Regions can apply for *variances* to the national system. Most points are allocated for highly matched kidneys, with a stepwise decrement in points for less well-matched kidneys. Points are also given for time spent waiting for a kidney, for a negative crossmatch in patients with a PRA greater than 79%, and for young children in whom a prolonged wait for a kidney can have a catastrophic effect on growth and development (see Chapter 15).

The Six-Antigen-Match Program

The UNOS six-antigen-match program provides evidence of the value of excellent HLA matching. In 1987, all the transplantation centers in the United States mutually agreed to match first every kidney donor with the national patient pool, and if a patient with all six HLA-A, -B, and -DR antigen matches was found, the kidney would be shipped to that recipient. In 1995, 0-A, B, and DR

Table 3.3.   United Network for Organ Sharing (UNOS) point system for allocation of cadaveric kidneys as of January 1999

Time waiting[a]	1 point for longest waiting patient in a blood group category
	fraction of a point for relative position on the list
	1 additional point for each additional year of waiting time
Quality of HLA match	0-A, B, DR mismatch[b]
	7 points 0-B or DR mismatch
	5 points 1-B or DR mismatch
	2 points 2-B or DR mismatch
Panel-reactive antibody	4 points for >80% and negative cross-match
Pediatric recipient	4 points for age <11 yr
	3 points for age 11–17 yr
Medical urgency	Physician judgment

[a] Defined from the time a patient is activated on the UNOS computer.
[b] All 0-A, B, DR mismatched organs are involved in the national mandatory sharing program (see text).
HLA, human leukocyte antigen.

mismatched kidneys were included in the national sharing program. This has increased the percentage of matched transplants to 15.5% from 2.5% prior to the six-antigen-match era. As of 1998, more than 7,000 kidneys have been shared through this program and their 1-year graft survival rate was 89%, which was significantly higher than the 83% for control transplants with at least one HLA mismatch. Overall, the shared HLA-matched kidneys had a better anticipated long-term survival rate as measured by transplant half-life (12.4 years) than locally transplanted HLA-mismatched kidneys (8.5 years).

FACTORS DETERMINING TRANSPLANTATION OUTCOME

Donor Type: Cadaveric Versus Live Donor

The type of donor kidney used is one of the most important predictors of both long-term and short-term allograft outcome. Figure 3.4 depicts allograft survival curves for HLA-identical siblings (two-haplotype match), parental donors (one-haplotype match), spousal (living-unrelated) donors (0 haplotype match), and first cadaveric donor and is based on the results of more than 80,000 transplantations performed between 1988 and 1998 and reported to UNOS. Kidney transplants from two-haplotype–matched siblings provide grafts with the highest survival rates. The long-term success of living-unrelated donor kidney transplants is comparable to that achieved with transplants from parent donors and is greater than that achieved with equivalently HLA-matched cadaveric donors. This may seem counterintuitive because living-unrelated donors share no HLA haplotypes with their recipients.

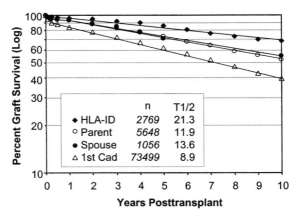

Figure 3.4.   Rate of graft loss for first kidneys transplanted between 1988 and 1998 and reported to the United Network for Organ Sharing. Note the difference in estimated half-life ($T_{1/2}$) depending on the source of the kidney. All sibling transplantations reported here are two-haplotype matches (HLA-ID). Parents are, by definition, one-haplotype matches, and spousal donors are zero-haplotype matches.

The high success rates for living-unrelated donor transplants is attributed, in part, to the overall excellent health of the donors, enhanced long-term compliance when a spouse donates, and avoidance of the multiple insults intrinsic to cadaveric harvesting and donation (see Chapter 5). Living donor kidney transplantations now account for more than 30% of kidney transplantations performed in the United States, compared with 20% just 10 years ago. The growing number of transplants from spouses and other living-unrelated donors has fueled much of this increase. Recipient candidates should be strongly encouraged to consider the option of a living donor (see Chapters 5 and 6).

It has been suggested that there is a graft survival benefit for recipients of living-related donor kidneys from one-haplotype–matched siblings when the donor has maternal HLA antigens not inherited by the recipient (Fig. 3.1). This has been attributed to the possibility that maternal antigens modulate the antigen-specific reactivity of the fetal (future recipient) immune system, leading to a lasting form of tolerance to future antigen challenge in the adult recipient.

Of the groups depicted in Fig. 3.4, the lowest graft survival rate is found in transplants from cadaveric donors. The 10-year graft survival rate for cadaveric donor transplants may be as low as 40%, compared with almost 70% for HLA-identical donor transplants. Because most of the transplantations performed today are from cadaveric donors, it is imperative that the issues leading to the lower short-term and long-term graft outcomes be addressed.

Improvements in immunosuppressive therapy have contributed to higher graft survival rates in recent years. In the cyclosporine era, 1-year living-related graft survival rates of greater than 90% and cadaveric graft survival rates of greater than 80% have become routine. Some centers have reported survival rates close to 100% for living-related transplants and 90% for cadaveric transplants. Figure 3.5 shows the improvement in cadaver donor kidney transplant survival that occurred between 1980 and 1998, including the nearly 20% improvement in the 1-year graft survival rate when cyclosporine use began in 1984. It should be noted that improvement has occurred despite a general lowering of the quality of cadaveric kidneys.

HLA-Matching Effect

HLA matching continues to have an effect on the long-term loss rate. As shown in Fig. 3.6, the 5-year graft survival rates decreased in a step-wise fashion from 69% for patients with 0-A, B, and DR mismatches (see HLA Matches and Mismatches) to 57% for completely mismatched grafts (five or six HLA-mismatched antigens). However, only a few percentage points separated the individual mismatch levels. The half-life of the transplanted kidneys also decreased in a step-wise fashion with increasing degrees of HLA mismatching. The half-life of zero-mismatched kidneys has increased in recent years despite the increased use of older donor kidneys in the national sharing program (see Donor Age) and the greater use of HLA-matched kidneys for highly sensitized patients. Sensitized patients have an inherently lower allograft survival rate.

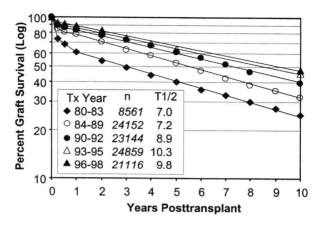

Figure 3.5. Graft survival rates for recipients of first cadaver kidney transplants improved steadily between 1980 and 1998. The largest improvement was associated with the introduction of cyclosporine in 1984. Graft half-lives have also improved from about 7 years in the early 1980s to more than 10 years in the 1993–1995 cohort. The short follow-up period for 1996–1998 transplantations may explain the slightly lower half-lives computed for these grafts.

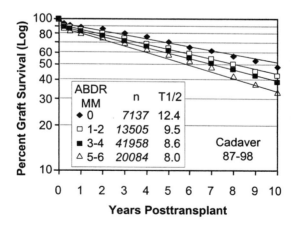

Figure 3.6. Impact of HLA-A, -B, and -DR mismatches on early and late graft survival of more than 28,000 first cadaveric transplants reported to the United Network for Organ Sharing from 1988 to 1992. $T_{1/2}$, half-life.

Sensitization

Broadly sensitized patients (more than 50% PRA before their transplants) have poorer graft survival rates than less sensitized patients. The reduced survival rate among broadly sensitized patients is apparent within the first 6 months after transplantation. Even those who survive the first posttransplantation year have a slightly accelerated rate of late graft loss compared with patients who are unsensitized. Because an important cause of the reduced survival rates of transplants in sensitized patients is the increased incidence of acute rejection episodes, more potent immunosuppressive protocols are often recommended for this patient population (see Chapter 4).

Racial Differences

The role of race in the success of kidney transplantation has been the subject of considerable debate. In the United States, allograft survival in black recipients tends to be about 10% to 20% less than for white recipients whether the transplant is from a living or cadaveric donor. Several factors have been proposed to explain the lower survival rate, including a transplantation center effect, noncompliance and socioeconomic factors, the prevalence of hypertension in blacks, and evidence of stronger immune responsiveness. The high prevalence of Duffy antigen receptor for chemokine (DARC, or Duffy blood group) negativity in black recipients has been associated with poor allograft outcome. DARC positivity may be beneficial, functioning as a "sink" for chemokines expressed during rejection episodes.

Differences in the frequencies of ABO blood groups (Table 3.2) and of HLA determinants (see Linkage Disequilibrium), as well as cultural and socioeconomic factors, may affect the rate of transplantation. Minorities may be more reluctant to donate organs. As a result, whites are represented disproportionately in the organ donor pool—a phenomenon that may favor white recipients when kidneys are allocated according to the blood group and tissue matching (see Kidney Allocation and Distribution). Efforts to encourage organ donation among minorities may help redress inequalities of allocation.

Despite the predominantly white donor pool, Asian recipients of renal allografts have superior graft survival rates. Asian recipients of cadaveric transplants have nearly 70% 5-year graft survival rates, compared with 60% for white recipients. The explanation for this difference in outcome is not clear.

Recipient Age

In general, the oldest and youngest recipients have the worst long-term allograft survival rates. The 5-year cadaveric graft survival rates range from 57% in patients older than 60 years of age to 65% in patients 31 to 45 years of age. The poor allograft survival rates for older recipients are due in part to the relatively high rate of graft loss because of patient death in this population. This underscores the importance of strict medical screening policies for older transplantation candidates.

There is, however, a growing trend toward more transplantations being performed in the older age groups. This is in part a reflection of the increasing average age of the dialysis population nationally (see Chapter 1). The mean age of recipients of cadaver donor kidneys increased from 42 to 46 years between 1991 and 1997 alone. During this same time period, the percentage of cadaver kidneys transplanted in recipients older than 60 years of age increased from about 5% to 15%. Though older patients have an intrinsically greater post-transplant mortality rate, the impact of age on graft survival may be counterbalanced by the fact that older patients tend to be less immunologically aggressive (see Chapter 4).

Donor Age

Increasing donor age has a pronounced negative effect on graft survival. The 5-year cadaveric graft survival rates range from 68% when the donor is 19 to 30 years of age to 44% when the donor is older than 60 years of age. This trend is also noted with living donor transplants. Because of the shortage of organs available for transplantation, however, older donor kidneys are being used more frequently. The percentage of kidneys from donors older than 60 years of age grew from 5% in 1991 to 8% in 1996. An increased incidence of delayed graft function among recipients of older donor kidneys and an overall decrease in "nephron dosing" for an average older donor may explain the poor long-term survival rates associated with this donor group. Because of the relatively poor long-term allograft survival rates for older donor kidneys, these kidneys are often allocated to older recipients who have a presumed shorter life span. Figure 3.7 depicts the effect of donor age on 5-year allograft survival by number of HLA mismatches. Overall, kidneys from older donors have poorer outcomes. Although the zero-mismatched kidneys from donors older than 60 years of age have the best outcome in that donor age group, their poor (52%) 5-year graft survival rate was comparable to that for completely mismatched kidneys from donors aged 46 to 50 years. It has been suggested that kidneys from older donors not be included in the

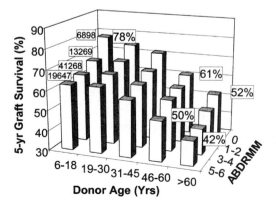

Figure 3.7. Interaction between donor age and HLA mismatches. The benefit of HLA matching is diminished with donors older than 60 years of age. ABDRMM, degrees of mismatched for A,B and DR loci.

national sharing program because the shipping process may add additional injury because of long cold ischemia times.

The Center Effect

Not all transplantation centers report similar results, and over-all transplant statistics are a conglomerate of results from centers with differing experiences. Numerous factors independent of immunosuppressive protocols or tissue typing may determine why a given center may have results better than another center or better than general experience. Results tend to be unfavorably influenced by a high proportion of older and younger patients (older than 45 or younger than 25 years of age), diabetic patients, African-Americans, retransplantation patients, and broadly sensitized patients. The center effect refers to the differences in results among transplantation centers.

Awareness of these factors is important in analyzing data from single-center reports, particularly when such data suggest benefits of therapeutic maneuvers or organ distribution criteria.

Other Factors

A number of other factors may play a role in determining allograft outcome. The presence of delayed graft function, long cold ischemia times, and acute rejection episodes are associated with a decrease in allograft survival. Diseases leading to end-stage renal disease, such as diabetes and hypertension, that have multiple organ system manifestations are associated with poorer long-term allograft survival rates than diseases not associated with systemic manifestations, such as polycystic kidney disease and IgA nephropathy. The length of time receiving dialysis treatment before transplantation may affect survival. Patients who are fortunate to receive a transplant before they need to start dialysis tend to do better; on the other hand, a prolonged duration of dialysis treatment tends to decrease the long-term survival of transplant recipients possibly by persistently exposing them to the morbid complications of dialysis (see Chapter 1).

SELECTED READINGS

Bodmer JG, Marsh SGE, Albert ED, et al. Nomenclature for factors of the HLA system, 1998. *Hum Immunol* 1999;60:361.

Bunce M, Young NT, Welsh KI. Molecular HLA typing: the brave new world. *Transplantation* 1997;64:1505.

Burlingham WJ, Grailer AP, Heisey DM, et al. The effect of tolerance to noninherited maternal HLA antigens on the survival of renal transplants from sibling donors. *N Engl J Med* 1998;339:1657.

Carpenter CB. Improving the success of organ transplantation. *N Engl J Med* 2000;342:647.

Cecka JM. The UNOS Scientific Renal Transplant Registry. In: Cecka JM, Terasaki PI, eds. *Clinical transplants 1999*. Los Angeles, UCLA Tissue Typing Laboratory, 2000.

Consensus conference on standardized listing criteria for renal transplant candidates. *Transplantation* 1998;66:962.

Feucht HE, Opelz G. The humoral immune response towards HLA class II determinants in renal transplantation. *Kidney Int* 1996;59:1464.

Hariharan S, Johnson CP, Bresnahan BA, et al. Improved graft survival after renal transplantation in the United States, 1988 to 1996. *N Engl J Med* 2000;342:65.

Lazda VA. Identification of patients at risk for inferior renal allograft outcome by a strongly positive B cell flow cytometry crossmatch. *Transplantation* 1994;57:964.

Martin S, Taylor CJ. The immunologically sensitised renal transplant recipient: the impact of advances in the technology on organ allocation and transplant outcome. *Transplant Rev* 1999;13:40.

McKenna RM, Takemoto SK. Improving HLA matching for kidney transplantation by the use of CREGs. *Lancet* 2000;355:1842.

Neylan JF, Sayegh MH, Coffman TM, et al. Allocation of cadaver kidneys for transplantation in the United States: consensus and controversy. *J Am Soc Nephrol* 1999;10:2237.

Parham P, Lawlor DA, Slater RD, et al. HLA-A,B,C: patterns of polymorphism in peptide-binding proteins. In: Tsuji K, Aizawa M, Sasazuki T, eds. *HLA 1991*. Oxford, UK, Oxford University Press, 1992:10–33.

Schnitzler MA, Hollenbeak CS, Cohen DS, et al. The economic implications of HLA matching in cadaveric renal transplantation. *N Engl J Med* 1999;341;1440.

Takemoto SK, Terasaki PI. Evaluation of the transplant recipient and donor: molecular approach to tissue typing, flow cytometry and alternative approaches to distributing organs. *Curr Opin Nephrol Hypertens* 1997;6:299.

4

Immunosuppressive Medications and Protocols for Kidney Transplantation

Gabriel M. Danovitch

A BRIEF HISTORY OF TRANSPLANT IMMUNOSUPPRESSION

To understand the construction of the immunosuppressive protocol and the use of immunosuppressive medications according to current standard transplantation practice, it helps to follow the development of organ transplantation and, in particular, kidney transplantation since the 1950s. Although sporadic attempts at kidney transplantation had been made throughout the first half of this century, the current era of transplantation was pioneered in the mid-1950s with live donor transplants from identical twins. The first attempts at immunosuppression used total-body irradiation; azathioprine was introduced in the early 1960s and was soon routinely accompanied by prednisolone. The polyclonal antibody preparations, antithymocyte globulin (ATG) and antilymphocyte globulin (ALG), became available in the mid-1970s. With azathioprine and prednisolone as the baseline regimen and ATG or ALG used for induction or for the treatment of steroid-resistant rejection, the success rate of kidney transplantation was about 50% at 1 year, and the mortality rate was typically 10% to 20%.

The situation was transformed in the early 1980s with the introduction of cyclosporine. Because the results of kidney transplantation were poor, it was not hard to recognize the dramatic benefit of cyclosporine that produced statistically significant improvement in graft survival rates to greater than 80% at 1 year. Mortality rates decreased with more effective immunosuppression, less use of corticosteroids, and overall improvements in surgical and medical care. The standard immunosuppressive regimen consisted of cyclosporine and prednisone, often combined with azathioprine, now used as an adjunctive agent in so-called 'triple therapy'. Although the benefits of cyclosporine were clear-cut, its capacity to produce both acute and chronic nephrotoxicity was soon recognized to be a major detriment. In 1985, OKT3, the first monoclonal antibody used in clinical medicine, was introduced based on its capacity to treat first acute rejection episodes, although the toxicity of the drug tended to restrict its use to episodes of rejection that were resistant to high-dose steroids and, in some programs, to use as an induction agent. With this limited armamentarium of medications—cyclosporine, azathioprine, corticosteroids, and the antibody preparations—the transplantation community entered the 1990s achieving, with justifiable pride, success rates of up to 90% in many centers and minimal mortality. Because the number of available immunosuppressive medications was low, there was relatively little variation between the protocol options used in different programs.

Two major developments then followed. Tacrolimus was introduced into liver transplantation and eventually into kidney transplantation as an alternative to cyclosporine with respect to its capacity to produce equivalent patient and graft survival, and mycophenolate mofetil (MMF) was found to be a more effective adjunctive agent than azathioprine by virtue of its capacity to reduce the incidence of acute rejection episodes when used with cyclosporine (and later with tacrolimus) and corticosteroids. Two new humanized monoclonal antibodies, basiliximab and daclizumab, have also been approved for use after kidney transplantation, also based on their capacity to reduce the incidence of acute rejection episodes, and a polyclonal antibody, thymoglobulin, available in Europe for several years, has been approved for use in the United States for the treatment of acute rejection. In late 1999, sirolimus was added to the immunosuppressive menu, and studies are in progress to evaluate several new chemical and biologic agents.

The therapeutic armamentarium for transplant immunosuppression thus continues to broaden and become more complex, as does the variety of potential drug combinations or protocols. To address this complexity, this chapter is divided into four sections. Part I reviews the drugs in current clinical use, emphasizing cyclosporine, tacrolimus, MMF, and sirolimus. Part II reviews the currently available biologic agents. Part III discusses the clinical trial process used to develop new immunosuppressive agents and reviews available data on promising new agents at different stages of development. Part IV discusses combinations of these drugs in the form of clinically applied immunosuppressive protocols.

PART I. IMMUNOSUPPRESSIVE AGENTS IN CURRENT CLINICAL USE

CALCINEURIN INHIBITORS
The term *calcineurin inhibitors* is a useful one that emphasizes the similarity in the mechanism of action of the two drugs, *cyclosporine* and *tacrolimus,* which currently serve as the backbone of solid organ transplant immunosuppression. Although they are biochemically distinct, they are remarkably similar, not only in their mechanism of action, but also in their clinical efficacy and side-effect profile. They are therefore considered together, and discrete differences between them are discussed in the text and summarized in Table 4.1. The choice of agent is discussed in Part IV.

Cyclosporine is a small cyclic polypeptide of fungal origin. It consists of 11 amino acids and has a molecular weight of 1,203. It is neutral and insoluble in water but soluble in organic solvents and lipids. The amino acids at positions 11, 1, 2, and 3 form the active immunosuppressive site, and the cyclic structure of the drug is necessary for its immunosuppressive effect. Tacrolimus, still often called by its nickname *Eff-Kay* from its laboratory designation *FK506,* is a macrolide antibiotic compound isolated from *Streptomyces tsukabaensis.*

Mechanism of Action
The calcineurin inhibitors differ from their predecessor immunosuppressive drugs by virtue of their selective inhibition of the

Table 4.1.   Some comparative features of cyclosporine and tacrolimus

	Cyclosporine	Tacrolimus
Mode of action	Inhibition of calcineurin	Inhibition of calcineurin
Daily maintenance dose	~3–5 mg/kg	~0.15–0.3 mg/kg
Administration	PO and IV	PO and IV[a]
Absorption bile dependent	Sandimmune, yes Neoral, no	No
Oral dose available (capsules)	100 mg; 25 mg	5 mg; 1 mg; 0.5mg
Therapeutic drug levels (high-performance liquid chromatography assay)	100–400 ng/mL[b]	5–20 ng/mL
Drug interactions	Similar	Similar
Capacity to prevent rejection[c]	+	++
Capacity to treat ongoing rejection	+	++
Use with MMF	+	+
Use with sirolimus	+	+[d]
Nephrotoxic	+	+
Steroid sparing	+	++?
Hypertension and sodium retention	++	+
Pancreatic islet toxic	+	++
Neurotoxic	+	++
Cosmetic side effects	++	+
Gastrointestinal side effects	–	+
Gastric motility	–	+
Hyperkalemia	+	+
Hypomagnesemia	+	+
Hypercholesterolemia	+	–

[a] IV rarely needed because oral absorption is good.
[b] See Table 4.8.
[c] See Table 4.5.
[d] Combination not formally approved.
Data are based on available literature and clinical experience.
+, known effect; ++, effect more pronounced; –, no or little effect; ++?, probable greater effect; MMF, mycophenoate mofetil.

immune response. They do not inhibit neutrophilic phagocytic activity as corticosteroids do, nor are they myelosuppressive as azathioprine is. Cell-surface events and antigen recognition also remain intact (see Chapter 2). Their immunosuppressive effect depends on the formation of a complex with their cytoplasmic receptor proteins, *cyclophilin* for cyclosporine and tacrolimus-binding protein (*FKBP*) for tacrolimus (see Plate 1). This complex binds with *calcineurin,* whose normal function is to act as a phosphatase that dephosphorylates certain nuclear regulatory proteins (e.g., *nuclear factor of activated T cells* [NF-AT]) and hence facilitates their passage through the nuclear membrane (see Chapter 2, Fig. 2.6). Inhibition of calcineurin thereby impairs the expression of several critical cytokine genes that promote T-cell activation. These include those for interleukin-2 (IL-2), IL-4, interferon-gamma (IFN-gamma), and tumor necrosis factor-alpha (TNF-alpha). The transcription of other genes, such as CD40 ligand and the protooncogenes H-*ras* and c-*myc*, is also impaired. The importance of these factors in T-cell activation is discussed in more detail in Chapter 2, but as a result of calcineurin inhibition, there is a quantitative limitation of cytokine production and downstream lymphocyte proliferation.

Cyclosporine enhances the expression of *TGF-beta,* which also inhibits IL-2 and the generation of cytotoxic T lymphocytes and may be responsible for the development of interstitial fibrosis, an important feature of calcineurin inhibitor nephrotoxicity. TGF-beta has also been implicated as an important factor in the proliferation of tumor cells, which may be relevant to the course of certain posttransplantation neoplasias (see Chapter 9). The *in vivo* effects of cyclosporine are blocked by anti–TGF-beta, indicating that TGF-beta may be central to the mediation of both the beneficial and detrimental effects of the calcineurin inhibitors.

Patients receiving successful calcineurin inhibitor–based immunosuppression maintain a degree of immune responsiveness that is still sufficient to maintain host defenses. This relative immunosuppression may be a reflection of the fact that at therapeutic levels of these drugs, calcineurin activity is reduced by only about 50%, permitting strong signals to trigger cytokine expression and generate an effective immune response. In stable patients receiving cyclosporine, CD4+ T cells have reduced IL-2 production to a degree that is inversely correlated to drug levels. The degree of inhibition of calcineurin activity and IL-2 production may be at the fulcrum of the delicate balance that exists between overimmunosuppression and underimmunosuppression.

Formulations and Pharmacokinetics

Cyclosporine

The original formulation of cyclosporine, the oil-based *Sandimmune,* has largely been replaced by the microemulsion formulation, *Neoral.* Both formulations are available in two forms: a 100 mg/mL solution that is drawn up by the patient into a graduated syringe and dispensed into orange juice or milk, or 25-mg and 100-mg soft gelatin capsules. Patients usually prefer the convenience of the capsule. The absorption of Sandimmune cyclosporine from the gastrointestinal (GI) tract is bile dependent and may be unreliable for patients with diabetic gastroparesis, diarrhea, biliary diversion, cholestasis, and malabsorption. The absorption of cyclosporine after an oral dose can be represented graphically in the form of a concentration–time curve (Fig. 4.1). The time to peak concentration of Sandimmune cyclosporine (t_{max},) is variable but averages 4 hours. A substantial proportion of transplant recipients exhibit a second peak. The bioavailability of Neoral (F) is better than that of Sandimmune, and there is less variability in cyclosporine pharmacokinetics. Peak cyclosporine levels (C_{max}) of Neoral cyclosporine are higher, and the trough concentration (C_{min}) correlates better with the systemic exposure, as reflected by the *area under the curve* (AUC).

The improved GI absorption of the microemulsion and lesser dependence on bile for absorption may reduce the necessity for intravenous cyclosporine administration. Compared with intravenous infusion, the bioavailability of the orally administered drug is in the range of 30% to 45%. Conversion between the oral and intravenous forms of the drug perioperatively requires a 3:1 dose ratio. Bioavailability of oral cyclosporine increases with time, possibly as a result of improved absorption by the previously uremic GI tract. As a result, the amount of cyclosporine required to achieve a given blood level tends to fall with time and typically reaches a steady level within 4 to 8 weeks. Food tends to enhance the absorption of cyclosporine (see Chapter 18).

Some studies have shown a reduction of up to 15% in the incidence of acute rejection with Neoral compared with Sandimmune, and the dose required to achieve an equivalent trough level may be reduced by about 10%. Chronic allograft loss appears similar for Sandimmune- and Neoral-treated patients.

The development of generic formulations of cyclosporine has been controversial because of the critical importance of this drug

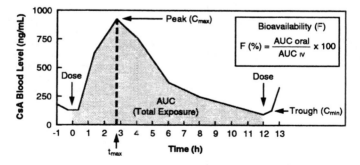

Fig. 4.1. Cyclosporine pharmacokinetic profile. t_{max}, the time to reach maximum cyclosporine concentration; C_{max}, the maximum cyclosporine concentration; C_{min}, the minimum cyclosporine concentration, or trough level; AUC, the area under the concentration–time curve, which approximates a patient's total exposure to cyclosporine over a dosage interval; F, percentage bioavailability of orally administered cyclosporine over a dosage interval. (From Grevel J, Kahan BD. *Ther Drug Monit* 1991;13:89, with permission.)

to the success of transplantation and the corporate and financial implications of their introduction. Cyclosporine is regarded as a drug with a *narrow therapeutic index,* and the standards for proving the *bioequivalence* of generic forms need to be rigorous. Generic formulations of cyclosporine, the liquid *SangCya,* the capsule *Cyclosporine USP* (Eon Labs), and the capsule *Gengraf,* have been approved for use in the USA; other generic formulations are available outside of the USA. The generic formulations are claimed to have an absorption profile that is very similar to that of Neoral. Sang Cya has been withdrawn from distribution because of lack of consistent bioequivalence. The capsules have received a so-called 'AB' rating by the US Food and Drug Administration (FDA), which means that in many states they can be substituted for Neoral cyclosporine without the approval of the prescriber. If conversions are made between the different formulations of cyclosporine, it is probably wise to monitor drug levels and renal function (see Part IV).

Tacrolimus

Tacrolimus (Prograf) is available in an intravenous formulation and as 5-mg, 1-mg, and 0.5-mg capsules; there are currently no generic formulations. Its GI absorption is independent of bile salts. Because of the effectiveness and relative consistency of its absorption, it is rarely necessary to use the intravenous formulation, and if necessary, the drug can be administered through a nasogastric tube. It is absorbed primarily from the small intestine, and its oral bioavailability is about 25% with large interpatient and intrapatient variability, particularly in patients with GI disease. Gastric emptying of solids is faster in patients taking tacrolimus than in those receiving cyclosporine, a property that may be beneficial for patients with gastric motility disorders.

Distribution and Metabolism

In the blood, one third of absorbed and infused cyclosporine is found in plasma, bound primarily to lipoproteins. Most of the remaining drug is bound to erythrocytes. Whole-blood drug levels (see Drug Level Monitoring) are thus typically three-fold higher than plasma levels. The binding of cyclosporine to lipoproteins may be important in the transfer of the drug through plasma membranes, and the toxic effects of cyclosporine may be exaggerated by low cholesterol levels and reduced by high cholesterol levels.

The binding of cyclosporine to the low-density lipoprotein receptor may account for the hyperlipidemia associated with its use. Tacrolimus also has a high affinity for formed blood elements, but it differs from cyclosporine in that, although it is highly protein bound, it is not significantly associated with lipoproteins, and it has a less unfavorable effect on the cholesterol level than does cyclosporine.

Both parent drugs have a half-life of about 8 hours and are metabolized to multiple metabolites by the cytochrome P450 IIIA (CYP3A) found in the GI and liver microsomal enzyme system. GI metabolism through CYP3A and *p*-glycoprotein produces a so-called first-pass metabolism, and the heterogeneity in intestinal CYP3A gene expression may explain some of the wide interpatient variability in drug kinetics. The liver is often considered the most important site of drug metabolism, but GI metabolism may account for up to half of cyclosporine metabolism. Some of the drug metabolites may have immunosuppressive and nephrotoxic potential, and the plasma levels of the most important cyclosporine metabolite, M17, may be similar to that of the parent compound.

Both drugs are excreted in the bile, with minimal renal excretion; therefore, drug doses do not need to be modified in the presence of kidney dysfunction. Neither drug is significantly dialyzed, and they can be administered during dialysis treatment without dose adjustment. The pharmacokinetic parameters of both drugs may vary among patient groups, and these variations may have clinical consequences. Pediatric and black transplant recipients may require relatively larger doses and short dosage intervals. Longer dosage intervals may be required in older patients and in the presence of liver disease.

Drug Level Monitoring

The measurement of cyclosporine and tacrolimus levels is an intrinsic part of the management of transplant patients because of variation in interpatient and intrapatient metabolism. There is also a relationship, albeit an inconsistent one, between blood levels of the drug and episodes of rejection and toxicity. Drug level monitoring is the source of much confusion because of the various assays available and the option of using different matrices (i.e., plasma or whole blood) for their measurement.

When Sandimmune was introduced, the trough level of cyclosporine (drawn immediately preceding the next dose), rather than the peak level, was measured because its timing was more consistent and appeared to correlate better with toxic complications. More sophisticated techniques of monitoring were suggested whereby a pharmacokinetic profile is constructed to calculate the AUC, which reflects the bioavailability of the drug and may theoretically allow for more precise and individualized patient management. Although attractive, these techniques never proved popular because of their cost and inconvenience, and most centers continue to rely on trough levels. With the introduction of Neoral, this trend has continued, although there is evidence to suggest that because of its more consistent absorption, its peak level (2 hours after dosing; Fig. 4.1) may correlate better with drug exposure than trough level. The trough level of tacrolimus is also used for monitoring, and this level is a good approximation of drug exposure.

Cyclosporine concentrations are routinely measured in plasma or whole blood. Whole blood is preferred because the plasma levels are temperature dependent. The clinician cannot begin to assess the significance of a cyclosporine level without knowing what kind of assay is being used. *High-performance liquid chromatography* (HPLC) is the most specific method for measuring unmetabolized parent cyclosporine and is considered the reference method. HPLC, however, is expensive and labor intensive and is not available at all centers. DiaSorin (Stillwater, Minnesota; new name for Incstar) has a *radioimmunoassay* that measures the parent compound and exhibits 30% cross-reactivity with inactive metabolites. Nonisotopic assays, such as the Abbot (Chicago, Illinois) fluorescence polarization immunoassay (FPIA), have become widely used because they are rapid, are technically simple, and yield reproducible results. Two forms of FPIA are available; it is very important to differentiate between them. The *polyclonal assay* employs antisera that measure both parent compound and metabolites; the *monoclonal assay* employs a mouse monoclonal antibody designed to be parent-compound specific; however, when compared with HPLC, it overestimates cyclosporine by up to 30% in kidney transplant recipients. Syva (Palo Alto, California) has an automated monoclonal *enzyme immunoassay* that cross-reacts less with metabolites and yields results more comparable with HPLC.

Two commercial kits are available to monitor tacrolimus concentrations. Both use a monoclonal antibody that detects the parent compound and an array of metabolites. The Abbot *microparticle immunoassay* (MEIA) is simpler and faster than the DiaSorin *enzyme-linked immunosorbent assay* (ELISA), but the ELISA has better analytic sensitivity. The MEIA is the most commonly used and permits accurate estimation of tacrolimus levels as low as 2 ng/dL. Target cyclosporine and tacrolimus levels are discussed in the section on immunosuppressive protocols.

Drug Interactions

The interaction of the calcineurin inhibitors with many commonly used drugs demands constant attention to drug regimens and cognizance of potential interactions. New drugs should be introduced with care, and patients should be warned to consult physicians familiar with the use of cyclosporine and tacrolimus before considering new pharmacologic therapy. Some of the drug interactions discussed below are consistent and well established (and are emphasized in **bold** lettering); others have been described in small series and case reports.

Unless a comment is made to the contrary, the drug interactions are common to both cyclosporine and tacrolimus, although more have been described with cyclosporine, which has been available longer. Drug interactions between calcineurin inhibitors and other immunosuppressive drugs are discussed in Part IV.

Drugs That Decrease Calcineurin Inhibitor Concentration by Induction of P450 Activity

ANTITUBERCULOUS DRUGS. **Rifampin** (and **rifabutin** to a lesser extent) markedly reduces cyclosporine and tacrolimus levels, and it may be difficult to achieve therapeutic levels for patients taking rifampin, the use of which should be avoided if at all possible. INH can be used with careful drug-level monitoring and is the preferred drug for tuberculosis prophylaxis if this proves essential (see Chapter 10).

ANTICONVULSANTS. **Barbiturates** reduce cyclosporine and tacrolimus levels to such an extent that their concomitant use may not be possible. **Phenytoin** reduces levels and should be used with care. The average requirement for cyclosporine or tacrolimus is about doubled for patients receiving phenytoin. **Carbamazepine** may also decrease cyclosporine levels, but the effect is less pronounced. Benzodiazepines and valproic acid do not affect drug levels, but the latter drug has been associated with hepatotoxicity. Patients taking anticonvulsants before transplantation should have a neurologic assessment with a view to discontinuing them when possible.

OTHER DRUGS. Several antibiotics, including nafcillin, intravenous trimethoprim, intravenous sulfadimidine, imipenem, cephalosporins, and terbinafine, have been described to reduce cyclosporine levels in isolated reports. An increased incidence of acute rejection episodes has been described after the introduction of ciprofloxacin. The antidepressant herbal preparation *Hypericum perforatum* (St. John's wort) may reduce cyclosporine levels by enzyme induction.

PROLONGED USE. If prolonged use of a drug that induces P450 activity is required, addition of a drug that inhibits or competes with the P450 system (e.g., diltiazem, ketoconazole) may facilitate the achievement of therapeutic calcineurin inhibitor levels. Administration of the calcineurin inhibitor on a thrice-daily basis rather than the usual twice-daily basis may also be effective.

Drugs That Increase Calcineurin Inhibitor Levels
by Inhibition of P450 or by Competition for Its Pathways

CALCIUM-CHANNEL BLOCKERS. **Verapamil, diltiazem,** amlodipine, and nicardipine may significantly increase calcineurin inhibitor levels. Diltiazem and verapamil are sometimes added routinely as adjuncts to the immunosuppressive regimen. Their use may safely permit a reduction in the cyclosporine dose of up to 40%. Careful monitoring of drug levels is required when these calcium-channel blockers are used for the management of hypertension or heart disease, and patients should be specifically warned that changing the dosage of these drugs is equivalent to changing the dosage of the calcineurin inhibitor. Brand-name and generic forms of these drugs (Cardizem, Dilacor, Tiazac, and Cartia are all forms of diltiazem) may have a different effect on calcineurin inhibitor levels. Nifedipine, isradipine, and felodipine have similar hemodynamic effects but have minimal effects on drug levels.

ANTIFUNGAL AGENTS. **Ketoconazole, fluconazole,** and itraconazole markedly elevate calcineurin inhibitor levels. The interaction with ketoconazole is a particularly potent one, which may permit a safe reduction in the cyclosporine or tacrolimus dose of up to 80%. Great care must be taken when stopping and starting these antifungal agents. An important interaction between ketoconazole and histamine blockers has also been described. The effective reabsorption of ketoconazole from the GI tract requires acidic gastric contents, and the addition of a histamine-2 receptor antagonist may reduce its absorption and thus indirectly produce a clinically significant fall in calcineurin inhibitor levels.

ANTIBIOTICS. **Erythromycin,** even in low doses, may increase calcineurin inhibitor levels. Other macrolide antibiotics (e.g., clarithromycin, josamycin, ponsinomycin) may also increase levels, although azithromycin does not. Because erythromycin is prescribed so ubiquitously, physicians, dentists, and patients should be warned about this interaction. The protease inhibitor saquanivir may increase cyclosporine levels, and new drugs in this class should be used with care. Chloramphenicol may increase tacrolimus levels.

HISTAMINE BLOCKERS. There are conflicting reports regarding the use of cimetidine, ranitidine, and omeprazole with calcineurin inhibitors. Cimetidine was initially reported to increase cyclosporine levels, but this effect has not been substantiated. These drugs may increase creatinine levels without reducing the glomerular filtration rate (GFR) by suppressing proximal tubular creatinine secretion. There may be increased hepatotoxicity when ranitidine and cyclosporine are used in combination.

HORMONES. Corticosteroids in high and low doses may increase calcineurin inhibitor levels by decreasing the clearance of their metabolites. This effect may be particularly pronounced during "pulse" steroid therapy and may result in a confusing picture of nephrotoxicity. In this circumstance, it is the drug levels as measured by nonspecific assay that rise and not levels of the parent compound; hence, dose modification may not be required. Oral contraceptives, anabolic steroids, testosterone, norethisterone, danazol, and somatostatin may also increase drug levels.

OTHER DRUGS. Amiodarone and carvedilol have been reported to increase cyclosporine levels. Grapefruit juice increases the absorption of calcineurin inhibitors (see Chapter 18). The interactions between psychotropic drugs and the calcineurin inhibitors is discussed in Chapter 16.

Drugs That May Exaggerate Calcineurin Inhibitor Nephrotoxicity

Any potentially nephrotoxic drug should be used with caution in combination with the calcineurin inhibitors because the vasoconstrictive effect of the drug tends to potentiate other nephrotoxic mechanisms. Well-substantiated enhanced renal impairment has been described after the introduction of **amphotericin** and **aminoglycosides,** and renal impairment may occur earlier than anticipated. **Nonsteroidal antiinflammatory drugs** should be avoided if possible. Calcineurin inhibitors may potentiate the hemodynamic renal dysfunction seen with **angiotensin-converting enzyme inhibitors** and **angiotensin receptor antagonists.** Metoclopramide may increase calcineurin inhibitor levels by increasing its intestinal reabsorption. A syndrome of diarrhea, hepatopathy, and renal dysfunction has been ascribed to the interaction between cyclosporine and colchicine, particularly when given to patients with familial Mediterranean fever.

Lipid-Lowering Agents

The HMG-CoA reductase inhibitors (HCRIs) are frequent accompaniments of the immunosuppressive protocol (see Part IV). **Lovastatin** has been implicated in several cases of acute renal failure. When used in full doses in combination with cyclosporine, lovastatin may cause rhabdomyolysis with elevated creatine phosphokinase levels and acute renal failure. Myopathy alone has been observed in up to 30% of recipients of the lovastatin–cyclosporine combination, with symptoms of muscle pain and tenderness developing 6 weeks to 16 months after commencement of therapy. The myopathic syndrome has not been observed when lovastatin is used in a daily dose of 20 mg or less. Even this dose should be used with caution, however, and patients should be made aware of the potential interaction. The coadministration of lovastatin with gemfibrozil further increases the likelihood of rhabdomyolysis. The newer HCRIs pravastatin, fluvastatin, simvastatin, and atorvastatin have not been described to produce this interaction, but they should be used with caution. Cholestyramine may interfere with cyclosporine absorption from the GI tract.

Side Effects

Nephrotoxicity

Nephrotoxicity is an important side effect of both calcineurin inhibitors and is the major detriment of these remarkable drugs. Theories linking the mechanism of immunosuppression and nephrotoxicity are discussed later. The terms *cyclosporine* and *FK toxicity* are often used loosely, and it is important to note that these terms encompass several distinct, overlapping syndromes produced by both functional and morphologic changes within the allograft (Table 4.2).

FUNCTIONAL DECREASE IN RENAL BLOOD FLOW AND FILTRATION RATE. The calcineurin inhibitors produce a dose-related, reversible renal vasoconstriction that particularly affects the afferent arteriole (Fig. 4.2). The glomerular capillary ultrafiltration coefficient (Kf) also decreases, possibly as a result of increased mesangial cell contractility. The picture is reminiscent of "prerenal" dysfunction, and in the acute phase, tubular function is intact. Most of the studies on the mechanism of this effect have used cyclosporine rather than tacrolimus.

The normal regulation of the glomerular microcirculation depends on a complex, hormonally mediated balance between vasoconstriction and vasodilation. Cyclosporine-induced vasoconstriction is due, at least in part, to alteration of arachidonic acid metabolism in favor of the vasoconstrictor thromboxane. Cyclosporine is also a potential inducer of the powerful vasoconstrictor endothelin, and circulating endothelin levels are elevated in its presence. Cyclosporine-induced changes in glomerular hemodynamics can be reversed by specific endothelin inhibitors and by anti-endothelin antibodies. The sympathetic nervous system is also activated.

Several *in vivo* and *in vitro* studies have suggested that alterations in the L-arginine nitric oxide (NO) pathway may be involved in calcineurin-induced renal vasoconstriction. NO causes relaxation of preglomerular arteries and improves renal blood flow. The constitutive enzyme endothelial nitric oxide synthase (NOS) is produced by renal endothelial cells and modulates vascular tone.

Table 4.2. Syndromes of calcineurin-inhibitor nephrotoxicity

Exaggeration of early posttransplantation graft dysfunction
Acute reversible decrease in GFR
Acute microvascular disease
Chronic nonprogressive decrease in GFR
Chronic progressive decrease in GFR
Hypertension and electrolyte abnormalities
    Sodium retention and edema
    Hyperkalemia
    Hypomagnesemia
    Hyperchloremic acidosis
    Hyperuricemia

GFR, glomerular filtration rate.

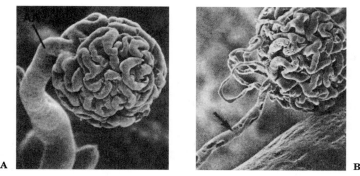

A   B

**Fig. 4.2. Cyclosporine-induced afferent arteriolar vasoconstriction.
A: Control rat showing afferent arteriole (AA) and glomerular tuft.
B: Constricted afferent arteriole *(arrow)* and glomerular tuft after
14 days of cyclosporine at 50 mg/kg/day. (From English J, Evan A,
Houghton DC. Cyclosporine-induced acute renal dysfunction in the
rat. *Transplantation* 1987;44:135 with permission.)**

Both acute and chronic cyclosporine toxicity can be enhanced by
NOS inhibition with *N*-nitro-L-arginine-methyl ester and amelio-
rated by supplementation with L-arginine. Interestingly, Sildenafil (Viagra) increases GFR in transplant patients, presumably by
reversing this effect.

Calcineurin inhibitor–induced renal vasoconstriction may manifest clinically as delayed recovery of early malfunctioning grafts or
as a transient, reversible, dose-dependent, blood level–dependent
elevation in serum creatinine concentration that may be difficult to
distinguish from other causes of graft dysfunction. Vasoconstriction may be a reversible component of chronic calcineurin inhibitor
toxicity, which may amplify the functional severity of the chronic
histologic changes seen with prolonged use. The vasoconstriction also helps to account for the hypertension and the tendency
for sodium retention that are commonly associated with cyclosporine use.

CHRONIC INTERSTITIAL FIBROSIS. Interstitial fibrosis, which may
be patchy or "striped" and associated with arteriolar lesions (see
Chapter 13), is a common feature of long-term calcineurin inhibitor
use. This lesion may produce chronic renal failure in recipients of
organ transplants; however, several long-term studies have shown
that in the dose regimens currently employed, kidney function
may remain stable, although often impaired, for many years. The
mechanism of calcineurin inhibitor–induced interstitial fibrosis
remains poorly defined. Evidence from experimental models suggests that chronic nephropathy involves an angiotensin-dependent
up-regulation of molecules that are important in the scarring process, such as TGF-beta and osteopontin. Enhanced production
of TGF-beta in normal T cells (see Mechanism of Action under Calcineurin Inhibitors) may provide the link between the immunosuppressive effects of the calcineurin inhibitors and their nephrotoxicity (Fig. 4.3), and variation in fibrogenic gene expression

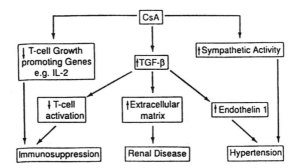

Fig. 4.3. Potential sequelae of cyclosporine-mediated augmentation of TGF-beta expression. In this scheme of events, the cyclosporine-associated increase in TGF-beta expression is hypothesized to contribute to the following: immunosuppression (because TGF-beta can prevent T-cell activation and generation of cytotoxic T cells); renal interstitial fibrosis (because TGF-beta can enhance extracellular matrix accumulation); and hypertension (because TGF-beta can increase endothelin production by vascular smooth muscle cells). In this formulation, TGF-beta represents the mechanistic link for the clinically desirable (immunosuppression) and deleterious (hypertension, fibrosis) consequences of cyclosporine use. (From Khanna A, Li B, Stenzel KH, et al. Demonstration of a transforming growth factor β-dependent mechanism of inhibition of cell growth. *Transplantation* 1994;57:577, with permission.)

may help explain the varying consistency of this effect. Interstitial fibrosis may also be a reflection of intense and prolonged vasoconstriction of the renal microcirculation. Cyclosporine may also impair the regenerative capacity of microvascular endothelial cells and induce apoptosis. The resulting chronic renal ischemia may enhance the synthesis and accumulation of extracellular matrix proteins in the interstitium.

ACUTE MICROVASCULAR DISEASE. Thrombotic microangiopathy (see Chapter 13 for pathology and Chapter 8 for clinical presentation and management) is a distinct form of calcineurin inhibitor vascular toxicity that may result from a direct toxic effect on vascular endothelium, possibly by interfering with the generation of endothelial prostacyclin. It produces a syndrome reminiscent of the hemolytic-uremic syndrome.

ELECTROLYTE ABNORMALITIES AND HYPERTENSION. Impaired sodium excretion is a reflection of the renal vasoconstrictive effect of the calcineurin inhibitors. Patients receiving long-term cyclosporine therapy tend to be hypertensive (see Chapter 9) and to retain fluid. Studies have shown activation of the renin-angiotensin-aldosterone system and sympathetic nervous system and suppression of atrial natriuretic factor, which results in attenuation of the natriuretic and diuretic response to an acute volume load. NO production is also impaired. Hypertension tends to be less marked (or the need for antihypertensive drugs may be less) in patients receiving tacrolimus, possibly because it produces less peripheral vasoconstriction than does cyclosporine. *Hyperkalemia* is common and occasionally requires treatment, although it is rarely life-threatening as long as kidney function remains good. It is not uncommon for patients taking calcineurin inhibitors to have potassium levels in the mid-fives. Hyperkalemia is often associated with a mild *hyperchloremic acidosis* and an intact capacity to excrete acid urine. The clinical picture is thus reminiscent of type IV renal tubular acidosis. Patients receiving cyclosporine may have an impaired capacity to excrete an acute potassium load, and there is evidence to suggest impaired production of aldosterone, an acquired impaired renal response to its action, and inhibition of cortical collecting duct potassium secretory channels. Hyperkalemia may be exaggerated by concomitant administration of beta blockers, angiotensin-converting enzyme inhibitors, and angiotensin receptor blockers. A defect of collecting tubule hydrogen ion secretion has been described with tacrolimus.

Both cyclosporine and tacrolimus are magnesuric, and hypomagnesemia is commonly associated with their use. In liver transplantation, hypomagnesemia may predispose patients to seizures; this has been observed rarely in kidney allograft recipients. The magnesuria is a manifestation of tubulotoxicity. Magnesium supplements are often prescribed but may be ineffective because of a lowered renal magnesium threshold (see Chapter 18).

METHODS OF AMELIORATION. The vexing issue of calcineurin inhibitor nephrotoxicity has spawned a variety of clinical and experimental approaches designed to modify the renal effects of these drugs and particularly their capacity to produce vasoconstriction. Low-dose dopamine is used in some centers in the early postoperative period to "encourage" urine output. Various calcium-channel blockers given to both the donor (see Chapter 5) and the recipient (see Part IV) may reduce the incidence and severity of delayed graft function. Omega-3 fatty acids in the form of 6 g of fish oil each day were initially thought to increase renal blood flow and GFR by reversing the cyclosporine-induced imbalance between the synthesis of vasodilator and vasoconstrictor prostaglandins, but long-term studies have shown no such benefit. The prostaglandin agonist misoprostol and thromboxane synthetase inhibitors may have a similar effect. Various protocol adjustments discussed later in this chapter may also be employed to minimize cyclosporine toxicity.

Nonrenal Calcineurin Inhibitor Toxicity

GASTROINTESTINAL. Episodes of hepatic dysfunction typically manifesting as subclinical, mild, self-limiting, dose-dependent elevations of serum aminotransferase levels with mild hyperbilirubinemia may occur in nearly half of all kidney transplant recipients taking cyclosporine and occur less frequently in those taking tacrolimus. No specific hepatic histologic lesion has been described in humans, and the hyperbilirubinemia is a reflection of disturbed bile secretion rather than hepatocellular damage. Cyclosporine does not itself produce progressive liver disease; other causes, most frequently one of the viral hepatitides, need to be considered when this occurs. Cyclosporine therapy is associated with an increased incidence of cholelithiasis, presumably resulting from an increased lithogenicity of cyclosporine-containing bile. Varying degrees of anorexia, nausea, vomiting, diarrhea, and abdominal discomfort occur in up to 75% of patients receiving tacrolimus and less frequently in patients receiving cyclosporine.

COSMETIC.   The cosmetic complications of cyclosporine, although not severe in a strict medical sense, must be treated seriously, particularly in women and adolescents, because of the misery they can produce and the temptation to resolve them through noncompliant behavior. Cosmetic complications are often exaggerated by concomitant use of corticosteroids. They are less prominent in patients receiving tacrolimus.

Hypertrichosis in varying degrees occurs in nearly all patients receiving cyclosporine and is particularly obvious in dark-haired girls and women. A coarsening of facial features is observed in children and young adults, with thickening of the skin and prominence of the brow. Tacrolimus may produce alopecia. Gingival hyperplasia, which can be severe, may develop in patients receiving cyclosporine and is exaggerated by poor dental hygiene and possibly by concomitant use of calcium-channel blockers. Azithromycin, a macrolide antibiotic that does not affect cyclosporine metabolism, may reduce gingival hyperplasia. Gingivectomy may occasionally be indicated, and switching from cyclosporine to tacrolimus is usually effective. Cosmetic complications tend to become less prominent with time. Sympathetic cosmetic counseling is required. Cyclosporine may increase prolactin levels, occasionally producing gynecomastia in men and breast enlargement in women.

HYPERLIPIDEMIA.   Cyclosporine has been implicated as one of the various factors responsible for the generation of posttransplantation hypercholesterolemia (see Chapter 9). The mechanism of this effect may be related to abnormal low-density lipoprotein feedback control by the liver, to altered bile acid synthesis, or to occupation of the low-density lipoprotein receptor by cyclosporine. Up to two-thirds of patients develop *de novo* hyperlipidemia in the first posttransplantation year. The effect is less marked with tacrolimus, and lipid levels may decrease when patients are switched from cyclosporine to tacrolimus.

GLUCOSE INTOLERANCE.   Posttransplantation glucose intolerance is discussed in Chapter 9. Both calcineurin inhibitors are toxic to pancreatic islets, although tacrolimus is more so. Morphologic changes include cytoplasmic swelling, vacuolization, and apoptosis, with abnormal immunostaining for insulin. In the randomized U.S. tacrolimus trial, the incidence of new-onset insulin requirement during the first posttransplantation year was 25% in patients receiving tacrolimus compared with 5% in those receiving cyclosporine, although the incidence tended to decrease with time. The problem was particularly notable in black patients receiving tacrolimus, close to 40% of whom required insulin at some stage during the first year.

NEUROTOXICITY.   A spectrum of neurologic complications has been observed in patients receiving calcineurin inhibitors; they are generally more marked with tacrolimus. Coarse *tremor,* dysesthesias, headache, and insomnia are common and may be dose related. More severe complications are uncommon in kidney recipients, although isolated seizures may occur in 1% to 2% of patients, and full-blown leukoencephalopathy has been described. Patients receiving Neoral may complain of *headache* 1 to 2 hours after taking the drug, presumably because of high peak levels. Patients receiving cyclosporine may complain of *bone pain.*

CARDIOTOXICITY. There have been case reports of prolongation of the QT interval and potentially dangerous arrhythmias associated with tacrolimus use. A reversible hypertrophic cardiomyopathy has been described in children receiving tacrolimus (see Chapter 15).

INFECTION AND MALIGNANCY. Infection and malignancy inevitably accompany immunosuppression and are discussed in detail in Chapters 9 and 10. Despite their immunosuppressive potency, the incidence of infections and most common *de novo* neoplasms has not significantly increased since the introduction of the calcineurin inhibitors, although the course of malignancies may be accelerated.

THROMBOEMBOLISM. *In vitro,* cyclosporine increases adenosine diphosphate–induced platelet aggregation, thromboplastin generation, and factor VII activity. It also reduces production of endothelial prostacyclin. These findings may be causally related to the somewhat increased incidence of thromboembolic events that have been observed in cyclosporine-treated kidney transplant recipients. The finding of glomerular microthrombi as part of calcineurin inhibitor–induced microangiopathy was discussed previously.

HYPERURICEMIA AND GOUT. Hyperuricemia, because of reduced renal uric acid clearance, is a common complication of calcineurin inhibitor therapy, particularly when diuretics are also employed. Episodes of gout have been reported in up to 7% of patients; its treatment is discussed in Chapter 9.

MYCOPHENOLATE MOFETIL

MMF (CellCept) was introduced into clinical transplantation in 1995 after a series of clinical trials (see Part III) showed that it was more effective than azathioprine for the prevention of acute rejection in recipients of cadaveric kidney transplants when used in combination with cyclosporine and prednisone. The active compound is mycophenolic acid (MPA), a fermentation product of several *Penicillium* species; the mofetil moiety serves to markedly improve its oral bioavailability. The role of MMF in clinical transplantation is discussed in Part IV.

Mechanism of Action

MPA is a reversible inhibitor of the enzyme inosine monophosphate dehydrogenase (IMPDH). IMPDH is a critical, rate-limiting enzyme in the so-called *de novo* synthesis of purines and catalyzes the formation of guanosine nucleotides from inosine. Depletion of guanosine nucleotides by MPA has relatively selective antiproliferative effects on lymphocytes; lymphocytes appear to rely on *de novo* purine synthesis more than other cell types that have a "salvage" pathway for production of guanosine nucleotides from guanine (Fig. 4.4).

In principle, MMF is thus a more selective antimetabolite. It differs radically in its mode of action from the calcineurin inhibitors and sirolimus in that it does not affect cytokine production or the more proximal events following antigen recognition. It differs from azathioprine by virtue of its selective effect on lymphocytes. *In vitro,* MMF blocks the proliferation of T and B cells, inhibits

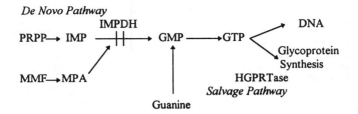

Fig. 4.4. **Mechanism of action of mycophenolate mofetil by inhibition of *de novo* purine synthesis. PRPP, 5-phosphoribosyl-1-phosphate; IMP, inosine monophosphate; MPA, mycophenolic acid; IMPDH, inosine monophosphate dehydrogenase; GMP, guanosine monophosphate; HGPRTase, hypoxanthine guanine phosphoribosyl transferase; GTP, guanosine triphosphate.**

antibody formation, and inhibits the generation of cytotoxic T cells. MMF also down-regulates the expression of adhesion molecules on lymphocytes, thereby impairing their binding to vascular endothelial cells. The capacity of MMF to treat ongoing rejection (see Part IV) may be a reflection of its ability to inhibit the recruitment of mononuclear cells into rejection sites and the subsequent interaction of these cells with target cells. MMF may also exert a preventive effect on the development and progression of proliferative arteriolopathy, a critical pathologic lesion in chronic rejection (see Chapter 13). In retrospective analysis MMF has been shown to reduce the rate of late allograft loss due to an effect that is both dependent and independent of its effect on the incidence of acute rejection.

Pharmacology and Toxicity

MMF is a generally well-tolerated and "user-friendly" compound that is available for clinical use in 250-mg and 500-mg capsules. The standard dose is 1 g twice daily. An intravenous preparation is available but is usually not required in kidney transplant recipients. Orally administered MMF is rapidly absorbed and hydrolyzed to MPA in the liver and is then glucuronidated to an inactive form (MPAG). Enterohepatic cycling of MPAG can occur, which may account for some of its GI side effects. Bioavailability of MMF in the capsule form is 90%, with a half-life of 12 hours. There is no unusual accumulation of MPA in hepatic or renal impairment, and neither MMF nor MPA is dialyzed.

Extensive safety data are available from the clinical trials of MMF. The most common adverse events are related to the GI tract, with diarrhea occurring in up to one third of patients and varying degrees of nausea, bloating dyspepsia, and vomiting in up to 20%. Frank esophagitis and gastritis with occasional GI hemorrhage occur in about 5% of patients and may be associated with cytomegalovirus (CMV) infection. The incidence of GI side effects may be higher if the dosage is greater than 1 g twice daily. Most of these symptoms respond promptly to transient reduction of drug dosage.

Despite the relatively specific action of MMF on lymphocytes, leukopenia, anemia, and thrombocytopenia occur with a frequency similar to that seen with azathioprine and may require dose adjustment. Prolonged leukocytosis may also occur. The incidence of lymphoproliferative disorders and opportunistic infections in all the various clinical trials of MMF is marginally greater than that seen in control groups and is a nonspecific reflection of its greater immunosuppressive potency. Nephrotoxicity, neurotoxicity, and hepatotoxicity have not been observed with MMF. Its safety in pregnancy has not yet been established.

Drug Interactions

MMF is not metabolized through the CYP3A enzyme system; thus, the multiple drug interactions seen with the calcineurin inhibitors do not occur. MMF and azathioprine should not be administered concomitantly because of the potential for combined hematologic toxicity. There is evidence for a pharmacokinetic interaction between MMF and tacrolimus. MPA trough levels increase when MMF is used with tacrolimus, and the MMF dose should not exceed 2 g daily and may need to be reduced further. The combination of MMF and sirolimus may be permissible, but dosage may be limited by combined toxicity. Interactions with other immunosuppressive drugs are discussed in Part IV. MMF should not be administered with antacids or cholestyramine. MMF, as opposed to azathioprine, can be administered with allopurinol without dose adjustment.

SIROLIMUS

Sirolimus (Rapamune), also known as *rapamycin,* is a macrolide antibiotic compound that is structurally related to tacrolimus. Sirolimus was introduced into clinical transplantation in 1999 after a series of clinical trials (see Part III) demonstrated that, when used in combination with cyclosporine and prednisone, it produced a significant reduction in the incidence of acute rejection episodes in the early posttransplantation period, compared with either azathioprine or placebo. Sirolimus has been used with prednisone without a calcineurin inhibitor, with or without MMF, and has been claimed to be about equivalent in immunosuppressive potency to cyclosporine. It has not been approved for use in this manner. Sirolimus has not been rigorously compared with MMF; it is probably a more potent but also a more toxic immunosuppressant. The place of sirolimus in clinical transplantation and dosing recommendations are discussed in Part IV. Its potential future clinical use in tolerance-generating protocols is discussed in Part III.

Mechanism of Action

The immunosuppressive activity of sirolimus appears to be mediated through a mechanism distinct from that of the calcineurin inhibitors. Like the calcineurin inhibitors, it binds to a cytoplasm-binding protein (the same one that binds tacrolimus, FKBP). The resultant sirolimus–FKBP ligand, however, does not block calcineurin (see Chapter 2, Fig. 2.6, and Mechanism of Action under Calcineurin Inhibitors), but rather engages a protein designated *target of rapamycin* (TOR). TOR is a key regulatory kinase, and its inhibition reduces cytokine-dependent cellular proliferation at the G_1 to S phase of the cell-division cycle. Both hematopoietic and non-hematopoietic cells are affected. Because sirolimus occupies the same binding protein as tacrolimus, it was originally presumed that it would impair the action of tacrolimus; the drug was thus developed as an adjunctive agent with cyclosporine. It now appears that the abundance of FKBP *in vivo* makes it unlikely that there would be inhibitive competition of tacrolimus and sirolimus for their receptor, and preliminary trials of their concomitant use in low dose suggest that the combination may prove to be extremely effective.

Pharmacology

The original formulation of sirolimus is an oral solution available in a concentration of 1 mg/mL either in a multidose bottle or in fixed-dose pouches to be dispensed into water or orange juice. A capsule will likely replace the oral solution when it becomes available. It is rapidly absorbed from the GI tract, reaching peak concentrations in 1 to 2 hours. It has a long half-life, averaging 62 hours, and a steady-state trough concentration can be achieved in most patients within 24 hours by administering a loading dose three times the size of the maintenance dose. It is largely metabolized by the liver by both CYP3A and p-glycoprotein; the native compound is the major component in human blood and contributes most of the immunosuppressive activity. Renal excretion is minimal, and dose adjustment is not required in renal dysfunction but is required in hepatic dysfunction. Therapeutic drug level monitoring is not required in most patients but may become necessary when the drug is used in a manner different from that in the trials that led to its introduction into clinical use. The target trough levels vary between 5–15 ng/dl, depending on the clinical circumstances, and are a good reflection of drug exposure. Because the drug has a long half-life, levels should be checked several days after a dosage adjustment is made.

Drug Interactions

Sirolimus and the calcineurin inhibitors are administered together and are metabolized by the same enzyme systems; therefore, the potential for interaction between them must be considered. In healthy volunteers, concomitant administration of sirolimus and the Neoral formulation of cyclosporine increased the AUC for sirolimus by 230% compared with administration of sirolimus alone; administration 4 hours after the cyclosporine dose increased the AUC by 80%. For this reason, it is recommended that sirolimus be administered consistently 4 hours after the morning cyclosporine dose. The effect of sirolimus on cyclosporine metabolism is less marked, but over time, lower doses of cyclosporine are required to maintain target trough levels. The pharmacologic interaction between sirolimus and tacrolimus has not been rigorously studied.

Available information suggests, not surprisingly, that sirolimus interacts with calcium-channel blockers, antifungal agents, anticonvulsants, and antituberculous agents in a manner similar to the calcineurin inhibitors. Careful surveillance for drug interactions

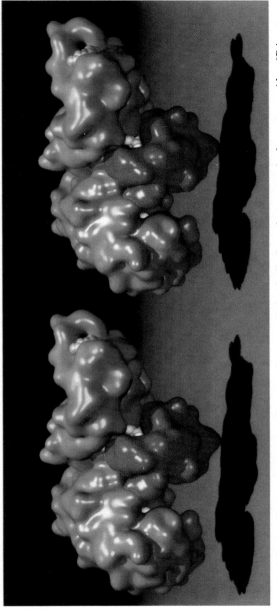

Plate 1. Parts A and B (next page) should be viewed consecutively, ideally through stereoscopic glasses to provide a 3D image. They show the x-ray structure at 2.5 Å resolution of the ternary complex of a calcineurin A fragment (CnA; blue), calcineurin B (CnB; green), tacrolimus-binding protein (FKBP; red), and tacrolimus (FK506; white). Note that the FKBP-FK506 complex does not directly contact the phosphatase active site on CnA that is more than 10 Å removed. Instead, the FKBP-FK506 complex is positioned so that it can inhibit the dephosphorylation of its substrates (e.g., nuclear factor of activated T cells [NFATpl]) by physically hindering their approach to the active site. (The bound phosphate in the phosphatase active site of CnA is shown in yellow.) A. The solvent accessible surface of the ternary complex.

A

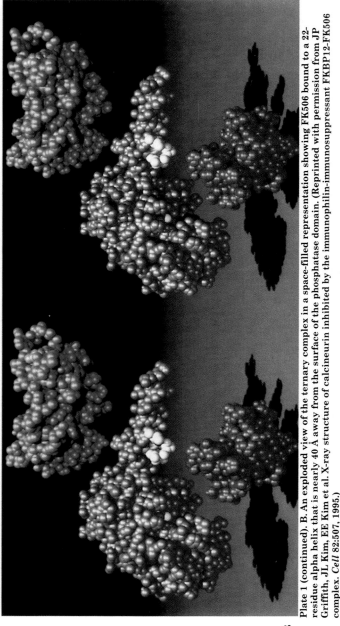

Plate 1 (continued). B. An exploded view of the ternary complex in a space-filled representation showing FK506 bound to a 22-residue alpha helix that is nearly 40 Å away from the surface of the phosphatase domain. (Reprinted with permission from JP Griffith, JL Kim, EE Kim et al. X-ray structure of calcineurin inhibited by the immunophilin-immunosuppressant FKBP12-FK506 complex. *Cell* 82:507, 1995.)

B

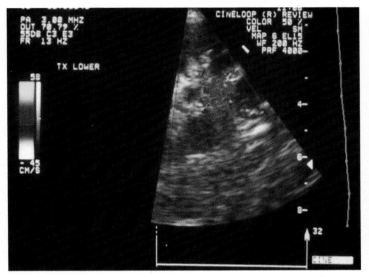

Plate 2. Postbiopsy arteriovenous fistula. Color Doppler image shows an area of random color assignment. Pulsed gate Doppler analysis revealed high-velocity, low-resistance arterial flow and arterialization of the venous waveform.

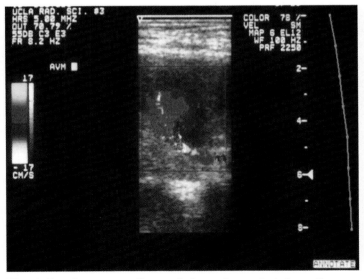

Plate 3. Pseudoaneurysm. Gray-scale image demonstrated a cystic lesion, and color Doppler image shows swirling internal flow.

with sirolimus will be required as the drug is introduced into clinical practice.

Side Effects

Despite the structural similarity of sirolimus to tacrolimus, it does not share its nephrotoxic potential, presumably because of its different mechanism of action. In the clinical trials using combinations of cyclosporine and sirolimus, however (see Part III), the GFR was about 10 mL/min lower and serum creatinine levels were slightly higher in the experimental groups than in the control group that received cyclosporine and azathioprine. This effect may be a manifestation of altered cyclosporine metabolism and should be considered if unexplained impairment of renal function occurs; it may also account for a somewhat increased incidence of hypertension. Sirolimus may be tubulotoxic, and hypokalemia and hypomagnesemia have been described.

Sirolimus causes hypercholesterolemia and hypertriglicceridemia, and in clinical trials, treatment of new-onset hyperlipidemia was required in about half of patients who received the drug. Patients with clinically significant hyperlipidemia before transplantation may not be candidates for sirolimus therapy. Treatment of hyperlipidemia is discussed in Chapter 9. Most patients respond adequately to HCRIs. Sirolimus can cause thrombocytopenia, leukopenia, and anemia, but only thrombocytopenia occurs at a rate more frequent than occurs with azathioprine.

All of these side effects are more marked with the 5-mg daily dose of sirolimus than with the 2-mg dose. The higher dose is more effective in reducing the incidence of acute rejection episodes but has also been associated with an increased incidence of thrombotic microangiopathy, skin ulcers, and lymphoceles. Wound healing may be impaired at high doses, presumably because of its antiproliferative effect, and occasional cases have been reported of a non-infectious pneumonitis that responds to drug withdrawal. Because of the dose dependency of the side effects, the 2-mg dose is the one that is recommended for standard clinical use.

AZATHIOPRINE

Azathioprine (Imuran) is an antimetabolite, an imidazole derivative of 6-mercaptopurine. It has been used in clinical transplantation for nearly 30 years. When cyclosporine was introduced, the role of azathioprine was largely relegated to that of an adjunctive agent in most circumstances (see Part IV), and with the introduction of MMF, its use has been discontinued in many programs.

Mode of Action

Azathioprine is a purine analogue that is incorporated into cellular DNA, where it inhibits purine nucleotide synthesis and interferes with the synthesis and metabolism of RNA. Unlike cyclosporine, it does not prevent gene activation, but it inhibits gene replication and consequent T-cell activation.

Azathioprine is a broad myelocyte suppressant. It inhibits the proliferation of promyelocytes in the bone marrow, and as a result, it decreases the number of circulatory monocytes capable of differentiating into macrophages. Thus, it is a powerful inhibitor of the primary immune response and is valuable in preventing the onset of acute rejection. It is not effective in the therapy of rejection episodes.

Side Effects

The most important side effects of azathioprine are hematologic. Patients first receiving the drug, particularly in higher dosages (2 mg/kg or more), should have complete blood counts performed, including a platelet count, at least weekly during the first month of therapy and less frequently thereafter. Delayed hematologic suppression may occur. In the event of significant thrombocytopenia or leukopenia, the drug can be discontinued for long periods if the patient is also taking cyclosporine, without great danger of inducing acute rejection. It is not necessary to maintain a low white blood cell count for the drug to be an effective immunosuppressant. The white blood cell count should be monitored with particular care when the corticosteroid dose is reduced or discontinued.

Azathioprine may occasionally cause hepatitis and cholestasis, which usually present as reversible elevations in transaminase and bilirubin levels. The azathioprine dose is usually reduced or stopped during episodes of significant hepatic dysfunction. Pancreatitis is a rare complication.

Azathioprine is converted to inactive 6-thiouric acid by xanthine oxidase. The inhibition of this enzyme by allopurinol demands that this drug combination be avoided or used with great care. When allopurinol is started, the azathioprine dose should be reduced to 25% to 50% of its initial level, and the white blood cell and platelet counts should be frequently monitored.

Dose and Administration

About half of orally administered azathioprine is absorbed; thus, the intravenous dose is equivalent to half the oral dose. Blood levels are not valuable clinically because its effectiveness is not blood level dependent. The drug is not significantly dialyzed or excreted by the kidney. Dose reduction is often practiced during kidney dysfunction, although it may not be necessary. When used as the primary immunosuppressant, the daily oral dose is 2 to 3 mg/kg. When used as adjunctive therapy with a calcineurin inhibitor, the dose is 1 to 2 mg/kg.

CORTICOSTEROIDS

Corticosteroids have commanded a central position in clinical transplantation since they were first used to treat rejection in the 1960s. Despite this long experience, there remains only a general consensus on their best therapeutic use, and changing protocols often reflect both fear of prescribing them and fear of not prescribing them. It is hoped that the new generation of immunosuppressants will eventually permit avoidance or withdrawal of corticosteroids for most patients, although this goal has not yet been reached.

The diffuse effects of corticosteroids on the body reflect the fact that most mammalian tissues have glucocorticoid receptors within the cell cytoplasm and can serve as targets for the effects of corticosteroids. The immunosuppressive actions of corticosteroids can be somewhat simplistically divided into their specific actions on macrophages and T cells and their broad, nonspecific immunosuppressant and antiinflammatory actions.

Mechanism of Action

Blockade of Cytokine Gene Expression

Corticosteroids exert their most critical immunosuppressive effect by blocking T-cell–derived and antigen-presenting cell–derived cytokine and cytokine-receptor expression. They inhibit the function of dendritic cells, which are the most important of the antigen-presenting cells (see Chapter 2). They are hydrophobic and can diffuse intracellularly, where they bind to cytoplasmic receptors found in association with the 90-kd heat-shock protein. As a result, the heat-shock protein becomes dissociated, and the steroid–receptor complex translocates to the nucleus, where it binds to DNA sequences referred to as *glucocorticoid response elements* (GREs). GRE sequences have been found in the critical promoter regions of several cytokine genes, and it is presumed that the binding of the steroid–receptor complex to the GRE inhibits the transcription of cytokine genes. Corticosteroids also inhibit the translocation to the nucleus of nuclear factor kappa-beta, a transcription factor that plays a major role in the induction of genes encoding a wide variety of cytokines.

Corticosteroids inhibit the expression of IL-1, IL-2, IL-3, and IL-6; TNF-alpha, and gamma-interferon. As a result, all stages of the T-cell activation process are inhibited. Cytokine release is responsible for the fever often associated with acute rejection. This fever typically resolves rapidly when high-dose corticosteroids are administered.

Nonspecific Immunosuppressive Effects

Glucocorticoids cause a lymphopenia that is due to the redistribution of lymphocytes from the vascular compartment back to lymphoid tissue. The migration of monocytes to sites of inflammation is also inhibited. Steroids block the synthesis, release, and action of a series of chemokines, permeability-increasing agents, and vasodilators, although these antiinflammatory effects are a relatively minor aspect of their efficacy in the prevention and treatment of acute rejection. The total white blood cell count may rise several-fold during high-dose steroid administration.

Complications

The ubiquitous complications of corticosteroids are familiar to medical practitioners and are not reviewed here in detail. They are a reflection of their profound immunosuppressive, antiinflammatory, and hormonal action on numerous target tissues. The most important complications are cosmetic changes, growth impairment, osteonecrosis, impaired wound healing and resistance to infection, cataracts, hyperlipidemia, glucose intolerance, and psychopathologic effects. There is marked variation in individual response to these drugs, presumably because of the varied concentration of tissue steroid receptors and individual variations in prednisone metabolism. In the dose regimens currently prescribed, untoward complications can be minimized but not totally prevented.

Commonly Used Preparations

In clinical transplantation, steroids are used in several different ways: as a high-dose intravenous or oral pulse given over 3 to

5 days, as a steroid cycle or taper with a gradually decreasing oral dose over days or weeks, or as a steady low-dose daily or every-other-day maintenance regimen. Corticosteroid dosage is discussed in Part IV.

Prednisolone, its 11-keto metabolite *prednisone,* and *methyl-prednisolone* (Solu-Medrol) are the corticosteroid preparations most commonly used in clinical transplantation. Prednisolone is the most active circulating immunosuppressive corticosteroid. Prednisone is the oral preparation usually used in the United States, whereas prednisolone is often preferred in Europe. Methyl-prednisolone is the most commonly used intravenous cortico-steroid. These preparations have a half-life that is measured in hours, but their capacity to inhibit lymphokine production persists for 24 hours; therefore, once-daily administration is adequate.

Corticosteroids are metabolized by hepatic microsomal enzyme systems. Drugs such as phenytoin, barbiturates, and rifampin, which induce these enzymes, may lower plasma prednisolone levels, whereas oral contraceptives and ketoconazole increase levels. Unfortunately, there is no readily available plasma pred-nisolone assay for clinical use, although empirical adjustments in dose may be advisable when potentially interacting drugs are administered.

PART II. BIOLOGIC IMMUNOSUPPRESSIVE AGENTS

MONOCLONAL AND POLYCLONAL ANTIBODIES

Polyclonal antibodies are produced by immunizing either horses or rabbits with human lymphoid tissue and then harvesting the resultant immune sera to obtain gamma-globulin fractions. Various polyclonal antibodies—ALG, antilymphoblast serum, and ATG— have been available for use in clinical transplantation since the 1970s. Currently, the only polyclonal antibodies widely available for clinical use are the antithymocyte globulins, Atgam and Thymoglobulin. The monoclonal antibody muromonab-CD3 (Ortho-clone OKT3, referred to here as simply *OKT3*) has been available for clinical use since 1987, and the humanized anti-Tac (HAT) monoclonal antibody preparations, daclizumab and basiliximab, became available in 1998. Biologic immunosuppressive agents can be used for induction immunosuppression and for the treatment of acute rejection; they are not used for maintenance immuno-suppression. Table 4.3 reviews their major indications, which are discussed in detail in Part IV.

OKT3

Mode of Action

OKT3 is an immunoglobulin G (IgG) globulin—a monoclonal anti-body produced by the hybridization of murine antibody-secreting B lymphocytes with a non-secreting myeloma cell line whose neo-plastic potential permits the secretion of antibody in perpetuity. Compared with the humanized monoclonal antibodies discussed later, OKT3 is *xenogeneic* because the whole antibody is of murine origin. OKT3 reacts with human T cells by binding to one of the 20-kd subunits of the CD3 complex, an intrinsic part of the T-cell receptor (see Chapter 2). The subsequent deactivation of the CD3

Table 4.3. Antibody preparations for renal transplant immunosuppression

Treatment	Indication	
Monoclonal	**Induction**	**Rejection**
OKT3	(+)	+
Basiliximab	+*	−
Daclizumab	+*	−
Polyclonal		
Atgam	+	+
Thymoglobulin	(+)	+

+, approved indication; (+) unapproved but commonly used indication; *, concomitant administration of calcineurin-inhibitor recommended.

complex causes the T-cell receptor to undergo endocytosis and be lost from the cell surface. The T cells become ineffectual, and within 1 hour, they become opsonized and are removed from the circulation into the reticuloendothelial system. OKT3 also blocks the function of killer T cells, which have an important role in generating the rejection response.

Concomitant with the initial depletion of CD3+ cells, there is depletion of T cells with other surface markers (CD4, CD8, CD11). Within a few days, T cells reappear in the circulation that carry CD4, CD8, and CD11 markers but are devoid of CD3 and are hence ineffectual, or so-called modulated, cells (Fig. 4.5). CD3+ functional cells may reappear later in the course of OKT3 and during a second course, possibly because of the production of neutralizing antibodies. The clinical importance of this reappearance is discussed later.

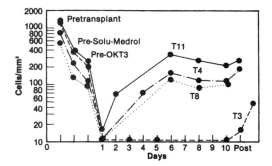

Fig. 4.5. Serial T-cell analysis during therapy with OKT3. The fall in T-cell count from pretransplantation levels before the use of OKT3 is due to routine immunosuppression and high-dose steroids. Note the appearance of "modulated" cells a few days after commencement of OKT3 therapy.

Dosage and Administration

The standard dose of OKT3 is 5 mg given as an intravenous bolus through a Millipore filter. The standard course consists of a daily dose for 10 days, although shorter (5 to 7 days) or longer (14 days or more) courses are sometimes given. Protocols using lower doses of OKT3 may be just as effective but are less well tested. OKT3 protocol recommendations are given in Table 4.4. The first few doses of OKT3 must be given in the hospital, preferably at an institution familiar with its use, side effects, and clinical indications. The first dose can be safely administered intraoperatively as long as the protocol recommendations are followed. If the drug is well tolerated, the course can be completed on an outpatient basis with substantial financial economy and patient convenience.

Monitoring

OKT3 monitoring refers to the repeated assessment of the effectiveness of the drug during a course because of the potential for the development of human antimurine antibodies, which may abrogate its action and allow for the reappearance of potent CD3+ T cells. Antibodies may be directed against the antibody site itself (antiidiotypic), against the IgG protein subclass (antiisotypic), and against the mouse protein of origin (antimurine).

Table 4.4.   Protocol recommendations for OKT3 use

1. Before administration of first dose, patient should be edema free, be within 3% of dry weight, and have a negative chest radiograph.
2. Use high-dose diuretics, dialysis, or ultrafiltration alone to achieve euvolemia in a volume-overloaded patient.
3. Administer premedication 15–60 minutes before first and second dose consisting of methylprednisolone, 5–8 mg/kg; diphenhydramine hydrochloride (Benadryl), 50 mg IV; and acetaminophen, 500 mg PO.
4. Before first and second dose, monitor vital signs every 15 minutes for 2 hours, then every 30 minutes for 2 hours.
5. Premedication is not required for remainder of the course; use acetaminophen p.r.n. for fever.
6. If OKT3 is stopped for more than one dose, repeat first-dose precautions.
7. Continue low dose of calcineurin-inhibitor, azathioprine, or MMF during the course.
8. If calcineurin-inhibitor is continued, use half dose; return to full dose 2 days before completion of the course and ensure therapeutic levels.
9. After first two doses, continue prednisone according to the protocol schedule.
10. Use antiviral and antibacterial prophylaxis (see Chap. 10).
11. During second course of OKT3, monitor CD3 levels at least twice weekly.
12. After the first two doses, encourage hydration for patient diuresis.
13. Consider outpatient administration after third dose in stable patients.

During an effective course of OKT3, the percentage of CD3+ T cells decreases precipitously within 24 to 48 hours, from about 60% to less than 5% (Fig. 4.5). The decrease may be somewhat slower in an effective second course. Failure of the CD3+ percentage to decrease or a decrease followed by a rapid rise indicates the appearance of blocking antibodies. Measurement of CD3 cells is available as a routine laboratory test in most immunology laboratories. Measurement of OKT3 blood levels is not yet routinely available. OKT3 antibodies can be measured by a time-consuming ELISA technique or by the more convenient Transtat OKT3 assay. The clinical value of these assays has yet to be clearly defined.

During an initial course of OKT3, CD3 monitoring is generally not required because it typically takes 2 weeks for antibody to develop. During retreatment, CD3 levels should be measured at least twice weekly. If CD3 levels are elevated, consideration should be given, depending on the overall clinical status of the patient, to doubling the OKT3 dose to overcome the antibody response. Two to 3 weeks after a course of OKT3 or before the next course, the presence of antibodies should be determined. A low-titer antibody response (less than 1 per 100) can be overcome by treatment. Such treatment, however, brings with it a significant risk for a high-titer response that may abrogate the effectiveness of all murine protein monoclonal antibodies. The concomitant use of low-dose calcineurin inhibitor, MMF, or azathioprine during a course of OKT3 (Table 4.4) serves to minimize the antibody response.

Side Effects

Significant, potentially life-threatening adverse reactions may occur during the first days of treatment with OKT3. These adverse reactions occur as the percentage of potent T cells plummets and a series of T-cell–derived cytokines, including TNF, IL-2, and gamma-interferon, are released into the circulation. The term *cytokine release syndrome* has been used to describe the clinical events that follow. Immediate complement activation may also play an important etiologic role. The OKT3 administration protocol (Table 4.4) is designed to minimize the severity of this syndrome. Other proposed techniques include use of indomethacin, anti-TNF antibodies, pentoxifylline, and administration of OKT3 over 2 hours as an infusion rather than as a bolus injection. A double-blind, randomized study of pentoxifylline, however, showed no measurable benefit.

Fever and Chills

After the first exposure to OKT3, nearly all patients become febrile, and many suffer rigors. The fever and rigors often occur "like clockwork" 45 minutes after the injection but may be delayed for hours. By the second or third dose, the fever typically abates, although some patients remain febrile for several days or throughout the whole course. Patients being treated with OKT3 are all immunosuppressed by definition; hence, infectious causes of fever should always be considered. If the fever is prolonged for more than two to three doses, a fever workup should be performed. The development of fever later in the course of OKT3 after an afebrile period is particularly suggestive of a infectious etiology (with CMV infection at the top of the differential diagnosis) and demands careful consideration of the wisdom of continuing the course.

Pulmonary Edema

A rapidly developing, potentially life-threatening noncardiogenic pulmonary edema may occur after the first or second dose of OKT3 if the patient is not euvolemic or is very close to his or her dry weight at the time of injection. Even euvolemic patients may wheeze and become dyspneic. Post-OKT3 pulmonary edema is a preventable syndrome as long as the precautions listed in Table 4.4 are adhered to compulsively. Clinical volume assessment is often unreliable, and patients may "hide" liters of fluid that are not clinically detectable. It is often wise and expeditious to dialyze or ultrafilter a patient before OKT3 administration to ensure that the required amount of fluid is removed.

After the first doses of OKT3, the fluid restrictions can be relaxed. Patients may, in fact, become hypotensive and dehydrated because of fever, diarrhea, and prior fluid restriction. The decision about whether to continue OKT3 in a hypotensive febrile patient may be difficult. In these circumstances, OKT3 can be continued safely as long as other causes of hypotension and fever are considered and excluded and hydration is maintained.

Nephrotoxicity

Renal function, as judged by serum creatinine levels, may deteriorate during the early days of an OKT3 course; a previously nonoliguric patient may even require dialysis. This deterioration of function is typically transient and is followed by a brisk diuresis. It may even be a harbinger of a successful course because it is presumably a manifestation of the hemodynamic abnormalities following cytokine release as the OKT3 takes its toll on the T cells. This transient nephrotoxicity probably accounts for the fact that the prophylactic use of OKT3 immediately after transplantation does not clearly reduce the frequency of delayed graft function as compared with postoperative use of calcineurin inhibitors, although the length of the oliguric period may be reduced (see later). Occasional cases of irreversible graft thrombosis have been described after OKT3 administration and may be due to OKT3-induced activation of the coagulation cascade.

Neurologic Complications

A spectrum of neurologic complications may occur during a course of OKT3, varying in severity from a commonly occurring mild headache to severe encephalopathy. The severe complications are more common when OKT3 is given for prophylaxis in patients with delayed graft function; diabetic patients may also be more susceptible.

The aseptic meningitis syndrome is self-limiting and typically resolves spontaneously without the necessity for discontinuing the OKT3 course. If a lumbar puncture is performed, a mild culture-negative leukocytosis with pleocytosis is often found. Clinicians may be more comfortable discontinuing the OKT3 for one or two doses while the results of lumbar puncture culture are awaited and the patient's clinical status is observed. About one third of patients with a diagnosis of aseptic meningitis have coexisting evidence of encephalopathy. OKT3 should be discontinued in severely encephalopathic patients.

Infection

Infection, most commonly with CMV, may be a late adverse sequela of OKT3 use. The frequency of infection varies with the number of courses of OKT3 and the overall amount of immunosuppression given. Most programs routinely employ CMV prophylaxis before or during a course of OKT3, with recipients of CMV-positive allografts representing a particularly high-risk population. Techniques of CMV prophylaxis are discussed in Chapter 10.

Rejection Recurrence

Episodes of rejection may occur after up to 60% of courses of OKT3. These episodes, which are typically mild, can usually be controlled with a low-dose prednisone pulse. They occur as potent CD3+ T cells reappear in the circulation. At the completion of a course of OKT3, it is important to ensure that calcineurin inhibitor blood levels are in the high therapeutic range (Table 4.4). It may be wise to increase the steroid dose routinely in the first 3 to 4 days after the course.

Hematologic Complications

The development of lymphoma in transplant recipients is a well-recognized, although infrequent, consequence of effective immunosuppression. Use of repeat courses of OKT3 or polyclonal antibodies has been associated with a particularly fulminant and typically rapidly fatal B-cell lymphoma that develops within the first few months after transplantation. Epstein-Barr virus (EBV) antibody–negative patients receiving a graft from an EBV-positive donor appear to be at greatest risk. The recognition, prevention, and management of posttransplantation lymphoma are discussed in Chapters 9 and 10.

Administration of OKT3 may be associated with coagulopathy manifested by occasional cases of allograft thrombosis, thrombotic microangiopathy, and thrombocytopenia.

POLYCLONAL ANTIBODIES: ATGAM AND THYMOGLOBULIN

Mode of Action

The relative benefits of Atgam and Thymoglobulin and indications for their use are summarized in Table 4.3 and discussed in Part IV. Atgam is made by the immunization of horses with human lymphoid material. Thymoglobulin is made by immunization of rabbits with human lymphoid tissue. The resultant gamma-globulin is then purified to remove irrelevant antibody material that may be responsible for some of the drugs' side effects. The precise mechanism of action of the polyclonal antibodies is not fully understood, but the immunosuppressive product contains cytotoxic antibodies directed against a variety of T-cell markers. After their administration, there is depletion of peripheral blood lymphocytes. The lymphocytes, T cells in particular, are either lysed or cleared by the reticuloendothelial system, and their surface antigens may be masked by the antibody. With the use of thymoglobulin, a prolonged lymphopenia may ensue, and the CD4 subset may be suppressed for several years. The prolonged immunosuppressive effect of these drugs may account for the relative infrequency of episodes of rejection recurrence compared with OKT3 (see Part IV).

Dose and Administration

Atgam is given in a dose of 10 to 15 mg/kg and Thymoglobulin in a dose of 1.5 mg/kg. Both drugs are usually given in a course lasting 7 to 14 days. Thymoglobulin may also be effectively dosed based on its impact on T-cell subsets. They are mixed in 500 mL of dextrose or saline and infused over 4 to 8 hours into a central vein or arteriovenous fistula. Use of a peripheral vein is sometimes followed by vein thrombosis or thrombophlebitis, although this may be prevented by adding hydrocortisone sodium succinate (Solu-Cortef), 20 mg, and heparin, 1,000 U, to the infusion solution.

To avoid allergic reactions, the patient should receive intravenous premedication consisting of methylprednisolone, 30 mg, and diphenhydramine hydrochloride (Benadryl), 50 mg, 30 minutes before injection. Acetaminophen should be given before and 4 hours after commencement of the infusion for fever control. Vital signs should be monitored every 15 minutes during the first hour of infusion and then hourly until the infusion is complete.

Azathioprine and MMF should generally be discontinued during the course of treatment so as not to exacerbate hematologic side effects. Cyclosporine or tacrolimus can be omitted during the course or given in a low dose, and oral prednisone is replaced by the methylprednisolone given in the premedication.

Side Effects

Most of the side effects of polyclonal antibodies relate to the fact that foreign protein is administered. Chills, fever, and arthralgias are common, although the severe first-dose reactions seen with OKT3 do not occur. There have been occasional cases of anaphylaxis. Serum sickness occurs rarely because the continued immunosuppression that follows the treatment course reduces the production of antiidiotypic antibodies and the consequent immune complex deposition.

Both preparations can produce thrombocytopenia and leukopenia, necessitating reduction or curtailment of drug dosage. Leukopenia is more frequent with Thymoglobulin and occurs in up to half of patients. The drug dose is usually halved for patients with a platelet count of 50,000 to 100,000 cells/mL or a white blood cell count of less than 3,000 cells/mL. Administration of the drugs should be stopped if the counts fall further. The infectious complications are similar to those described for OKT3. The incidence and severity of CMV infection is clearly more common with all of these agents but can be minimized with the prophylactic measures included in the protocol (see Chapter 10).

HUMANIZED ANTI-TAC MONOCLONAL ANTIBODIES

Mechanism of Action

The HAT monoclonal antibodies basiliximab and daclizumab are targeted against the alpha chain (also referred to as CD25, or Tac) of the interleukin-2 (IL-2) receptor. The receptor is up-regulated only on activated T cells (see Chapter 2), and as a result of the binding of the antibody, IL-2 mediated responses are blocked. The HAT monoclonal antibodies thus complement the effect of the calcineurin inhibitors, which reduce the production of IL-2. They are designed to prevent, but not treat, episodes of acute rejection.

Basiliximab (Simulect) and *daclizumab* (Zenapax) are two similar compounds that were introduced into clinical transplantation by virtue of their capacity to reduce the incidence of acute rejection episodes when used in combination with cyclosporine and corticosteroids (see Part III). They both originate as murine monoclonal antibodies, which are then genetically engineered so that large parts of the molecule are replaced by human IgG. The resulting compounds have low *immunogenicity* because they do not induce production of significant amounts of human antimurine antibody. As a result, they have a prolonged half-life in the peripheral blood, and they do not induce a first-dose reaction. The compounds thus differ from the fully xenogeneic OKT3 that has a short half-life, generates a strong antimurine response, and has a pronounced first-dose reaction.

In the case of basiliximab, the entire variable region of the murine antibody remains intact, whereas the constant region originates from human IgG; the resulting compound is strictly deemed *chimeric* and is of 75% human and 25% murine origin. In the case of daclizumab, only the antibody binding site is of murine origin, and the resulting compound is deemed *humanized* and is of 90% human and 10% murine origin. This discrete difference between the compounds accounts for the fact that the affinity of basiliximab for the IL-2 receptor is greater than the affinity of daclizumab for the receptor. This difference appears to have little clinical significance but explains the fact that the dose of daclizumab is greater than the dose of basiliximab.

Dosage and Administration

The immunosuppressive potency of both drugs is presumed to be related to their capacity to produce complete and consistent binding to the IL-2 receptor alpha sites on T cells. Both drugs have a half-life of greater than 7 days, which permits a long dosage interval. The dosing protocols used in the clinical trials leading to their introduction into clinical transplantation (see Part IV) were designed to produce binding of the receptor sites during the early posttransplantation period when the incidence of acute rejection episodes is highest. In the case of basiliximab, two intravenous doses of 20 mg are given, the first dose preoperatively and the second dose on postoperative day 4; this regimen produces saturation of the IL-2 alpha receptor sites for 30 to 45 days. In the case of daclizumab, five doses of 1 mg/kg are given, starting preoperatively and then at 2-week intervals, producing saturation of the IL-2 alpha sites for up to 12 weeks. Shorter courses of daclizumab have also been used effectively.

Side Effects

Both drugs are remarkable by virtue of the absence of significant side effects. Their largely human origin accounts for the absence of anaphylaxis or a first-dose reaction. In the clinical trials leading to their introduction, the incidence of typical transplantation-related side effects was not greater in the treatment groups than in the control groups.

PART III. CLINICAL TRIALS AND NEW
IMMUNOSUPPRESSIVE AGENTS

During the 1990s, a series of promising new immunosuppressive agents underwent laboratory and clinical evaluation in a successful attempt to broaden and improve the immunosuppressive therapeutic armamentarium. This process continues apace, and several promising new immunosuppressive candidates are at various stages of development. The race for their introduction into clinical transplantation practice can be likened to an obstacle course. Some drugs have passed the finishing line (e.g., tacrolimus, MMF, sirolimus, the HATs), some have already faltered and fallen from current clinical consideration in organ transplantation (e.g., brequinar sodium, cyclosporine G, leflunomide, deoxyspergualin, and the anti-adhesion molecule antibodies), and some are still in the race with obstacles ahead (e.g., FTY720 and the new antibody preparations).

The great success of organ transplantation that was achieved in the 1990s with currently available agents is, paradoxically, making it exceedingly difficult (and enormously expensive) to prove the added benefit of new agents. In clinical trials of new agents, as discussed later, the use of the traditional marker of drug or protocol superiority—patient or graft survival—is now proving to be impractical and has largely been replaced by alternative end points. Examples of such alternative end points include reduced incidence of acute rejection episodes, improved renal function, and more cost-effective immunosuppression.

CLINICAL TRIALS

Before any clinical trials can be performed with an investigational agent, an *investigational new drug* (IND) application has to be submitted to the *U.S. Food and Drug Administration* (FDA) or equivalent regulatory body outside of the United States. Approval of the IND application is based on the evaluation of preclinical studies that suggest potential therapeutic benefits of a new agent and on the evaluation of studies in a variety of animals that suggest its safety.

Phase 1 clinical studies are performed in healthy human volunteers or patients to evaluate human metabolism, pharmacokinetics, dosage, safety, and, if possible, effectiveness. Phase 2 includes controlled, open-labeled, clinical studies conducted to evaluate the effectiveness of the drug for a particular indication or indications and to determine dose regimens, common side effects, and risks. Phase 3 studies are expanded trials based on preliminary evidence from the previous phases that suggest efficacy and safety. They are sometimes called *pivotal trials* because they are critical for FDA-approved licensing. They typically involve large, usually *multi-centered,* clinical trials that are *randomized* and, if possible, *double blinded* using *placebo controls.* These studies serve to refine dosage, determine benefit, and further evaluate the overall risk-to-benefit ratio of the new drug. In organ transplantation, particular care has to be taken to ensure that any potential benefit of a new agent is not outweighed by the consequences of overimmunosuppression or by organ-specific toxicity. Successful completion of phase 3 should provide an adequate basis for product labeling and permit approval of the drug for its defined indications.

Any human use of an experimental drug is strictly governed by the predetermined rules of the experimental protocol under which the drug is administered. Patients must read, understand, and sign an informed consent form that clearly defines the nature of the experiment in which they are involved and its potential risks and benefits. They must also receive a copy of the *patient's bill of rights,* which clearly defines the nature of their commitment. The experimental protocol and consent form must have been approved by an *institutional review board* or *human subjects protection committee,* and the medical staff administering the protocol must feel totally comfortable with it. After a drug is licensed, it is often used "off label" for indications, or in doses, different from those precisely defined. Such use does not require a formal consent procedure, although it is wise to inform the patient that the drug is being given for an unapproved use.

Clinical Trial Design in Transplantation

Immunosuppressive practitioners must understand the way in which new agents are introduced because clinical trials of new immunosuppressive agents not only have led to their clinical use but also have largely determined the way in which these agents are used. It is also particularly important to appreciate what primary *end points* were used to determine the efficacy of the new agents. The choice of primary end point, the frequency with which this end point occurs in the control population, and the anticipated capacity of the new agent to change the incidence of the end point (estimated from phase 2 studies), permits a statistical evaluation of the number of patients required to be enrolled in the study so that the study has sufficient statistical power to determine the effectiveness of the new agent. Secondary end points usually include side-effect comparisons, renal function estimations, and long-term effects on patient and graft survival. Studies may not have the *statistical power* to provide answers to the questions posed by the secondary end points.

When the clinical trials for cyclosporine use in kidney transplantation were designed in the late 1970s and early 1980s, the primary end point used was improvement of patient and graft survival, which cyclosporine indeed achieved. Tacrolimus was introduced based on its capacity to produce results equivalent to cyclosporine. OKT3 was introduced based on its superior capacity, when compared with corticosteroids, to reverse episodes of acute rejection, and Thymoglobulin was introduced for its superiority in reversing acute rejection when compared with Atgam. All the remaining new drugs (MMF, sirolimus, HAT monoclonal antibodies) have been introduced based on their capacity, when combined with cyclosporine and prednisone, to reduce the incidence of acute rejection episodes.

Incidence of Acute Rejection Episodes as an End Point for Studies of New Immunosuppressive Drugs

The incidence of acute rejection episodes, typically biopsy-proven (see Chapter 13), has become the most frequently used marker of the effectiveness of new immunosuppressive drugs for the following reasons:

1. The excellent results of kidney transplantation with currently available immunosuppressants, with 1-year graft survival of close to 90% in most centers and minimal mortality, make it statistically extremely difficult to prove benefit of new agents or protocols in terms of patient or graft survival.

2. Acute rejection is a potent risk factor for the development of chronic allograft failure (see Chapter 9). In retrospective analyses, patients who have suffered episodes of acute rejection have a long-term graft survival rate that is 20% to 30% less than the graft survival rate of patients who have not suffered acute rejection.

3. Acute rejection episodes are morbid events in themselves, requiring intensification of immunosuppression and sometimes hospital admission.

4. Most acute rejection episodes take place within the first few months of transplantation, and their presence can be proved on biopsy. This permits a rapid evaluation of the effectiveness of a new agent or protocol (a "luxury" that is not available when immunosuppressive drug trials are performed in other clinical circumstances, such as systemic lupus erythematosus or rheumatoid arthritis).

Figure 4.6 provides an example of the way in which the incidence of biopsy-proven acute rejection episodes is used to show the effectiveness of a new agent from one of the pivotal trials leading to the introduction of MMF. This trial was a randomized, double-blind, placebo-controlled, multicenter, phase 3 study to evaluate the efficacy of MMF for the prevention of acute rejection

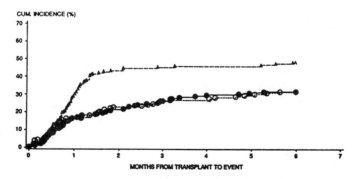

Fig. 4.6.   Effects of mycophenolate mofetil on the cumulative incidence of biopsy-proved acute rejection and treatment failure during the first 6 months after transplantation. A, azathioprine group; O, mycophenolate mofetil, 1.0 g bid; •, mycophenolate mofetil, 1.5 g bid. (From Sollinger HW, for the U.S. Renal Transplant Mycophenolate Mofetil Study Group. Mycophenolate mofetil for the prevention of acute rejection in primary cadaveric renal allograft recipients. *Transplantation* 1995;60:225, with permission.)

episodes during the first 6 months after transplantation. In this trial, standard therapy consisted of cyclosporine, prednisone, and azathioprine. The study compared two doses of MMF (1.0 g given twice daily and 1.5 g given twice daily) or azathioprine in combination with cyclosporine and prednisone. In the United States, the study involved 500 recipients of a first cadaveric transplant (very similar studies involving another 1,000 patients were performed in Europe, Canada, and Australia). Figure 4.6 illustrates the clear-cut benefit of MMF with respect to the primary end point. There was a statistically significant reduction in the incidence of acute rejection episodes from 41% in the azathioprine group to about 20% in both the MMF groups. Use of high-dose steroids and OKT3 was also markedly reduced in the MMF groups. In this particular study, however, there was no statistically significant benefit of MMF with respect to patient or graft survival when estimated at either 1 or 3 years.

Table 4.5 summarizes the results of the pivotal clinical trials leading to the introduction of MMF, sirolimus, and the HAT monoclonal antibodies. Readers are referred to the Selected Readings for detailed descriptions of these trials. A statistically significant reduction in the incidence of acute rejection episodes was achieved for each of these drugs, which permitted their introduction into

Table 4.5.   Incidence of biopsy-proven acute retention episodes from selected randomized clinical trials using standard dose of experimental agent[a]

Agents Compared		Acute Rejection (%)		
Control	Experimental	Control	Experimental	Reference
CyA, Aza	FK, Aza	46	31	Pirsch et al., 1997 (Part I)
CyA, Aza	CyA, MMF 2g	41	20	Cho et al., 1999 (Part I)
CyA	CyA, basiliximab	48	23	Kahan et al., 1998 (Part I)
CyA, Aza	CyA, daclizumab	43	27	Nashan et al., 1999 (Part II)
CyA, Aza	CyA, Rapa 2 mg	29	16	Kahan et al., 1999 (Part II)

CyA, cyclosporine; Aza, azathioprine; FK, tacrolimus; MMF, mycophenolate mofetil; Rapa, sirolimus.

[a] All trials included standard dosage of corticosteroids.

clinical transplantation. A significant effect on patient and graft survival was not achieved, probably because the studies did not have the statistical power to show such an effect.

As new immunosuppressive drugs and protocols are introduced and the incidence of acute rejection decreases, it is becoming increasingly difficult to prove the statistically significant benefit of newer drugs. In the pivotal trials leading to the introduction of MMF, sirolimus, and the HAT monoclonal antibodies, the incidence of acute rejection in the patients receiving the experimental drug protocol was compared with the incidence of acute rejection in patients receiving *standard therapy* with cyclosporine, prednisone, and azathioprine. The success of MMF in reducing the incidence of acute rejection led to it becoming part of an updated standard therapy protocol in many centers (see Part IV). In future, trials of newer agents, MMF, or possibly sirolimus, will represent standard therapy, and statistical proof of further reduction in the incidence of acute rejection will likely be more difficult to achieve. Similarly, it is becoming more difficult to introduce new drugs based on their capacity to reverse episodes of acute rejection because these episodes are becoming less frequent.

NEW IMMUNOSUPPRESSIVE DRUGS

A variety of new immunosuppressive drugs are at different stages of development. Some of these may produce modest improvements of drugs that are already available (e.g., fewer side-effects, better therapeutic index), and some, if their clinical development proves successful, may radically alter the way immunosuppression is practiced in the near future. Many of these drugs are still known by their laboratory designations.

Modifications of Available Drugs

SDZ RAD is a derivative of sirolimus. RAD has a hydroxyethyl chain at position 40 that renders the molecule more polar and improves its oral bioavailability. It may be administered simultaneously with cyclosporine, whereas it is usually recommended that administration of sirolimus be separated from administration of cyclosporine by several hours. Its half-life is shorter than that of sirolimus. Phase 3 trials are in progress in which it is being compared to standard therapy with cyclosporine, prednisone, and MMF.

ERL080A is an enteric-coated form of MMF that may produce less in the way of troublesome GI side effects and permit a somewhat reduced dose.

Indolyl-ASC is related to tacrolimus and may have an improved therapeutic index.

FTY720

FTY720 is a novel immunosuppressive compound with a mechanism of action not previously encountered. It reduces the number of T and B cells in the peripheral blood while increasing their numbers in lymph nodes and Peyer's patches. This redirected cell "homing" is thought to be due to modification by FTY720 of chemokine receptors on lymphocytes. As a result, there is suppression of lymphocyte infiltration into allografts and prolonged lymphopenia. Immunologic memory is not impaired and granulocyte number and function are not affected. The drug may potentiate the immuno-suppressive effects of cyclosporine. Phase 2 clinical trials are in progress.

New Monoclonal Antibodies

HuM291 is a humanized form of OKT3 that may be as effective but is less toxic because it does not induce cytokine release. Clinical trials are in progress.

Anti-CD3 immunotoxin is a conjugate of a murine anti-CD3 monoclonal antibody with mutant diphtheria toxin. The conjugate is directed predominantly at T cells through the antibody's high affinity for the CD3 receptor. It promotes allograft tolerance in nonhuman primates. Preclinical studies are in progress.

OKT4A is a murine anti-CD4 monoclonal antibody that may inhibit the costimulatory function of the CD4 molecule (see Chapter 2). A low rejection rate and favorable toxicity profile were achieved in phase 1 trials.

Antibodies targeted against adhesion molecules (see Chapter 2) have potential for both the prevention of rejection and the prevention of delayed graft function, presumably because of their capacity to reduce cell–cell interactions. Phase 3 trials of the anti-LFA molecule *odulimomab* and the anti-ICAM-1 molecule *enlimomab*, however, showed no significant reduction in the incidence of either acute rejection or delayed graft function, and further clinical development has been halted.

T-Cell Costimulatory Blockade

The most promising approach to the induction of clinically relevant donor-specific graft tolerance comes from the studies manipulating the two major signals required for T-cell activation. Optimal and sustained T-cell response after antigen recognition (signal 1) requires costimulatory signals (signal 2) delivered through accessory T-cell–surface molecules (see Chapter 2). The best understood of the costimulatory pathways are CD28:B7 and CD154:CD40. CTLA-4–Ig is a fusion protein, a homologue of CD28, which binds the B7 molecule with high affinity and blocks the interaction with CD28. Both CTLA-4–Ig and anti-CD154 antibodies, used alone or in combination, have been shown to be effective in preventing rejection in small animal models. In nonhuman primates, a combination of the agents produced prolonged survival of kidney transplants without additional immunosuppression.

In small animal models, the tolerogenic effect of costimulatory blockade is enhanced by the induction of apoptosis in the responding T cells. The calcineurin inhibitors impair this effect by blocking the induction of apoptotic signals, whereas sirolimus promotes apoptosis and improves graft tolerance (Fig. 4.7). These observations have important clinical implications because they may permit an advance from the global immunosuppression produced by combinations of the agents currently at our disposal to a more selective immunosuppression produced by the apoptotic cell death of activated T cells.

Immune Modulation

Immune modulation is a somewhat vague term used to describe attempts to modify the immune response in a nonspecific fashion

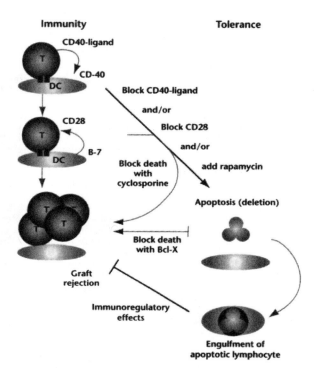

Fig. 4.7.   Apoptosis promotes graft acceptance. Graft antigens, including allogeneic major and minor histocompatability molecules, are presented to the T-cell receptors of specific T cells by dendritic cells (DC).
CD40 ligand on the T cells stimulates CD40 on the DC, causing the DC
to express costimulatory molecules, such as B-7, which in turn binds to
CD28 on the T cell. The combination of the T-cell receptor ligation and
CD28 costimulation results in immunity (and in this case, graft rejection). Blockade of the costimulatory signal, either through the use of
antibodies that bind CD40 ligand or with CTLA-4-Ig, which binds B-7,
results in activation of T-cell unresponsiveness and, ultimately, apoptosis. Rapamycin promotes this apoptosis and improves graft tolerance. Cyclosporine blocks the induction of apoptotic signals, and
blocks tolerance. Bcl-x$_1$, which specifically inhibits apoptosis, also
blocks tolerance induction. The deletion of the responding T cells
creates the tolerant state, which may then be maintained through the
immunoregulatory effects of the apoptotic cells and the cells that
engulf them. (From Ferguson TA, Green DR. T cells are just dying to
accept grafts. *Nature Med* 1999;5:1231, with permission.)

in order to facilitate allograft acceptance without impairing effector cells or mechanisms. Several techniques fall within this category.

Infusion of *donor-specific bone marrow,* in combination with short-term nonspecific immunosuppression, has produced long-term graft survival in the absence of immunosuppressive therapy in experimental and clinical organ allografts. The donor bone marrow provides an as yet unidentified signal for tolerance. *Blood transfusions* are known to exert beneficial effects on animal and human allograft survival through a variety of potential mechanisms. The tolerogenic effect of bone marrow and blood may also be a result of the development of a state of microchimerism (see Chapter 2). A randomized trial of perioperative donor-specific blood transfusions in live donor transplants showed no practical benefit.

Infusions of *intravenous immunoglobulin* (IVIG) may provide blocking or antiidiotypic antibodies that can reduce the production of anti-HLA antibodies and can be used to reduce the formation of preformed anti-HLA antibodies in the pretransplantation period (see Chapter 3). There is also limited experience in the use of IVIG to augment standard immunosuppression or act as a single agent for the treatment of allograft rejection.

Plasmapheresis has been used with inconsistent success to treat episodes of humoral rejection. *Photopheresis* is a new form of extracorporeal photochemotherapy used for the treatment of cutaneous T-cell lymphomas and a variety of autoimmune diseases. In a multicenter trial, it was effective in reducing the frequency of rejection in cardiac transplant recipients without increasing infection risk. Several case reports have shown benefits in the treatment of renal transplant rejection, although the results of large clinical trials are not yet available. Photopheresis may serve to down-regulate autoreactive and alloreactive T-cell clones.

PART IV: IMMUNOSUPPRESSIVE PROTOCOLS

GENERAL PRINCIPLES OF PROTOCOL DESIGN

The variety of immunosuppressive drugs available for use in clinical transplantation permits permutations that make up immunosuppressive protocols. Transplantation centers tend to be loyal to their own protocols, which have often been developed in response to local needs and experience. Protocols should be regarded as guides for therapy that need not necessarily be adhered to slavishly and may require modification from patient to patient and with new knowledge and experience. In an era in which short-term success rates for cadaveric transplantations of greater than 85% are commonplace, it may take experience with hundreds of patients followed for prolonged periods to prove the benefit of a new or modified approach. There are still few data on the effects of different protocols on 5- and 10-year graft survival.

The components of a standard immunosuppressive protocol are shown in Table 4.6 and are relevant to all recipients with the possible exception of two-haplotype matched living-related donors. Because the risk for acute rejection is highest in the first weeks and months after transplantation (*induction phase*) and diminishes thereafter (*maintenance phase*), immunosuppression should be at its highest level in this early period and should be reduced

Table 4.6.   Components of the immunosuppressive protocol

Class of Agent	Options
Calcineurin inhibitor	Cyclosporine, tacrolimus
Corticosteroids	Dose and regimen
Adjunctive agent	Azathioprine, MMF, sirolimus
Antibody induction	OKT3, Atgam, thymoglobin
HAT monoclonal antibody	Basiliximab, daclizumab
Supplementary agents	CCB, HCRI
Infection prophylaxis	Bactrim, antivirals

CCB, calcium-channel blocker; HAT, human anti-Tac; HCRI, HMGCoA reductase inhibitor.

for long-term therapy. The most feared side effects of immunosuppression—opportunistic infection and malignancy—tend to reflect the total amount of immunosuppression given rather than the dose of a single drug. The total quantity of immunosuppression should thus be monitored and considered in all stages of the posttransplantation course.

Cyclosporine or Tacrolimus?
Calcineurin inhibitors remain the backbone of transplant immunosuppression. Although much has been made of discrete differences between cyclosporine and tacrolimus, the fact is that these drugs are remarkably similar, and both are highly effective. Table 4.1 summarizes their similarities and differences. These differences may guide the choice of agent in individual patients. For example, cyclosporine may be preferred in some centers for black patients because of the increased incidence of posttransplantation glucose intolerance in patients who receive tacrolimus; tacrolimus may be preferred in adolescents and other patients concerned about cosmetics because of the more marked cosmetic changes associated with cyclosporine; cyclosporine may be preferred in some patients because of the generally milder neurologic side effects; tacrolimus may be preferred in recipients of simultaneous kidney and pancreas transplants because of its somewhat greater immunosuppressive potency despite its greater islet toxicity (see Chapter 14). In the United States, about 70% of programs base their immunosuppression on cyclosporine and the remainder on tacrolimus.

Which Adjunctive Agent?
In this discussion, the term *adjunctive agent* is used to describe the immunosuppressive drugs that are used in combination with a calcineurin inhibitor to enhance the potency of the immunosuppressive protocol as reflected by a decreased incidence of acute rejection episodes. Most programs use an adjunctive agent for prophylactic purposes starting from the immediate posttransplantation period; some programs choose to introduce adjunctive therapy only in the event of an acute rejection episode. Azathioprine

(used in combination with cyclosporine and prednisone in so-called 'triple therapy') has been replaced by MMF in most centers because of its superior capacity to reduce the incidence of acute rejection (Fig. 4.7 and Table 4.5) as compared with azathioprine. Sirolimus became available for clinical use in late 1999. It is unclear, at this time, to what extent transplantation programs will choose to prescribe it as a replacement for MMF or to what extent it will be used with a standard or low-dose of a calcineurin inhibitor.

Antibody Induction

In this discussion, *antibody induction therapy* refers to the use of OKT3 or a polyclonal antibody in the first 7 to 10 days after transplantation. The calcineurin inhibitor is withheld or its dose is kept to a minimum until 2 to 3 days before the antibody course is completed. Induction protocols with OKT3 or a polyclonal antibody represent the major alternative to the use of a calcineurin inhibitor in the early posttransplantation period and are therefore different from induction using an HAT monoclonal antibody, in which concomitant use of a calcineurin inhibitor is recommended. In *sequential* therapy, OKT3 or the polyclonal antibody is administered and the calcineurin inhibitor is introduced only when renal function has reached a predetermined level (e.g., a plasma creatinine level of 3 mg/dL). The antibody is discontinued as soon as adequate calcineurin inhibitor levels are achieved. A patient with a well-functioning graft may thus receive only a few days of antibody treatment.

The comparative advantages and disadvantages of antibody induction are listed in Table 4.7. The availability of improved adjunctive therapy and the HAT monoclonal antibodies has reduced the use of antibody induction in most centers, and it is often reserved for immunologically high-risk recipients or for patients with delayed graft function. Antibody induction may also be indicated for patients requiring anticonvulsant drugs that may make it difficult to achieve therapeutic levels of calcineurin inhibitors in the early posttransplantation period.

Table 4.7. Potential advantages and disadvantages of antibody induction therapy

Potential Advantages	Potential Disadvantages
1-yr cadaveric function of 90% reported	Risk for first-dose reaction with OKT3
Period of delayed graft function may be foreshortened	May prolong hospital admission stay
Onset of first rejection is delayed	Greater cost
Obviates early use of calcineurin inhibitor	Higher incidence of CMV infection
May permit less aggressive maintenance regimen	Occasional limitation of future treatment options

High-Risk and Low-Risk Groups

All patients are not equal with respect to the chances of rejection or graft loss, and protocols should take this into account. Patients undergoing multiple-organ transplantation and patients with high levels of preformed antibodies may require more intense therapy. In several clinical trials, black patients have required higher doses of immunosuppressive drugs to achieve the same immunosuppressive benefit, and some programs take this into account routinely in protocol design. Young patients tend to be immunologically aggressive; protocol design for children is discussed in Chapter 15. Older patients may not tolerate heavy immunosuppression. Recipients of transplants from living-related donors, particularly from two-haplotype–matched donors, may require less immunosuppression.

How Long to Continue Immunosuppression?

Kidney allografts have long memories! Immunosuppression is required for the functional life of the graft even if it has lasted 20 years or more, and discontinuation of immunosuppressive drugs, even many years after transplantation, may lead to late acute rejection or accelerated chronic rejection. In stable patients, carefully monitored reduction or even discontinuation of individual components of the immunosuppressive protocol may be safe (see Immunosuppressive Drug Withdrawal).

When to Stop Immunosuppression?

The minimal mortality that is now associated with kidney transplantation is to a large degree the result of an appreciation of when to minimize or stop immunosuppression and abandon a kidney. Discontinuation of immunosuppression may be necessary in patients with resistant opportunistic infection or malignancy (see Chapters 9 and 10). Patients with deteriorating graft function despite more than two or three appropriately treated rejections are better allowed to return to dialysis and seek another transplant. With the constant introduction of new immunosuppressive agents into clinical practice, great care and judgment will be needed to avoid the temptation of excessively adding or exchanging new agents.

SPECIFIC PROTOCOL RECOMMENDATIONS

Cadaveric Transplants

Cyclosporine

Cyclosporine, 8 to 12 mg/kg/day orally (3 to 4 mg/kg/day intravenously), is given as a single dose or twice daily starting immediately before transplantation. The intravenous infusion is given over at least 4 hours or can be given as a constant infusion over 24 hours. Some programs prefer to omit the preoperative dose or avoid intravenous cyclosporine altogether. In patients who receive antibody induction, oral cyclosporine is usually started several days before the completion of the course of therapy so that drug levels will be therapeutic at the time of the final antibody dose. Doses are then adjusted to maintain levels within the ranges given in Table 4.8. It is wise to continue to monitor trough levels of cyclosporine, although the degree of reliance on these levels varies from program to program. The desired dose and target level are influ-

Table 4.8. Approximate therapeutic ranges for cyclosporine (ng/mL)

Months After Transplantation	HPLC and Monoclonal RIA	Monoclonal FPIA	Polyclonal FPIA
0–2	150–350	250–500	500–900
2–6	100–250	175–350	400–700
>6	~100	~150	300–840

HPLC, high-performance liquid chromatography; FPIA, fluorescent polarization immunoassay; RIA, radioimmunoassay.

enced by the concomitant use of adjunctive agents and history of rejections. By 3 months after transplantation, most patients are receiving cyclosporine in a dose of 3 to 5 mg/kg/day.

There is still no clear consensus regarding the best dose or drug level for long-term cyclosporine use, and it is unfortunate that prospective randomized trials comparing cyclosporine dose ranges are not available. Fear of progressive nephrotoxicity has tempted many clinicians to permit low levels, yet such a policy may allow for the insidious development of chronic rejection. Retrospective studies have shown that continued use of cyclosporine is conducive to prolonged adequate graft function and that, within the range of the recommended doses, higher doses may be better than lower doses.

WHICH CYCLOSPORINE FORMULATION? Most patients are started and maintained on Neoral. Patients who were started on Sandimmune may choose to switch from Sandimmune to Neoral; however, there is no overriding medical reason to do so. The switch requires care because of the different pharmacokinetics of the two formulations (see Cyclosporine under Formulations and Pharmacokinetics). Although a 1:1 dose ratio is recommended, some patients require somewhat less Neoral than Sandimmune. Even in stable patients, cyclosporine blood levels should be monitored more carefully in the month after the switch and dose adjustments made. An elevation of the creatinine level soon after a switch is more likely to be a result of nephrotoxicity than of rejection. The decision to use a generic formulation is a financial rather than a medical one. Any switching of formulations requires careful monitoring.

Tacrolimus

The recommended starting dose of oral tacrolimus is 0.15 to 0.30 mg/kg/day administered in a split dose each 12 hours. Intravenous tacrolimus is rarely required in kidney transplantation. Doses are adjusted to maintain tacrolimus drug levels at between 10 to 20 ng/dL during the first few posttransplantation months and between 5 and 15 ng/dL thereafter. There is marked patient-to-patient variation in the dose of tacrolimus required to achieve these levels, with some patients receiving as little as 2 mg daily and some patients receiving 10 times that dose. Some programs use the toxicity of tacrolimus to gauge its dose and will permit drug levels to rise until there is evidence of nephrotoxicity or neurotoxicity (usually manifested as headache or tremulousness). The relationship between drug levels and manifestations of toxicity also varies considerably between patients.

Corticosteroids

Methylprednisolone is given intraoperatively in a dose of up to 1 g. The dose is then reduced rapidly from 150 mg on day 1 to 20 to 30 mg on day 14. Some programs avoid the steroid cycle altogether, modifying it or starting at 30 mg daily or even less. The maximal oral dose of prednisone at 1 month should be 20 mg and 15 mg at 3 months. After a year, many patients tolerate an every-other-day regimen. The low long-term maintenance doses that patients typically receive (5 to 7.5 mg daily) should be regarded with great care and respect. Rejection episodes may occasionally occur when even very small dose reductions are made (see Immunosuppression Drug Withdrawal). High-maintenance-dose protocols of steroids sometimes used for collagen vascular disease and vasculitides are unnecessary and contraindicated in kidney transplantation.

Adjunctive Agents

The dose of azathioprine is 1 to 3 mg/kg. Drug levels are not measured, and the dose is usually fixed with adjustments made for hematologic toxicity. The standard dose of MMF in adults is 1,000 mg twice daily, although black patients may benefit from a higher dose (1,500 mg twice daily). Some evidence suggests that measurement of blood levels of mycophenolic acid may be useful in predicting the effectiveness of MMF; however, blood levels are generally not measured, and a clinical assay is not routinely available. The dose of MMF can be safely reduced or held for short periods in the event of side effects as long as calcineurin inhibitor and prednisone doses are maintained.

The standard dose of sirolimus is 2 mg administered once daily 4 hours after the morning dose of cyclosporine. A loading dose of 6 mg is given on the first day of treatment. Black patients may benefit from a 5-mg/day maintenance dose with a 15-mg loading dose. In nonblack patients, it may be possible to use a lower dose of cyclosporine when sirolimus is used. Routine measurement of drug levels is not required when the drug is used according to the FDA labeling. It may be beneficial for children, for patients with hepatic impairment, and for patients in whom potentially interacting drugs are introduced. In the clinical trials of sirolimus, the mean 24-hour whole-blood trough level for the 2-mg daily dose was 9 ng/mL, and a therapeutic trough level of 5 to 15 ng/mL is usually recommended.

The HAT monoclonal antibodies are designed to be given (see Part II for specific dose recommendations) with standard doses of cyclosporine and prednisone. They may also be given with other adjunctive agents to produce a further reduction in the incidence of acute rejection. Their use is not associated with a significant increase in side effects; hence, the decision to use them is often based on an assessment of whether their extra cost can be justified.

Supplementary Agents

The inclusion of *calcium-channel blockers,* usually either diltiazem or verapamil, in the standard immunosuppressive regimen has several potential advantages. In addition to their antihypertensive properties, both drugs may minimize calcineurin inhibitor–induced vasoconstriction and protect against ischemic graft injury and nephrotoxicity. Both drugs compete with the calcineurin inhibitors for excretion by the P450 enzyme system, raising drug levels and permitting safe administration of lower doses. Calcium-channel blockers may also possess some intrinsic immunomodulatory activity of their own related to the role of cytosolic calcium levels or gene activation. The routine inclusion of calcium-channel blockers in the posttransplantation protocol may improve 1-year graft survival by 5% to 10%.

The HCRIs have been shown to lower cholesterol levels safely in transplant recipients and to reduce the incidence of clinically severe rejection in cardiac transplant recipients. A similar beneficial effect has been observed in preliminary studies in kidney transplant recipients. The mechanism of this effect may be related to the capacity of HCRIs to suppress the cytotoxic activity of natural killer cells (see Chapter 2). HCRIs may have benefits in the immunosuppressive regimen that are not directly related to their effect on the lipid profile.

Protocols for Live Donor Transplants

Excellent results were achieved for two-haplotype–matched living-related transplants immunosuppressed with azathioprine and prednisone alone before the introduction of cyclosporine into routine clinical practice. Despite this experience, most transplantation programs now use calcineurin inhibitor–based protocols for these patients because of the lesser incidence of acute rejection. Two-haplotype–matched transplant recipients receiving calcineurin inhibitors may be good candidates for eventual steroid withdrawal. MMF or sirolimus could potentially be used to replace the calcineurin inhibitor. For all other live donor transplants, a calcineurin inhibitor–based protocol should be employed similar to that described for cadaveric transplants.

Immunosuppressive Drug Withdrawal

The availability of multiple immunosuppressive agents has stimulated attempts to minimize or avoid the most toxic components of the standard protocol. The most obvious targets for such efforts are corticosteroids and the calcineurin inhibitors, because of their nephrotoxicity.

Steroid withdrawal implies the discontinuation of steroid administration after transplantation and needs to be differentiated from steroid avoidance, in which steroids are administered only in the event of rejection. Steroid avoidance has never been popular in the United States, although it has been applied in Europe. Many patients who avoid steroids end up receiving them for rejection anyway. Steroid avoidance, or early withdrawal, is being reevaluated using combinations of immunosuppressive agents.

Steroid withdrawal is a tempting ploy that may be considered in selected patients, although the anxiety associated with withdrawal (for both the patients and their physicians!) has tended to dampen its popularity. A randomized, blinded trial of steroid withdrawal 4 months after transplantation was performed in a group of patients with good graft function who had not suffered rejection episodes and who were receiving cyclosporine and MMF in standard doses. The trial was discontinued because of a 20% incidence of acute rejection in the withdrawn group compared with a 5% incidence in the control group. Most of the rejection episodes occurred in the black patients. Steroid withdrawal should thus be considered only at least several months after transplantation in patients who have not suffered recent or recurrent rejections and who have excellent graft function. Black patients may not be suitable candidates for withdrawal, and all patients should be warned of a small but finite increased incidence of rejection. A clear-cut benefit of withdrawal, in terms of certain steroid-related side effects (e.g., bone disease, hyperlipidemia), has not been demonstrated, presumably because most of the familiar steroid-related problems are produced by the high doses used in the early posttransplantation period. There may be long-term deterioration in graft function patients after steroid withdrawal; these patients should be forewarned.

In the pivotal trials leading to the introduction of cyclosporine, tacrolimus, MMF, and sirolimus, the drugs were continued long-term and the safety of their discontinuation was not studied in a rigorous fashion. Several studies have shown that it may be possible to withdraw these drugs or reduce their dose in some stable patients, and randomized trials are in progress to provide a definitive answer to the safety of this approach. Trials are also in progress using low doses and blood levels of the calcineurin inhibitors in various combinations with MMF, sirolimus, and the HAT monoclonal antibodies. The potential advantage of these protocols is that they may maintain immunologic effectiveness while minimizing short-term and long-term nephrotoxicity. Until the results of these trials become available, withdrawal or dose reduction should be carried out only after a careful evaluation of risk and benefit, particularly with respect to the calcineurin inhibitors.

Management of Acute Rejection

First Rejection

PULSE STEROIDS. High doses of pulse steroids reverse about 75% of first acute rejections. There are numerous ways to pulse a patient, and there is no good evidence that the higher-dose pulses (500 to 1,000 mg methylprednisolone for 3 days) are necessarily more effective than the lower-dose pulses (120 to 250 mg oral prednisone or methylprednisolone for 3 to 5 days). Most programs still prefer to use intravenous methylprednisolone, which is given over 30 to 60 minutes into a peripheral vein. Pulse therapy is suitable for outpatient use when clinically indicated. The dose of prednisone can be continued at its previous level when the pulse is completed, although some programs elect to *recycle* the prednisone dose after the pulse has been completed.

ANTIBODY TREATMENT. OKT3 is a highly effective therapy for the management of a first acute rejection, and about 90% of such rejections will be reversed. Similar results can be achieved with Thymoglobulin, which is more effective than Atgam. Despite the greater effectiveness of these agents, most programs still prefer to use pulse steroids as their first-line acute rejection therapy because of their convenience, lesser risks of side effects, and lower costs. OKT3 or Thymoglobulin may be a better first-line option for particularly severe or vascular rejections (Banff grade IIB or greater; see Chapter 13). The HAT monoclonal antibodies are not designed to be used in the treatment of established acute rejection.

Recurrent and Refractory Rejections

Repeated courses of pulse steroids may be effective in reversing acute rejections, but it is probably not wise to administer more than two courses of pulse therapy before resorting to OKT3 or polyclonal antibodies. Many programs use antibody treatment for all second rejections unless the rejection is clinically mild or separated from the first by at least several weeks. Antibody treatment is particularly valuable for rejection episodes that are steroid resistant and may succeed in reversing a high percentage of such rejections. Some programs commence antibody treatment if there is not an immediate response to pulse therapy, whereas others wait several days. If renal function is deteriorating rapidly in the face of pulse steroids, it is probably wise to start antibody treatment early.

The term *refractory rejection* is not well defined. It usually refers to ongoing rejection despite treatment with pulse steroids and antibody. The management of these patients is problematic. Second courses of OKT3 or polyclonal antibodies can be given in selected patients, and long-term graft function can be achieved in 40% to 50% of such patients. When deciding whether to give a second course of an antibody preparation, the clinician should bear in mind the severity and potential reversibility of rejection on biopsy; the increased risk for infection and malignancy that ensues, particularly if two courses are given close together; and the possibility of generating high levels of anti-OKT3 antibodies that might limit treatment options for a future transplantation.

Switching from cyclosporine to tacrolimus, or adding MMF in patients who have not previously received it, have both been shown to be effective treatments for refractory rejections. About 75% of such rejections can be reversed in this manner. If a decision is made to change to tacrolimus, it is important that cyclosporine is discontinued, and it is generally recommended that levels be allowed to decrease to less than 100 ng/mL on a specific assay before tacrolimus is introduced. It may be wise to "cover" the period between adequate cyclosporine and tacrolimus levels with high-dose steroids. Preliminary trials of sirolimus in patients with recurrent rejections and nephrotoxicity suggest that it may be effective, but it must be given with great care because of the dangers of overimmunosuppression. Protocol guidelines for switching from calcineurin inhibitors to sirolimus are not yet available.

Late Rejections

The terms *early* and *late rejection* are not well defined. The differentiation between early and late rejection is not just semantic; each may respond differently to therapy. For practical purposes, a late rejection is one that occurs more than 3 to 4 months after transplantation and may be a first, or more frequently, a recurrent rejection. Late rejections can also be divided into those that occur in the face of apparently adequate immunosuppression and those that occur as a result of obviously inadequate immunosuppression, typically in noncompliant patients. Late rejections are often a prelude to chronic rejection and accelerated graft loss.

The initial treatment of a late rejection is pulse steroids. The effectiveness of OKT3 for acute rejection treatment tends to diminish with time, so that by 3 to 4 months after transplantation, only 40% to 50% of episodes respond to OKT3 treatment. By 1 year after transplantation, this figure may be only about 20%, and at this stage, it may not be worth the risks associated with therapy. There is evidence that late rejections associated with noncompliance are more likely to respond to therapy. Use of polyclonal antibodies for late steroid-resistant rejection has not been systematically studied.

Thus, there are limited therapeutic options for late steroid-resistant rejection, which often occurs in a background of chronic rejection. It may often be wiser to accept graft dysfunction or loss rather than use potent high-dose immunosuppression in an already chronically immunosuppressed patient.

The management of chronic allograft failure is discussed in Chapter 9.

SELECTED READINGS

Part I

Cho S, Danovitch G, Deierhoi M, et al. Mycophenolate mofetil in cadaveric renal transplantation. *Am J Kidney Dis* 1999;34:296.

Danovitch GM. Immunosuppressant induced metabolic toxicities. *Transplant Rev* 2000;14:65.

Groth CG, Bäckman L, Morales JM, et al. Sirolimus (rapamycin)-based therapy in human renal transplantation. *Transplantation* 1999;67:1036.

Halloran P, Mathew T, Tomlanovich S, et al. Mycophenolate mofetil in renal allograft recipients. *Transplantation* 1997;63:39.

Henry ML. Cyclosporine and tacrolimus (FK506): a comparison of efficacy and safety profiles. *Clin Transplant* 1999;13:209.

Kahan BD, for the Rapamune U.S. Study Group. Sirolimus is more effective than azathioprine to reduce the incidence of acute allograft rejection episodes when used in combination with cyclosporine and prednisone: a phase III US multicenter study. Abstracts 1999:68.

Khanna AK, Cairns VR, Becker CG, et al. Transforming growth factor (TGF)-β mimics and anti-TGF-β antibody abrogates the in vivo effects of cyclosporine. *Transplantation* 1999;67:882.

Ojo A, Meier-Kriesche H, Hanson JA, et al. Mycophenolate mofetil reduces late renal allograft loss independent of acute rejection. *Transplantation* 2000;69:2405.

Pirsch JD, Miller J, Deierhoi MH, et al. A comparison of tacrolimus (FK506) and cyclosporine for immunosuppression after cadaveric renal transplantation. *Transplantation* 1997;63:977.

Sabatini S, Ferguson RM, Helderman JH, et al. Drug substitution in transplantation: a National Kidney Foundation white paper. *Am J Kidney Dis* 1999;33:389.

Sehgal SN. Rapamune (RAPA, rapamycin, sirolimus): mechanism of action immunosuppressive effect results from blockade of signal transduction and inhibition of cell cycle progression. *Clin Biochem* 1998;31:335.

Shah MB, Martin JE, Schroeder TJ, et al. The evaluation of the safety and tolerability of two formulations of cyclosporine: Neoral and Sandimmune. *Transplantation* 1999;67:1411.

Solez K, Vincenti F, Filo RS. Histopathological findings from 2-year protocol biopsies from a U.S. multicenter kidney transplant trial comparing tacrolimus versus cyclosporine. *Transplantation* 1998; 66:1736.

Trimarchi HM, Truong LD, Brennan S, et al. FK506-associated thrombotic microangiopathy. *Transplantation* 1999;67:539.

Veenstra DL, Best JH, Hornberger J, et al. Incidence and long-term cost of steroid-related side effects after renal transplantation. *Am J Kidney Dis* 1999;33:829.

Part II

Gaber AO, First MR, Tesi RJ, et al. Results of the double-blind, randomized, multicenter, phase III clinical trial of thymoglobulin versus ATGAM in the treatment of acute graft rejection episodes after renal transplantation. *Transplantation* 1998; 66:29.

Jordan SC, Tyan D, Czer L, et al. Immunomodulatory actions of intravenous immunoglobulin (IVIG): potential applications in solid organ transplant recipients. *Pediatr Transplant* 1998; 2:92.

Kahan BD, Rajaagopalan PR, Hall M. Reduction of the occurrence of acute cellular rejection among renal allograft recipients treated with basiliximab, a chimeric anti-interleukin-2-receptor monoclonal antibody. *Transplantation* 1999;67:276.

Kamath S, Dean D, Peddi VR, et al. Efficacy of OKT3 as primary therapy for histologically confirmed acute renal allograft rejection. *Transplantation* 1997;64:1428.

Müller TF, Grebe SO, Neuman MC, et al. Persistent long-term changes in lymphocyte subsets induced by polyclonal antibodies. *Transplantation* 1997;64:1432.

Nashan B, Light S, Hardie IR, et al. Reduction of acute renal allograft rejection by daclizumab. *Transplantation* 1999;67:110.

Szczech LA, Berlin JA, Feldman HI, et al. The effect of antilymphocyte induction therapy on renal allograft survival. *Ann Intern Med* 1998;128:817.

Part III

Abrams JR, Lebwohl MG, Guzzo CA, et al. CTLA4Ig-mediated blockade of T-cell costimulation in patients with psoriasis vulgaris. *J Clin Invest* 1999;103:1243.

Contreras JL, Eckhoff DE, Cartner S, et al. Tolerability and side effects of anti-CD3-immunotoxin in preclinical testing in kidney and pancreatic islet transplant recipients. *Transplantation* 1999;68:215.

Cole MS, Stellrecht KE, Shi JD, et al. HuM291, a humanized anti-CD3 antibody, is immunosuppressive to T cells while exhibiting reduced mitogenicity in vitro. *Transplantation* 1999;68:563.

Dall'Amico R, Murer L, Montini G, et al. Successful treatment of recurrent rejection in renal transplant patients with photopheresis. *J Am Soc Nephrol* 1997;9:121.

Delmonico FL, Cosimi AB, Colvin R, et al. Murine OKT4A immunosuppression in cadaver donor renal allograft recipients. *Transplantation* 1997;63:1243.

Dumont FJ, Koprak S, Staruch M, et al. A tacrolimus-related immunosuppressant with reduced toxicity. *Transplantation* 1998;65:18.

Gudmundsdottir H, Turka LA. T cell costimulatory blockade: new therapies for transplant rejection. *J Am Soc Nephrol* 1999;10: 1356.

Gummert JF, Ikonen T, Morris RE. Newer immunosuppressive drugs: a review. *J Am Soc Nephrol* 1999;10:1336.

Halloran PF. Immunosuppressive agents in clinical trials in transplantation. *Am J Med Sci* 1997;313:283.

Kirk AD, Burkly LC, Batty DS, et al. Treatment with humanized monoclonal antibody against CD154 prevents acute renal allograft rejection in nonhuman primates. *Nature Med* 1999;5:686.

Li Y, Li XC, Zheng XX, et al. Blocking both signal 1 and signal 2 of t-cell activation prevents apoptosis of alloreactive T cells and induction of peripheral allograft tolerance. *Nature Med* 1999;5:1298.

Murphy B, Krensky AM. HLA-derived peptides as novel immunomodulatory therapeutics. *J Am Soc Nephrol* 1999;10:1346.

Salmela K, Wramner L, Ekberg H, et al. A randomized multicenter trial of the anti-ICAM-1 monoclonal antibody (enlimomab) for the prevention of acute rejection and delayed onset of graft function in cadaveric renal transplantation. *Transplantation* 1999;67:729.

Troncoso P, Stepkowski SM, Wang M, et al. Prophylaxis of acute renal allograft rejection using FTY720 in combination with subtherapeutic doses of cyclosporine. *Transplantation* 1999; 67:145.

Part IV

Best JH, Sullivan SD. The changing cost-effectiveness of renal transplantation: the impact of improvements in immunosuppressive therapy. *Transplant Rev* 1998;12:34.

Danovitch GM. Choice of immunosuppressive drugs and individualization of immunosuppressive therapy for kidney transplant patients. *Transplant Proc* 1999;31 suppl. 8A:2.

Danovitch GM. Cyclosporin or tacrolimus: which agent to choose? *Nephrol Dial Transplant* 1997;12:1566.

Denton MD, Magee CC, Sayegh MH. Immunosuppressive strategies in transplantation. *Lancet* 1999;353:1083.

Fassi A, Sangalli F, Colombi F, et al. Beneficial effects of calcium channel blockade on acute glomerular hemodynamic changes induced by cyclosporine. *Am J Kidney Dis* 1999;33:267.

Hollander AA, Hene RJ, Hermans J, et al. Late prednisone withdrawal in cyclosporine-treated kidney transplant patients: a randomized study. *J Am Soc Nephrol* 1996;7:293.

Johnson EM, Canafax DM, Gillingham KJ, et al. Effect of early cyclosporine levels on kidney allograft rejection. *Clin Transplant* 1997;11:552.

Roth D, Colona J, Burke GW, et al. Primary immunosuppression with Tacrolimus and Mycophenolate mofetil for renal allograft recipients. *Transplantation* 1998;665:248.

Shapiro R, Jordan ML, Scantlebury VP, et al. A prospective, randomized trial of tacrolimus/prednisone versus tacrolimus/prednisone/mycophenolate mofetil in renal transplant recipients. *Transplantation* 1999; 67:411.

Shinn C, Malhotra D, Chan L, et al. Time course of response to pulse methylprednisone therapy in renal transplant recipients with acute allograft rejection. *Am J Kidney Dis* 1999;34:304.

Stegall MD, Wachs M, Everson GT, et al. Corticosteroid withdrawal in solid organ transplantation. *Transplant Rev* 1998;12:140.

Vanrenterghem YF. Impact of new immunosuppressive agents on late graft outcome. *Kidney Int* 1997;52:S-81.

Vu MD, Qi S, Xu D, et al. Tacrolimus (FK506) and sirolimus (Rapamycin) in combination are not antagonistic but produce extended graft survival in cardiac transplantation in the rat. *Transplantation* 1997;64:1853.

Living and Cadaveric Kidney Donation

H. Albin Gritsch, J. Thomas Rosenthal,
and Gabriel M. Danovitch

Kidney transplantation cannot proceed without kidney donors, and although much emphasis is given to posttransplantation patient management, the appropriate identification and preparation of donors contribute critically to the success of the transplantation endeavor on both the individual and the national levels. Tables 5.1 and 5.2 list the potential advantages and disadvantages of living and cadaveric transplantation. Living donors are used for about 33% of all kidney transplantations performed in the United States, and most transplantation centers regard them as the preferred donation modality despite the potential morbidity associated with them.

Figure 1.1 in Chapter 1 illustrates graphically the inexorably widening gap between the demand for donor kidneys and their supply. The number of cadaver donors has remained steady in recent years, whereas the number of potential recipients has risen steadily each year. The inevitable effect of this discrepancy is an increase in the waiting time for cadaveric kidneys, which is now measured in years (see Chapter 3). Surveys suggest that although almost all Americans are aware that kidney transplantations are performed and as many as 75% express willingness to donate an organ after death, only about 40% of all potential cadaveric organ donors actually become donors. Some possible reasons for this discrepancy are discussed later. The transplantation community now finds itself critically reexamining some long-held tenets regarding the suitability of certain types of living and cadaveric donors and carefully reevaluating the manner in which potential donors and their loved ones are approached.

LIVING KIDNEY DONATION

Who Can Be a Living Donor?

For many years, only first-degree relatives (parents, children, and siblings who were at least one-haplotype matches [see Chapter 3]) were deemed suitable living kidney donors. This policy was largely based on the premise that the matching of these kidneys compared with all others so improved their prognosis, or "utility," for the recipient that the risk to the donor was justified. The advent of cyclosporine and the widening gap between the supply and demand for cadaveric kidneys are changing this attitude. It is now clear that the results of transplantation with zero-haplotype–matched sibling transplants and transplants from more distant relatives and biologically unrelated donors are excellent and are similar or even better than those of six-antigen–matched cadaveric transplants (see Chapter 3). This suggests that it is not just the matching of

Table 5.1.   Potential advantages of living versus cadaveric kidney donation

1. Better short-term results (about 95% versus 90% 1-yr function; see Chap. 3)
2. Better long-term results (half-life of 12–20 yr versus 8–9 yr; see Chap. 3)
3. More consistent early function and ease of management
4. Avoidance of brain death stress; see Chap. 8
5. Minimal incidence of delayed graft function; see Chap. 8
6. Avoidance of long wait for cadaveric transplant; see Chap. 3
7. Capacity to time transplantation for medical and personal convenience
8. Immunosuppressive regime may be less aggressive; see Chap. 4
9. Helps relieve stress on national cadaver donor supply
10. Emotional gain to donor; see Chap. 18

the live donor kidney that determines its benefits for the recipient but also the excellent condition of the kidney at the time of its transplantation. There is also a widespread realization that it is highly unlikely that the cadaveric organ supply will ever keep pace with the need for organs. As a result, there has been a gradual broadening of the definition of who can be a living donor.

Most transplantation centers now routinely accept as donors zero-haplotype–matched siblings and second-degree relatives (e.g., cousins, uncles, aunts; see Fig. 5.1). Biologically unrelated transplant donors are most frequently spouses or individuals who have an emotional relationship to the recipient (e.g., adopted siblings, significant others, best friends). The term *emotionally related donor* is a good one because it emphasizes the importance of the relationship between the donor and the recipient. Some transplantation centers are more liberal in their definition of an emotionally related donor and will accept a "friend of a friend," member of a club, or religious affiliation for whom the relationship is less personal. Some centers accept *altruistic donors* where there is no personal relationship with the recipient. As of 1997, donors who were not first-degree relatives accounted for 21% of all living

Table 5.2.   Potential disadvantages of live donation

1. Psychological stress to donor and family (see Chap. 16)
2. Inconvenience and risk of evaluation process (i.e., intravenous contrast)
3. Operative mortality (about 1 in 2000 patients)
4. Major postoperative complications (about 2% of patients)
5. Minor postoperative complications (up to 50% of patients)
6. Long-term morbidity (possibly mild hypertension and proteinuria)
7. Risk for traumatic injury to remaining kidney
8. Risk for unrecognized covert chronic renal disease

Living Donor / Recipient Relationships

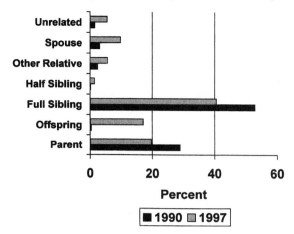

Fig. 5.1. **Changes in the relationship between living kidney transplant donor and recipient.**

donors in the United States. *Paired donor exchange* has been proposed as a solution for donor–recipient pairs for whom there is ABO incompatibility, although experience with the practical and emotional aspects of such practice is limited.

A careful family history should be a routine part of the evaluation of all potential transplant recipients, and the advantages and disadvantages of living donation should be discussed when relevant. A brief screening excludes obviously inappropriate donors. Patients should not be pressured into approaching family members for donation when they are uncomfortable doing so, nor should potential donors be pressured into the evaluation process. It is often a good prognostic sign when the donor accompanies the recipient to his or her pretransplantation evaluation appointments. The first approach to the potential donor should ideally come from the patient and not from the patient's nephrologist, transplantation physician, or surgeon. Some patients find it difficult to approach family members, and the nephrologist and transplantation team should be prepared to facilitate the discussion of donation. Written material explaining the donation process can often help to alleviate the fears and anxiety of potential donors.

Donor Evaluation
Evaluation of living donors is a stepwise process that progresses from initial screening through noninvasive to invasive evaluation and surgery. A practical scheme for the process is shown in Table 5.3. Certain basic principles are consistent in the manner that all programs approach and evaluate donors, although details of policy may differ. The donors, who must appreciate that the process is

**Table 5.3. Suggested evaluation process
for potential live donors**

Donor screening

Educate patient regarding cadaveric and live donation.
Take family and social history and screen for potential donors.
Review ABO compatibilities of potential donors.
Tissue-type and crossmatch ABO-compatible potential donors.
Choose primary potential donor with patient and family.
Educate donor regarding process of evaluation and donation.

Donor evaluation

Complete history and physical examination
Comprehensive laboratory screening to include complete blood count,
    chemistry panel, human immunodeficiency virus, very-low-density
    lipoprotein, hepatitis B and C serology, cytomegalovirus, glucose
    tolerance test (for diabetic families)
Urinalysis, urine culture, pregnancy test
24-hr urine collection for protein[a]
24-hr urine collection for creatinine[a]
Chest radiograph, cardiogram, exercise treadmill for patients older
    than 50 years of age
Helical computed tomography urogram[b]
Psychosocial evaluation
Repeat crossmatch before transplantation.

[a] Done twice in some programs.
[b] May be replaced by intravenous pyelogram and renal angiogram in some centers (see Chap. 12).

not irreversible, should determine the pace of the evaluation. The donor can withdraw at any time, although clearly it is wasteful to do so at the more advanced stages of evaluation. Precise definition of renal anatomy with spiral computed tomography (CT) scan or intravenous pyelogram and angiography (see Chapter 12) is the final step in the process and should follow completion of the recipient workup.

Careful psychosocial evaluation (see Chapters 16 and 19) should be part of the evaluation of all living donors to assess the degree of motivation and voluntarism. This is particularly important when the nature of the motivation is not clear-cut. Live kidney donation, biologically or not biologically related, is an extraordinary act of altruism and love by one individual for another. Follow-up studies of donors show that most are satisfied and gratified by the process, although dissatisfaction is more likely if the donor is not biologically related and if the outcome of the transplantation is unfavorable. Financial incentives for donation are illegal in the United States and in most countries, although the ethical underpinnings of this policy have been questioned in the case of countries in which the therapeutic options for patients with end-stage renal disease are limited. The donor who has second thoughts about donation should be provided, if he or she wishes, with a medical alibi to justify his or her hesitation to the family.

Exclusion Criteria

Potential donors are excluded on medical grounds when it is believed that there may be a risk for unrecognized kidney disease or an increased risk for short-term or long-term morbidity and mortality from the operative procedure. Table 5.4 reviews some common criteria for excluding potentially compatible donors. Many of these criteria are not absolute, and when findings are borderline, it is always wise to err on the side of donor safety because the donor, unlike the recipient, does not need the operation to improve his or her health. Some centers adhere rigidly to an upper age limit, whereas other centers attempt to judge biologic rather than chronologic age. A glomerular filtration rate (GFR) of 80 mL/min or more has generally been believed to be adequate to permit donation, although older donors, women with low muscle mass, and vegetarians may have a GFR of less than 80 mL/min with no evidence of renal disease. To avoid conflict of interest, it is preferable for a physician other than the one caring for the recipient to determine donor suitability. It must be clear to all concerned that donors are not to be sacrificed for recipients even in circumstances (particularly parents to children) in which the donor is prepared to make the sacrifice.

Hereditary Kidney Disease

The issue of donation in families with hereditary kidney disease occurs most frequently in families with adult polycystic kidney disease (PKD) or hereditary nephritis. In families with PKD, a negative ultrasound or CT scan in a potential donor older than 30 years of age safely excludes the disease and permits donation. Because the PKD gene is a dominant one, the children of such a donor will not inherit the disease. Use of genetic testing in PKD is complicated by the fact that testing is available only for one of

Table 5.4.   Exclusion criteria for live-related donors

Age <18 yr or >65–70 yr
Hypertension (>140/90 mm Hg or necessity for medication)
Diabetes (abnormal glucose tolerance test or hemoglobin A_{1c}
Proteinuria (>250 mg/24 hr)
History of recurrent kidney stones
Abnormal glomerular filtration rate (< 80 mL/min)[a]
Microscopic hematuria
Urologic abnormalities in donor kidneys
Significant medical illness (e.g., chronic lung disease, recent malignancy)
Obesity (30% above ideal weight)
History of thrombosis or thromboembolism
Psychiatric contraindications (see Chap. 16)
Strong family history of renal disease, diabetes, and hypertension

[a] Measured by either creatinine clearance or a radiolabeled filtration marker.

the abnormal genes. In hereditary nephritis, the situation may be more complex. A patient in the third decade of life who is free of urinary abnormalities could be deemed free of disease and hence be a donor. It is not inconceivable, however, that the offspring of such a donor could suffer kidney disease; this possibility may be a consideration in the potential donor's decision, particularly when the family history is a strong one.

There may also be familial aggregation of renal disease in excess of that predicted by clustering of diabetes and hypertension within families, suggesting that either genetic susceptibility or environmental exposures shared within some families increase the risk for end-stage renal disease. The risk is much higher when two or more first-degree relatives have renal disease, and in such families, it may be wise to avoid live donation, particularly from young donors. In North America, this situation is most frequently encountered in Hispanic and Native American families with a high incidence of non–insulin-dependent diabetes.

Which Donor to Choose?

If there is more than one donor in a family, it is logical to commence work-up on the relative who is best matched (i.e., a two-haplotype match versus a one-haplotype match). If the donors are of the same match grade (i.e., a one-haplotype–matched parent and a one-haplotype–matched sibling), it may be advisable to choose the older donor with the thought that the younger donor would still be available for donation if the first kidney eventually fails. When more than one one-haplotype–matched sibling is available, it may be worthwhile to check the tissue typing of one parent to determine which sibling shares the noninherited maternal antigens (see Chapter 3). Such sharing may improve long-term graft survival. Women of childbearing age are not at increased risk for obstetric problems after donation. Biologically related donors are generally preferred over emotionally related donors.

Surgical Evaluation of the Donor

Preoperative spiral CT urography provides both functional and sufficiently sensitive anatomic detail to detect most polar renal arteries. This less invasive imaging modality has replaced intravenous urography and renal arteriography in most centers (see Chapter 12). Usually, the left kidney is selected for donation because the left renal vein is longer than the right vein and thus easier to transplant. If there are multiple arteries to the left kidney and a single artery to the right kidney, the right kidney can be used. If there are two arteries bilaterally, a kidney may still be used, employing one of several surgical techniques to handle multiple renal arteries. Occasionally, the donor has minor unilateral renal abnormalities, such as renal cysts, or even more severe problems, such as ureteropelvic junction obstruction. In these situations, the most prudent approach, if such abnormalities are not too severe, is to transplant the abnormal kidney, leaving the donor with the normal one. The unexpected finding of unilateral or bilateral fibromuscular dysplasia in a normotensive potential donor presents a difficult dilemma. In the absence of definitive data regarding natural history of this condition, most programs have avoided using such donors.

Donor Nephrectomy

The standard method for removing a kidney from a living donor is through a flank incision. Most donor surgeons use an extrapleural and extraperitoneal approach, just above or below the 12th rib. The kidney must be carefully dissected to preserve all renal arteries, renal veins, and the periureteral blood supply. Excessive traction on the renal artery should be avoided to prevent vasospasm. The donor should be well hydrated, and intraoperative mannitol is administered to ensure a brisk diuresis. After the renal vessels are securely ligated and divided, the kidney is removed and placed in a basin of frozen saline slush to decrease renal metabolism. The renal arteries are cannulated and flushed with cold heparinized Collins solution in lieu of systemic heparinization of the donor.

Endoscopically assisted nephrectomy techniques provide an alternative to the standard method, and the procedures are gaining in availability and popularity. For a fully *laparoscopic nephrectomy,* the donor is placed in the flank position, and the abdominal cavity is insufflated with carbon dioxide gas. Three or four tubes are inserted through small incisions in the abdominal wall, and a miniature video camera and instruments are then manipulated through these ports (Fig. 5.2). The colon is reflected away, and the renal artery and vein are then carefully identified and isolated by observing the instruments on a video monitor. The perinephric tissue and ureter are then mobilized and manipulated into a plastic sack. The renal vessels are divided with a vascular stapler, and an incision is made that is just large enough (usually in the midline below the umbilicus) to allow removal of the kidney and sack. The kidney is then placed in the frozen saline slush, the vascular staples are removed, and the renal artery is flushed with heparinized preservation solution. The hand-assisted laparoscopic technique employs a relatively small abdominal incision to allow the introduction of the surgeon's hand to supplement the laparoscopic procedure and permit rapid atraumatic removal of the kidney. Laparoscopic techniques can be rapidly converted to open nephrectomy in the event of uncontrolled bleeding or unforeseen anatomic abnormalities.

There are advantages and disadvantages to each of the nephrectomy procedures (Tables 5.5 and 5.6), and these should be reviewed with the potential donor and recipient. The major impetus for the development of the laparoscopic techniques has been the pain and discomfort suffered after standard nephrectomy. The relatively prolonged hospital stay and delay in return to work have been disincentives to living donation even among motivated donors. Programs with a long experience of laparoscopic techniques have an excellent safety record, comparable to that of the open operation. There has, however, been some understandable reticence regarding widespread introduction of laparoscopic techniques because of concern regarding donor safety and graft function. This concern is particularly relevant during the period of the "learning curve" when the procedure is first introduced by a program. Endoscopic procedures require an experienced laparoscopic surgeon and a transplant recipient surgeon that can handle shorter and multiple renal vessels. As endoscopically assisted nephrectomy techniques become more popular, it is hoped that their safety

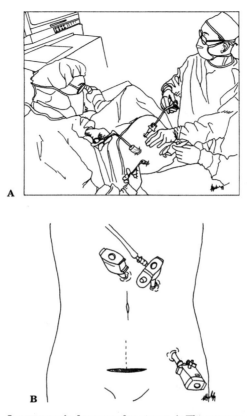

Fig. 5.2.   Laparoscopic donor nephrectomy. A: The surgeon and assistants perform the operation by viewing instruments placed through the abdominal wall using a miniature television camera. B: After the kidney has been completely mobilized and the ureter and renal vessels have been divided, the kidney is removed through a small incision in the lower abdomen.

record will be maintained and that rates of living kidney donation will increase as a result of reduced pain and suffering of the donor.

Postoperative Management

A chest radiograph is obtained in the recovery room if a pneumothorax is suspected, and if necessary, the air is evacuated or a chest tube is placed. A nasogastric tube is not routinely inserted. If a flank incision has been made, most patients are able to eat 24 to 48 hours after surgery. Early ambulation is encouraged, as is aggressive pulmonary toilet. The average hospital stay is 2 to 4 days. Most donors can return to all but the most strenuous exercise or work by 3 to 4 weeks. Complete recovery takes 6 to

**Table 5.5.   Advantages and disadvantages
of open nephrectomy**

Advantages

Long-term international record of safety
Retroperitoneal approach minimizes potential abdominal
    complications
Shorter operative time
Minimal warm ischemia time to remove kidney
Excellent early graft function

Disadvantages

Postoperative pain
Requires 6–8 weeks of recovery to return to work
Long surgical scar with potential for hernia and abdominal wall
    asymmetry

8 weeks, although some donors complain of incisional pain for
2 to 3 months. Laparoscopic nephrectomy donors are usually in
the hospital for 1 to 2 days and report less postoperative pain and
a full recovery in 4 to 5 weeks.

Postoperative Complications
Operative mortality is minimal but has been reported. In a series
of more than 8,000 living donors, there were 5 deaths due to
myocardial infarction, pulmonary embolus, and hepatitis. The rate
of major complications was 1.8%, which consisted of pulmonary
emboli, myocardial infarctions, sepsis, pneumonia, wound infec-

**Table 5.6.   Advantages and disadvantages
of laparoscopic nephrectomy**

Advantages

Less postoperative pain
Minimal surgical scarring
Rapid return to full activities and work (approx. 4 weeks)
Shorter hospital stay
Magnified view of renal vessels

Disadvantages

Impaired early graft function
Graft loss or damage during "learning curve"
Pneumoperitoneum may compromise renal blood flow
Longer operative time
Tendency to have shorter renal vessels and multiple arteries
Added expense of specialized instrumentation

tions, pancreatitis, and injuries to the spleen or the adrenal gland. There are also risks due to arteriography, such as femoral artery pseudoaneurysm or thrombosis. Careful and compulsive medical evaluation of the donor with adherence to strict donation criteria is the key to minimizing postnephrectomy complications.

Long-term morbidity has not proved to be a major problem; follow-up data for up to 45 years (after traumatic wartime uninephrectomy) suggest that having only one kidney does not have a significant health impact. There is a statistically higher risk for low-grade proteinuria. When large numbers of kidney donors have been followed, however, no increase in incidence of hypertension or deterioration of kidney function has been shown. Serum creatinine levels generally remain about 20% higher and clearance rates 20% lower than predonation values. Occasional cases of chronic renal failure have been observed after donation, but it is unclear whether the pretransplantation work-up of these donors was adequately compulsive or whether the cases are a reflection of the incidence of *de novo* renal disease in the general population. Long-term mortality is not affected by kidney donation, and most life insurance companies do not penalize donors. The main risk for kidney failure in kidney donors is from trauma to the remaining kidney or unrecognized familial kidney disease.

CADAVERIC KIDNEY DONATION

The process of cadaveric transplantation, from recognition of a potential donor to the operation itself, is complex (Table 5.7). It represents the epitome of coordinated teamwork and institutional cooperation. It is orchestrated by regional *organ procurement organizations* (OPOs) (see Chapter 3) that provide a nationally integrated 24-hour service. The quality of the cadaveric kidneys that are harvested by this process has a major effect on the short-term and long-term outcome of the whole transplantation endeavor (see Chapters 8 and 9).

The responsibility for identifying potential donors and notifying the OPOs belongs to every health professional and hospital involved in acute patient care; it has been legally established in *required request legislation* (see Chapter 17). The benefits of this legislation have been less than expected, however. It has been estimated that more than 25% of the families of potential cadaveric donors are not approached, and more than half of the families that are approached decline to permit donation. Trained organ procurement professionals should handle the most difficult and sensitive part of the donation process, the approach to the recently bereaved family. Family members are more likely to permit donation if they are given time to accept the fact that their relative is brain dead before organ donation is discussed. *Uncoupling* of the discussion of death and donation significantly increases the likelihood of family consent. Although organ donor cards are in themselves valid legal documents, all OPOs request specific permission from families to maintain a high degree of public trust and acceptance. Discussion among family members of their attitudes toward organ donation should be encouraged so that the wishes of the deceased can be respected in the event of a catastrophe. Ongoing education by the transplantation commu-

Table 5.7.   Sequence of events preceding cadaveric donor transplantation[a]

1. Recognition of potential donor (see Table 5.8)
2. Notification of organ procurement organization
3. Diagnosis of brain death made by attending physicians; family informed
4. Suitability of donor ascertained
5. Permission for organ donation obtained from family
6. Tissue typing and ABO blood typing of donor[b]
7. Kidneys removed and stored
8. Local and national computer listing of all potential recipients reviewed
9. Top recipient selected by ABO blood type and United Network for Organ Sharing scoring system[b]
10. Transplantation program to review clinical indication for transplantation for recipients of marginal kidneys
11. Top recipient patient notified and admitted to hospital
12. "Backup" recipient prepared if recipient panel-reactive antibodies are high
13. Donor lymphocytes and recipient serum crossmatched[b]
14. Preoperative history and physical examination
15. Preoperative chest radiograph, electrocardiogram, ABO blood typing, and routine chemistry
16. Dialysis performed if necessary
17. Transplantation performed

[a] The precise sequence may vary in individual cases.
[b] See Chapter 3.

nity of both health care professionals and the lay public is central to the maintenance of the cadaveric organ supply.

Who Is a Donor?

Most solid organ donors are brain-dead cadavers whose hearts are still beating; these are often victims of head trauma, vascular catastrophes, cerebral anoxia, and nonmetastasizing brain tumors. It is best to regard all such patients as potential donors and then to exclude inappropriate candidates (Table 5.8). Many governmental agencies have implemented legislation to increase awareness of the need for organ donation. In the United States, current law requires hospitals to report all deaths to the local OPO; the OPO staff can then determine the potential for organ donation and approach the family for consent. The criteria for donor acceptance are not all absolute, and some are controversial.

Donor Age

In response to the organ donor shortage, there has been a broadening in the age limits traditionally applied to organ donors. The use of kidneys from donors younger than 5 years of age is associated with an increased risk for surgical complications and impaired tolerance to episodes of graft dysfunction. Some programs have reported favorable results by transplanting both infant

Table 5.8.   Contraindications to cadaveric donation

Absolute

Chronic renal disease
Age > 70 yr
Potentially metastasizing
    malignancy
Severe hypertension
Bacterial sepsis
Current intravenous
    drug abuse
Hepatitis B surface
    antigen positive
Human immunodeficiency
    virus positive
Prolonged warm ischemia
Oliguric acute renal failure

Relative

Age > 60 yr
Age < 5 yr
Mild hypertension
Treated infection
Nonoliguric acute tubular necrosis
Positive hepatitis B and C serology
Donor medical disease (diabetes,
    systemic lupus erythematosus)
Intestinal perforation with
    spillage
Prolonged cold ischemia
High-risk behavior

kidneys with their attachment to the great vessels, so-called *pediatric en bloc* transplantation (see Chapter 7, Fig. 7.4). With advances in immunosuppression, the success of pediatric donor kidney transplantation has improved. If rejection can be avoided, the pediatric kidney will grow to nearly adult size within the first year.

There is a consistent trend to use organs from older donors, and as of 1999, about one third of all kidney donors were older than 50 years of age. Organs from donors in their 60s may be acceptable, although the long-term outcome of these kidneys may be significantly impaired, particularly if the cause of the donor's death was vascular rather than traumatic. Donor age and cause of death as a determinant of long-term graft function are discussed in Chapter 3. Older kidneys may be more susceptible to delayed graft function, particularly if the cold ischemia time is prolonged (see Chapter 8). A biopsy of the potential allograft can be performed to aid in the decision to transplant it. The degree of glomerular sclerosis is relatively easy to measure; some programs do not accept kidneys if more than 20% of glomeruli are sclerosed. The extent of interstitial fibrosis and atrophy and vascular changes may be more important than a numeric value for glomerulosclerosis (see Chapter 13). A borderline or "marginal" kidney (e.g., from a 62-year-old donor with mild hypertension and a cold ischemia time of 30 hours) may be regarded as acceptable for a patient with a high percentage of panel-reactive antibodies and failing dialysis access but unacceptable for a young patient in good medical condition without antibodies. The final decision to offer a kidney to a patient is made by a transplantation clinician equipped with information on the donor characteristics, the tissue match grade, and the recipient's clinical status.

Kidneys from donors who are male, nonblack, of intermediate age, with immediate postoperative function, and a good tissue match may be less susceptible to chronic allograft failure than kidneys from poorly matched, female, black donors who are older than 60 years of age or younger than 3 years of age with delayed initial function (see Chapter 9). The common factor explaining these findings may be the relative "nephron dose" that is transplanted (see Chapter 3). No systematic attempt is made to match the kidney size and nephron number to the size of the patient, and retrospective analysis suggests that such a policy would not necessarily be beneficial.

Contraindications to Donation

Contraindications to cadaveric transplantation are summarized in Table 5.8. Positive serology for the human immunodeficiency virus (HIV) is a contraindication to the use of a cadaver kidney. Concern regarding transmission of HIV and the possibility of a false-negative HIV test result is such that HIV-negative donors are excluded if they are deemed to be at high risk for HIV infection because of intravenous drug use or because of high-risk sexual behavior. The use of donors with serologic evidence of hepatitis B and C infection is discussed in Chapter 11.

Cancer can be transmitted by donor organs and, other than for some specific exceptions, is a contraindication to donation. Rare but well-documented cases of transplanted cancer have been described as a result of covert malignancy in the donor. Primary brain tumors are generally not regarded as a contraindication to transplantation because, in the absence of a systemic shunt, they rarely metastasize. Confirmation of histology is mandatory to ensure that the tumors are not metastases.

Ideally, donors have excellent graft function at the time of harvesting, but nonoliguric acute renal failure is common. In such cases, it is crucial to review the clinical circumstances carefully to determine whether the cause of acute renal failure is consistent with reversible renal failure, often called *acute tubular necrosis* (ATN). The kidney function of young donors with ATN typically recovers rapidly after transplantation, whereas with older donors, recovery may be delayed or incomplete. The combination of donor ATN and prolonged cold ischemia time may be particularly unfavorable, and it may be wise to discard such kidneys.

Non–Heart-Beating Cadaver Donors

To reduce the shortage of kidneys for transplantation, attempts have been made to use organs from non–heart-beating donors

(NHBDs). Before criteria for the declaration of brain death in 1968 (see later), all cadaveric organs were recovered from patients with cardiac arrest. Use of these organs decreased substantially, however, because of the fear of irreparable ischemic damage. Some trauma centers have developed protocols to minimize ischemia by rapid placement of intravenous cannulas to cool the organs after death by irreversible cardiac arrest has been declared. In these cases of "uncontrolled" NHBD, the option to donate has been preserved until the family can be informed of the death and then counseled by the organ procurement staff. If consent to donate is obtained, the organs must be recovered quickly to prevent further ischemic injury.

In reality, the practical obstacles to this process for most cases of unexpected cardiac arrest are overwhelming. Use of NHBDs has proved practical, however, in cases of brain-injured patients who are not expected to survive but in whom brain-death criteria are not met before hemodynamic deterioration. In these "controlled" NHBD circumstances, in which the decision to withdraw supportive care has been made by the family and primary medical team, consent can be obtained, and potentially well-functioning organs can be harvested. Ventilator support is discontinued, cardiac function is monitored, death is pronounced by standard cardiac criteria, and the patient is then quickly moved to the operating room for organ recovery. If NHBD protocols were maximized, it is estimated that the supply of cadaveric donor organs would increase by about 25%. Protocols for NHBDs must respect the feelings of donor families and avoid the appearance of conflicts of interest.

Diagnosis of Brain Death

Cadaveric solid organ transplantation requires that the organ to be transplanted is maintained in a state of good function until the moment of harvest. Somatic death and cardiac standstill tend to follow brain death by 2 to 3 days, and by this time, organ function is often irreversibly impaired. Societal acceptance and the legal and medical establishment of brain-death criteria are essential components of cadaveric transplantation (see Chapter 17); countries that do not have such criteria do not have well-developed cadaveric transplantation programs.

The diagnosis of brain death should be made by a physician who is independent of the transplantation team and thus free of conflict of interest. Clinically, the diagnosis requires irrefutable documentation of the irreversible absence of cerebral and brainstem function (Table 5.9). Electroencephalogram and isotope or dye angiography can be used to support the diagnosis, but they are not mandatory. After the diagnosis of brain death has been made in a potential donor, steps must be taken to maintain adequate circulatory and respiratory function until permission for donation is given. Harvesting should then be performed as expeditiously as possible.

Management of the Brain-Dead Donor

Maintenance of cardiovascular stability becomes more difficult the longer the period of brain death. At the time of diagnosis, patients are often relatively hypovolemic because of prior thera-

Table 5.9.   Clinical criteria for diagnosis of brain death

Irreversibility
    No sedating, paralyzing, or toxic drugs
    No gross electrolyte or endocrine disturbances
    No profound hypothermia
Absent cerebral function
    No seizures or posturing
    No response to pain in cranial nerve distribution[a]
Absent brain-stem function
    Apnea in response to acidosis or hypercarbia
    No pupillary or corneal reflexes
    No oculocephalic or vestibular reflexes
    No tracheobronchial reflex

[a] Spinal reflexes may be present.

peutic attempts to minimize brain swelling by inducing dehydration. A diabetes insipidus–like state may accompany head injuries and brain death, resulting in obligatory urine outputs of up to 1 L/hour. Brain death is associated with a massive release of cytokines, a so-called *cytokine storm,* which has the potential to injure the donated kidney and make it more susceptible to ischemic and immunologic injury (see Chapter 8).

Blood pressure should be maintained at greater than 100 mm Hg by aggressive administration of crystalloids, colloids, or blood products. Central venous pressure should be monitored and maintained at greater than 10 mm Hg. If urine output decreases to less than about 40 mL/hour in a well-hydrated donor, furosemide or mannitol may be given. Insulin administration may be necessary to minimize hyperglycemia and glycosuria. If, despite good hydration, blood pressure remains low, low-dose dopamine and other inotropic agents, such as dobutamine or norepinephrine, are sometimes required. If a hypotonic diuresis ensues, suggesting a diagnosis of diabetes insipidus, a hypotonic infusion should be used to replace the urine output. Dextrose infusion, which may induce an additional osmotic diuresis, should be avoided; a vasopressin infusion may be required if the hypotonic urine volume is massive (more than 500 mL/hour).

Technique of Cadaveric Organ Harvesting

The principles of the harvesting operation are similar regardless of the organs to be removed. Wide surgical exposure is obtained. Each organ to be removed is dissected with its vasculature intact. There is no dissection into the renal hila, in order to avoid damage to the vasculature and to prevent delayed graft function caused by vasospasm. Cannulas are placed for *in situ* cooling. At the time of aortic cross-clamping, flush and surface cooling is begun. The organs are removed in an orderly fashion. The kidneys are removed *en bloc* with the aorta and vena cava (Fig. 5.3). If multiple organs are to be removed, the preferred sequence is heart or lung first, liver or pancreas second, and kidneys last. The kidneys are pro-

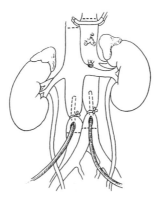

Fig. 5.3. *En bloc* **dissection for cadaveric kidney donation with cannulas in place for in situ perfusion. Perihilar and periureteral fat are left in place.**

tected against ischemia by the cold flush and surface cooling during the 10 to 15 minutes that it takes to remove the other organs.

One variation of this approach is a rapid infusion technique whereby cannulas are placed immediately, the aorta cross-clamped, and the dissection is completed under cold infusion. This technique is used primarily when the donor is hemodynamically unstable.

Kidneys Alone

Fewer than 5% of all organ donations are for kidneys only. In these circumstances, either a long midline incision from pubic notch to sternal notch can be used, splitting the sternum, or a cruciate midline incision can be made. The right colon and duodenum are mobilized, exposing the great vessels. The aortic bifurcation is isolated. The inferior mesenteric artery and vein are ligated. The aorta is controlled above the take-off of the celiac trunk. Exposure can be achieved either by mass ligation of the porta hepatis to expose the superior mesenteric and celiac arteries or by mobilization of the left lateral segment of the liver, splitting the diaphragmatic crus, controlling the aorta, and mass-clamping the superior mesenteric and celiac arteries. The supraceliac aorta can also be controlled in the left chest behind the heart before the thoracic aorta enters the abdomen. The ureters are divided deep in the pelvis, maintaining a long segment and leaving all periureteral tissue. The aorta is cannulated at the bifurcation of the iliac arteries, and the proximal aorta is cross-clamped. An ice flush solution is begun. The kidneys are then widely mobilized, leaving Gerota's capsule intact, and removed *en bloc* with the abdominal aorta and vena cava.

If the heart and kidneys are being donated, the procurement is similar, except that the heart team mobilizes the heart before cross-clamping the aorta, and the heart is removed first. The kidneys are separated in slush on a back table. The left renal vein is taken off the cava with a small cuff of vena cava. The remainder of the vena cava is left with the right kidney. The aorta is divided longitudinally, leaving the renal arteries attached to cuffs of aorta on each side.

Kidneys With Other Abdominal Organs

If the liver and pancreas are removed, their removal precedes kidney removal. The lower border of their dissection is the vena cava, just above the insertion of the renal veins, and the aorta, at or just below the take-off of the superior mesenteric artery. After their removal, the abdominal landmarks are usually obscured. *En bloc* kidney removal as described in the previous section on kidneys alone is carried out by dissecting widely around the kidneys to avoid damage to the important hilar structures.

Pharmacologic Adjuncts

Most cadaver donors are given large doses of corticosteroids to deplete circulating donor lymphocytes. Mannitol in doses of up to 1 g/kg is also given to ensure diuresis and possibly to minimize ischemic injury. There is some evidence that alpha-blockers or calcium-channel blockers given intravenously before kidney manipulation may lower the rate of delayed graft function. Phentolamine (Regitine), 10 to 15 mg, may be used just before cross-clamping of the aorta; earlier use would cause significant hypotension. Systemic heparinization is carried out at the time of cannula placement with doses of 10,000 to 30,000 units.

Ischemia Times

Warm ischemia time refers to the period between circulatory arrest and commencement of cold storage. With modern *in situ* perfusion techniques, the warm ischemia time is essentially zero, although there is warm ischemia if hemodynamic deterioration or cardiac arrest occurs before harvest. A kidney may function after up to 20 minutes of warm ischemia, but rates of delayed function and nonfunction increase markedly thereafter.

Cold ischemia time refers to the period of cold storage or machine perfusion (see later section on cold storage versus machine perfusion). *Rewarm time* is the period from removal of the kidney from cold storage or perfusion to completion of the renal arterial anastomosis. Rewarm time can be minimized by cooling the kidney during surgery (see Chapter 7).

Cadaveric Kidney Preservation

Cold Storage Versus Machine Perfusion

Harvested kidneys must be stored for a period of time before transplantation, either by cold storage on ice or by machine perfusion. For cold storage, the kidneys are flushed and separated and then placed on ice in sterile containers for transport. For machine perfusion, they are flushed and separated and then placed on specially designed perfusion machines that pump a cold colloid solution continuously through the renal artery until the time of transplantation. Machine perfusion may allow a longer preservation time. Rates of delayed graft function of about 25% are obtained with simple static cold storage with cold ischemia times of up to 30 hours. After 30 hours, the rate of delayed graft func-

Table 5.10.   Comparison of contents of flush solutions for kidney preservation

University of Wisconsin Solution	Collins Solution
Modified hydroxyethyl starch	Potassium phosphate
Lactobionic acid	Potassium chloride
Potassium phosphate	Sodium bicarbonate
Magnesium sulfate	Glucose
Raffinose	Magnesium sulfate
Adenosine	
Allopurinol	
Glutathione	

tion increases significantly. Most centers prefer not to use kidneys that have been in cold storage for longer than 48 hours. Delayed graft function rates of about 25% are obtainable with up to 48 hours of machine perfusion. Machine preservation is expensive and complex, and most transplantation centers prefer simple static cold preservation, attempting to keep cold ischemia times under 30 hours.

Collins Solution Versus University of Wisconsin Solution

For many years, kidneys have been flushed with modifications of a solution called *Collins solution* during harvesting to achieve rapid cooling and blood wash-out. This solution is high in potassium, is hyperosmolar, and has an intracellular-like composition to stabilize cell membranes and prevent cell swelling.

The University of Wisconsin (UW) solution for flushing cadaveric organs is clearly superior to Collins solution for liver and pancreas preservation. It may also be preferable for kidneys with prolonged preservation times. UW solution contains a number of components, and the importance of each has not been fully resolved (Table 5.10). Glutathione may serve to facilitate the regeneration of cellular adenosine triphosphate (ATP) and maintain membrane integrity, and adenosine may provide the substrate for regeneration of ATP during reperfusion. The introduction of UW solution has had a major effect on nonrenal solid organ transplantation by allowing much longer cold ischemia times.

SELECTED READINGS

Beasley CL. Maximizing donation. *Transplant Rev* 1999;13:31.

Gaston RS, Hudson S, Julian BA, et al. Impact of donor/recipient size matching on outcomes in renal transplantation. *Transplantation* 1996;61:383.

Gonwa TA, Atkins C, Zhang YA, et al. Glomerular filtration rates in persons evaluated as living-related donors: are our standards too high? *Transplantation* 1993;55:983.

Kasiske BL, Bia MJ. The evaluation and selection of living kidney donors. *Am J Kidney Dis* 1995;26:387.

Kavoussi L. Laparoscopic donor nephrectomy. *Kidney Int* 2000;57:2175.

Lu CY. Management of the cadaveric donor of a renal transplant: more than optimizing renal perfusion. *Kidney Int* 1999;56:756.

Matas AJ, Gillingham K, Payne WD, et al. Should I accept this kidney? *Clin Transplantation* 2000;14:90.

Nogueira JM, Cangro CB, Fink JC, et al. A comparison of recipient renal outcomes with laparoscopic versus open live donor nephrectomy. *Transplantation* 1999;67:722.

Peters TG, Shaver TR, Ames JE, et al. Cold ischemia and outcome in 17,937 cadaveric kidney transplants. *Transplantation* 1995; 59:191.

Potts JT. Non-heart-beating organ transplantation: medical and ethical issues in procurement. Washington, DC: National Academy Press, 1998.

Pratschke J, Wilhelm MJ, Kusaka M, et al. Brain death and its influence on donor organ quality and outcome after transplantation. *Transplantation* 1999;67:343.

Randhawa PS, Minervini MI, Lombardeno M, et al. Biopsy of marginal donor kidneys: Correlation of histologic findings with graft dysfunction. *Transplantation* 2000;69:1352.

Rosenthal JT. Expanded criteria for cadaver organ donation in renal transplantation. *Urol Clin North Am* 1994;21:283.

Siminoff LA, Arnold RM, Caplan AL, et al. Public policy governing organ and tissue procurement in the United States. *Ann Intern Med* 1995;123:10.

Terasaki PI, Cecka JM, Gjertson DW, et al. High survival rates of kidney transplants from spousal and living unrelated donors. *N Engl J Med* 1995;333:333.

Veller MG, Botha JR, Britz RS, et al. Renal allograft preservation: a comparison of University of Wisconsin solution and of hypothermic continuous pulsatile perfusion. *Clin Transplant* 1994;8:97.

Evaluation of the Transplant Recipient

Elizabeth Kendrick

The potential kidney transplant recipient must be evaluated by the transplantation team to determine whether he or she is a suitable candidate. The patient must also make a personal evaluation of the transplantation option, and the transplantation team must see to it that this evaluation is an educated one. The excellent statistics achieved by most transplantation centers for graft survival and morbidity have changed the attitude of both physicians and patients regarding the appropriateness of transplantation. Whereas transplantation was once reserved for "ideal" candidates who were either particularly brave or particularly desperate, nearly all patients with end-stage renal disease (ESRD) can now be regarded as potentially acceptable candidates for transplantation. Instead of denying the option to broad groups of patients, such as the elderly or those with diabetes mellitus and coronary artery disease, each person's candidacy should be evaluated individually. As part of the evaluation, factors that need to be corrected before the transplantation takes place need to be identified.

Clinical practice guidelines for the evaluation of renal transplantation candidates have been developed by the Patient Care and Education Committee of the American Society of Transplantation. These guidelines provide a detailed algorithmic approach to the process of transplantation evaluation (Kasiske et al., 1995).

CONTRAINDICATIONS TO KIDNEY TRANSPLANTATION

Malignancy

There are two major reasons for excluding patients with malignant disease. The first is that immunosuppressive drugs may unfavorably influence the natural history of the malignancy. The second is that it is not reasonable for someone whose life expectancy is significantly curtailed by the presence of malignant disease to undergo transplantation. Much of the data on which transplantation recommendations have been made have come from the Cincinnati Transplant Tumor Registry, an international registry for malignancy in solid organ transplant recipients. Most centers require at least a 2-year disease-free interval after the treatment of a malignant tumor, although a 5-year waiting period would exclude most patients who would develop recurrence. The precise waiting period, however, should be determined by the nature of the tumor; oncologic consultation may be wise. Guidelines for waiting periods for commonly encountered tumors in potential transplant recipients are shown in Table 6.1.

Chronic Infection

The presence of chronic infection precludes transplantation and the use of immunosuppressive therapy. Osteomyelitis should be

Table 6.1. Guidelines for recommending tumor-free waiting periods for common pretransplantation malignancies

Site	Waiting Period
Renal	
Incidental, asymptomatic	None
Large, infiltrating	At least 2 yr
Wilms' tumor	At least 2 yr
Bladder	
In situ	None
Invasive	At least 2 yr
Uterus	
In situ cervical	None[a]
Invasive cervical	5 yr
Uterine body	At least 2 yr
Testis	At least 2 yr
Thyroid	At least 2 yr
Breast	At least 5 yr[b]
Colorectum	At least 2 yr[b]
Prostate	At least 2 yr
Lymphoma	At least 2 yr
Skin	
Melanoma	At least 5 yr[b]
Squamous cell	2 yr
Basal cell	None

[a] Routine cytologic screening required.
[b] In situ lesions may not require a waiting period.

treated, and, if necessary, the infected part should be removed surgically to prepare the patient for transplantation. Diabetic foot ulcers must be healed before transplantation. Tuberculosis requires a full course of therapy and preferably 1 year of subsequent observation for relapse. Infection with the human immunodeficiency virus (HIV) has been considered an absolute contraindication to kidney transplantation, but with improvement of survival of HIV-infected patients with newer antiretroviral therapy, this approach is being reconsidered in some centers. Patients with a low viral load and a normal CD4 count who are able to adhere to their antiviral regimen therapy may be considered candidates for transplantation. Recurrent urinary tract infection and peritonitis are discussed in the section on urologic evaluation and candidates on peritoneal dialysis.

Severe Extrarenal Disease

Most patients who have evidence of extrarenal disease are acceptable transplantation candidates. In certain circumstances, however, extrarenal disease may preclude transplantation either because the patient is not an operative candidate or because the transplant and associated immunosuppression may accelerate disease progression. Chronic liver disease and advanced uncorrectable heart disease are contraindications to kidney transplantation alone, although these patients may benefit from combined organ transplantation. Chronic lung disease may preclude safe general anesthesia. Severe peripheral vascular disease may make arterial anastomosis technically difficult or endanger limb viability.

Noncompliance
Any patient with a history of repeated noncompliance with previous medical therapy should be considered at extremely high risk for graft loss. It is wise to demand a period of acceptable compliance as a condition for being placed on the waiting list. Assessment of compliance is discussed in Chapters 16 and 19.

Psychiatric Illness
Organic mental syndromes, psychosis, and mental retardation of a degree that seriously impairs the patient's capacity to understand the transplantation procedure and its complications may be contraindications to transplantation. Patients with significant mental retardation who have excellent social support and a long life expectancy appear to do well after transplantation. Any patient addicted to alcohol or any other drug should enter and successfully complete a rehabilitation program before being offered a transplant (see Chapter 16).

RECIPIENT EVALUATION
General Medical Evaluation
All patients referred to a transplantation center should provide details of their medical history at the time of the initial evaluation. Particular emphasis should be placed on preexisting cardiovascular disease. Every effort should be made to determine the cause of the underlying renal disease, because of its potential relevance to the posttransplantation course. If a native kidney biopsy has been performed, the report should be available. Many patients present with a diagnosis of *ESRD of uncertain etiology,* and if a precise diagnosis cannot be made, at the very least an ultrasound should confirm that the kidneys are small and echogenic. Such a diagnosis in young patients should elicit suspicion for underlying urologic abnormalities. The family history is very important because it may provide information regarding the nature of the kidney disease and also allows the physician to introduce a discussion about potential living-related donors.

The physical examination must be equally thorough. The presence of femoral bruits may be a clue to the presence of iliac atherosclerosis, and poor peripheral pulses and a history of claudication warrant an evaluation for potentially correctable peripheral vascular disease. Care should be taken to document the presence of dental disease. Colonoscopy should be performed in patients older than 50 years of age and in those with guiaic-positive stool tests. In men, the prostate must be palpated, and the prostate-specific antigen level should be routinely checked in men older than 40 years of age. Many patients are oliguric or anuric and may not be aware of prostatic hypertrophy. All women should have a Papanicolaou smear and pelvic examination, and women older than 40 years of age should have a mammogram. If a recent renal ultrasound is not available, one should be done to assess for evidence of renal cancer in acquired cystic disease. A careful infectious disease history should be done, including assessment of possible endemic exposure, and appropriate studies should be done as well as serologies for specific chronic or latent infections to assess risk for reactivation with immunosuppressive therapy. A screening tuberculin skin test (PPD) should be done as well as a screening chest radiograph to assess for evidence of prior tuberculosis exposure or infection.

Patients with a positive skin test or an abnormal chest radiograph should be assessed for the need for preventative therapy with isoniazid. Patients who are anergic to tuberculin and control antigens and who have risk factors for tuberculosis infection, such as history of residence or travel to endemic areas, prior exposure, or prior treatment, should also be assessed for the need for preventative therapy. Suggested laboratory and radiologic tests are listed in Table 6.2. Diabetic patients, patients older than 50 years of age, and patients with multiple risk factors for coronary artery disease should undergo exercise stress testing. Cardiac catheterization should be done depending on the results. Some centers advocate routinely performing cardiac catheterization in all patients with insulin-dependent diabetes mellitus even in the absence of angina, electrocardiograph changes, or evidence of prior myocardial infarction. Figure 14.1 in Chapter 14 provides an algorithmic approach to the evaluation of coronary artery dis-

Table 6.2. Routine and elective pretransplantation evaluations

Routine	Elective
Full history and physical exam	Voiding cystourethrogram
Complete blood count and chemistry panel	Exercise treadmill
Prothrombin time and partial thromboplastin time	Echocardiogram
Blood type	Coronary angiogram
HBsAg, HBsAB, HepCAb, VDRL, HIV, HSV, and CMV titers	Mammogram
Pelvic exam and Papanicolaou smear	Noninvasive vascular studies
Chest radiograph	Right upper quadrant ultrasound
Electrocardiogram	Upper gastrointestinal series and upper endoscopy
Tissue typing and cytotoxic antibodies	Barium enema and lower endoscopy, prostate-specific antigen test
	Immunoelectrophoresis
	EBV, VZV, HSV, toxoplasmosis titers
	Lipid profile
	PPD

CMV, cytomegalovirus; EBV, Epstein-Barr virus; HIV, human immunodeficiency virus; HSV, herpes simplex virus; PPD, purified protein derivative (tuberculin); VZV, varicella-zoster virus.

ease in diabetic patients but is also relevant to nondiabetic high-risk patients. Cigarette smokers should be encouraged to break the habit and offered professional help to do so. Some centers will not perform transplantation in patients who continue to smoke in the presence of high vascular risk.

Urologic Evaluation

Ideally, the lower urinary tract should be sterile, continent, and compliant before transplantation. Urinalysis and urine culture should be performed in all urinating patients, and some programs obtain bladder washings from anuric patients. A voiding cystourethrogram should be performed in patients in whom a voiding or genitourinary abnormality is suspected.

Graft implantation into the native bladder is always preferred. Diverted urinary tracts should be undiverted when possible to make the lower urinary tract functional before transplantation. Even a very small bladder may develop normal compliance and capacity after transplantation. Transplantation is possible in patients whose urinary tracts have been diverted into ileal conduits and cannot be undiverted. The rate of urologic complications is high, but the overall patient and graft survival is not different from that of patients with intact urinary tracts.

Indications for pretransplantation native nephrectomy are listed in Table 6.3. If nephrectomy is performed, it should be done at least 6 weeks to 3 months before transplantation.

Older men frequently have prostatic enlargement and may develop outflow tract obstruction after transplantation. In general, if patients are still passing sufficient volumes of urine, the prostate should be resected preoperatively. Otherwise, the operation should be postponed until after the transplantation has been successfully performed. These patients may require an indwelling bladder catheter or be prepared to self-catheterize, until the prostate has been resected.

Patient Education

At the time of the evaluation, the physician or transplantation nurse coordinator should inform the patient of the risks of the operation and of the side effects and risks associated with immunosuppression. The surgical procedure and its complications should

Table 6.3.   Indications for pretransplantation native nephrectomy

Chronic renal parenchymal infection
Infected stones
Heavy proteinuria
Intractable hypertension
Polycystic kidney disease[a]
Acquired renal cystic disease[b]
Infected reflux[c]

[a] Only when the kidneys are massive, recurrently infected, or bleeding.
[b] When there is suspicion of adenocarcinoma.
[c] Uninfected reflux does not require nephrectomy.

be discussed in lay terms. The nature of rejection should be explained and mention made of the increased risk for infection and posttransplantation malignancy and the occasional mortality from these complications. Patients need to understand that immunosuppressive therapy must be continued for as long as the graft survives. The benefits of live donor transplantation and cadaveric transplantation should be compared and contrasted (see Chapter 5). Graft survival and morbidity statistics should be shared with the patient (see Chapters 1 and 3).

Patients should be warned that even successful transplantations do not last forever and that they may, at some point, require a return to dialysis or repeat transplantation. The importance of compliance with dialysis and dietary prescriptions while waiting for a transplant should be emphasized. The possibility of posttransplantation pregnancy should be discussed with women of childbearing age (see Chapter 9).

Special Features Related to the Primary Kidney Disease

The effects of recurrent renal disease on the posttransplantation course are discussed in Chapter 9. The following section considers the aspects of the primary kidney disease that are relevant to the pretransplantation work-up.

Diabetes Mellitus

Diabetic nephropathy accounts for about 40% of cases of ESRD in the United States. The evaluation of patients with type 1 diabetes for both kidney alone and simultaneous pancreas–kidney transplantation is discussed in Chapter 14. Potential candidates for combined pancreas–kidney transplantation must be thoroughly educated about the additional risks and benefits of the double-organ procedure. Patients with type 2 diabetes are generally not offered this procedure. The differentiation between the two types can usually be made with confidence from the history of onset, necessity for insulin, and use of oral hypoglycemic agents. The C-peptide level can be measured for confirmation. Both coronary artery and peripheral vascular disease are frequently present in these patients and must be rigorously assessed.

Systemic Lupus Erythematosus

Clinically active systemic lupus erythematosus (SLE) typically improves with development of renal failure but may not do so in some patients, particularly black women. Patients with clinically active disease are generally not candidates for transplantation. Patients should be taking doses of less than 10 mg of prednisone before transplantation. Evidence of serologic activity in the absence of clinical activity does not contraindicate transplantation. Some studies have shown poorer graft survival in patients with SLE than in matched controls, whereas others have shown equivalent survival rates. Graft loss due to acute and chronic rejection appears to account for the differential survival rather than recurrent disease, which is uncommon. Superior outcome of living-related over cadaveric grafts has been suggested. SLE patients who have been heavily immunosuppressed during the course of their illness may be at increased risk for posttransplantation opportunistic infection or lymphoma.

Thrombophilic Disorders

Antiphospholipid antibodies, as detected by inhibition of phospholipid-dependent blood coagulation (prolonged partial thromboplastin time), false-positive VDRL, or as anticardiolipin antibodies, have been found in up to half of SLE patients and may be associated with antiphospholipid antibody syndrome. There may also be a history of recurrent spontaneous abortion and thrombotic events. These patients are at higher risk for allograft loss as well as other thrombotic complications compared with controls, whether or not there is a history of prior thrombotic episodes. Careful questioning of patients for these events, as well as screening for antiphospholipid antibodies, is warranted.

Antiphospholipid antibodies have been reported in up to 28% of non-SLE ESRD patients, who are also at increased risk for thrombotic complications. Patients with other coagulation abnormalities, such as antithrombin III, protein S, and protein C deficiency, as well as the factor V Leiden mutation, may be at risk, as may patients with very high levels of homocysteine. Pretransplantation screening of patients for a history of recurrent thrombotic episodes is warranted. Prophylactic postoperative anticoagulation should be considered, although controlled studies are lacking.

Focal Glomerulosclerosis

Primary focal glomerulosclerosis differs from other potentially recurrent nephropathies in that it may recur rapidly and aggressively after transplantation, presumably as the result of an unidentified serum factor that affects the permselectivity of the glomerular basement membrane (GBM). About 25% of patients develop recurrence, usually within days or weeks of transplantation. Recurrence is more common in younger patients, in patients whose initial presentation was florid, and in patients whose initial biopsy also showed mesangial hypertrophy (see Chapter 15). Patients should be forewarned of the possibility of recurrence, the chances of which are high in a second transplant if the first was affected. The specter of recurrence may make a cadaveric transplant the preferred donor source, particularly if the first transplant was affected. There may be some benefit to plasma exchange before transplantation to reduce the risk for recurrent disease; posttransplantation management is discussed in Chapter 15.

Goodpasture's Syndrome

When the primary disease is the result of antibodies directed against the GBM, transplantation should be deferred until the patient is clinically stable and anti-GBM antibody levels are undetectable. If these guidelines are followed, this group of patients does well after transplantation, and recurrence is rare. Pretransplantation native nephrectomy was once recommended for these patients but is no longer regarded as necessary.

Alport's Syndrome

Patients with Alport's syndrome have a hereditary abnormality of the GBM that lacks the Goodpasture antigen. When exposed for the first time to a normal basement membrane in the allograft, they may develop *de novo* anti-GBM antibody disease, with a crescentic glomerulonephritis characterized by linear immunofluorescence staining of the GBM. Aggressive treatment has been tried with protocols similar to those used for primary anti-GBM disease, including plasmapheresis. The outcome is poor. The incidence of this catastrophic complication is probably less than 10%. Most patients with Alport's syndrome who do not develop this complication do well after transplantation. The presence of inherited kidney disease mandates intensive family screening before consideration of living-related donation.

Amyloidosis

Patients with amyloidosis have a higher-than-average mortality rate after transplantation. The rate may be as high as 45% at 1 year and depends on the extent to which amyloid has been deposited in the heart, liver, spleen, and gastrointestinal (GI) tract. Infectious and cardiac complications are common. Some patients without severe extrarenal disease may be considered acceptable candidates, particularly if the amyloidosis is due to chronic inflammation. An echocardiogram should be performed to assess the extent of myocardial infiltration. The subgroup of patients with amyloidosis complicating familial Mediterranean fever may not tolerate cyclosporine therapy as a consequence of systemic and GI symptoms. Patients with primary amyloidosis, a manifestation of a plasma cell dyscrasia, have a poor prognosis no matter what form of therapy is used.

Paraproteinemia

In patients older than 60 years of age and in those with ESRD of uncertain etiology, the pretransplantation evaluation should include plasma immunoelectrophoresis to screen for the presence of a paraprotein. When a benign monoclonal gammopathy is identified, serial evaluations should be performed during the next 12 months to exclude the development of myeloma or macroglobulinemia. If the patient is free of myeloma or macroglobulinemia after the 12 months, it is probably safe to progress with transplantation, although surveillance should continue. Immunosuppression may increase the risk for progression of benign monoclonal gammopathy to myeloma. There are reports of successful transplantation in patients whose original kidney disease was due to myeloma, light-chain disease, or macroglobulinemia. These patients may be at particular risk for infection in the posttransplantation period and for other causes of renal impairment, such as dehydration, nephrotoxicity, hypercalcemia, and hyperuricemia. Some programs regard frank paraproteinemia as a contraindication to transplantation. At the least, patients should be apprised of their high-risk status, and they may elect to remain on dialysis.

Polycystic Kidney Disease

The transplant prognosis of patients with polycystic kidney disease is not different from that of other "low-risk" groups. Occasionally, the polycystic kidneys are so large that a pretransplantation nephrectomy must be performed to create a space for the allograft. Recurrent infection or hemorrhage may be an indication for pretransplantation nephrectomy. There may be an increased risk for GI complications after transplantation, usually related to diverticular disease. Patients with headaches or other central nervous system symptoms or with a family history of aneurysms in affected relatives should undergo noninvasive screening for intracranial aneurysms. The possibility of living-related donation in families afflicted with polycystic kidney disease is discussed in Chapter 5.

Fabry's Disease

Some programs exclude patients with Fabry's disease from transplantation, although it is best to consider patients on an individual basis. Early hopes that the underlying defect in glycosphingolipid metabolism would be reversed by transplanting the missing enzyme have not been fulfilled. Infection, poor wound healing, and progression of the disease contribute to a high mortality rate.

Scleroderma

There is little documented experience of transplantation outcome in patients with scleroderma. As in patients with amyloidosis and Fabry's disease, the extent of generalized systemic involvement must be assessed in each patient. Wound healing is not usually impaired, and extrarenal complications may improve after transplantation. Cyclosporine is being investigated as a therapeutic agent for the treatment of scleroderma. Tight control of blood pressure is required, and the early use of angiotensin-converting enzyme inhibitors may be indicated.

Hyperoxaluria

Primary hyperoxaluria type 1 is an inborn error of metabolism with an autosomal recessive inheritance. The underlying defect is a deficiency of the peroxisomal enzyme alanine glyoxylate aminotransferase, which is found primarily in the liver. Deposition of oxalate leads to ESRD, and, after transplantation, rapid deposition of oxalate in the allograft leads to graft failure. Failure of the graft usually occurs despite intensive therapy with perioperative plasma exchange, intensive dialysis, high-dose pyridoxine, and oral phosphates, which are designed to minimize oxalate deposition. Bilateral native nephrectomy, by decreasing total-body oxalate load, may reduce oxalate deposition in the renal allograft. A more rational approach may be to consider combined liver–kidney transplantation for the management of these patients (Table 6.4). The new liver provides the missing enzyme.

Secondary hyperoxaluria is most commonly of intestinal origin and may also lead to recurrence in the allograft. If the underlying defect is reversible (e.g., intestinal bypass for obesity), consideration should be given to surgical reversal before transplantation.

Thrombotic Thrombocytopenic Purpura

The rate of recurrence of thrombotic thrombocytopenic purpura (TTP) or hemolytic-uremic syndrome after transplantation is variable. Most patients with the so-called 'non-diarrheal' form of TTP will suffer recurrence (see Chapter 15), and patients in whom the condition recurs usually lose their grafts. Both cyclosporine and tacrolimus may produce a glomerular capillary thrombotic lesion similar to that of TTP (see Chapter 4); and it is probable that their use increases the rate of recurrence. There is evidence to suggest that the risk for relapse is greater when the graft comes from a

**Table 6.4. Indications for combined
kidney and liver transplantation**

OLT candidate with severe[a] irreversible renal dysfunction due to:
1. Polycystic kidneys with massive hepatomegaly
2. Glomerulonephritis (typically IgA nephropathy)
3. Failing kidney transplant with end-stage liver disease
   (typically HCV or HBV related)
4. Repeat OLT with cyclosporine nephrotoxicity
5. Oxalosis
6. Prolonged pre-OLT dialysis dependence[b]
7. Diabetic nephropathy

OLT, orthotopic liver transplantation; HBV, hepatitis B virus; HCV, hepatitis
C virus.
[a] "Severe" indicates that the patient is or would become dialysis dependent after
transplantation.
[b] Hepatorenal syndrome may become irreversible after weeks of dialysis
dependence.

living-related donor; and some programs avoid lung donation
when the rise of recurrence is judged to be high. Removal of the
native kidneys may reduce the recurrence rate.

Systemic Vasculitis and Wegener's Granulomatosis

Systemic symptoms of vasculitis should be quiescent before transplantation. Pretransplantation antineutrophil cytoplasmic antibody (ANCA) levels appear to have no predictive value for recurrence in patients without symptoms, and positive values do not
preclude transplantation. The rate of relapse of vasculitis after
transplantation can be substantial, but relapses usually respond to
treatment with cyclophosphamide and high-dose prednisolone.
Patient and graft survival rates are comparable to those of patients
with other causes of ESRD. Close monitoring of hematuria, early
renal biopsy, and possibly monitoring of ANCA titers is warranted
to detect recurrent disease.

Sickle Cell Disease

Sickle cell anemia and sickle cell disease produce a variety of
renal abnormalities that may occasionally cause ESRD. The
transplantation experience with these patients has been a mixed
one. There is an increased incidence of severe and potentially
lethal sickling crises after transplantation, presumably related to
the improving hematocrit. Exchange transfusions may be effective treatment. Some programs regard sickle cell anemia as a contraindication to kidney transplantation. A trend toward improved
survival of patients who undergo transplantation compared with
those continuing dialysis treatment has been reported, but long-
term graft outcome appeared to be diminished.

Risk Factors Related to Organ System Diseases

Cardiovascular Disease

Cardiovascular disease is the leading cause of death in the years
after kidney transplantation. Diabetic patients frequently suffer

from covert coronary artery disease and should be specifically evaluated with this in mind (see Chapter 14). Older patients and patients with multiple risk factors for coronary artery disease should undergo stress testing and, when indicated, coronary angiography. Prior angioplasty or coronary artery bypass grafting is not a contraindication to transplantation so long as the patient has a current nonischemic treadmill test and adequate myocardial function.

Symptoms and signs of peripheral and cerebrovascular disease should be elicited, evaluated, and, if indicated, corrected before transplantation. Patients who have suffered a cerebrovascular accident with significant fixed neurologic deficit may be poor transplantation candidates in terms of both their perioperative risk status and the rehabilitative potential of the transplantation. Patients who have required intraabdominal reconstructive arterial surgery represent a formidable surgical challenge, and transplantation may be contraindicated.

Some dialysis patients manifest symptomatic heart failure of nonischemic origin. The term *uremic cardiomyopathy* has been applied to this condition, and cardiac function may improve markedly after transplantation. Symptomatic heart failure of nonischemic origin is not an absolute contraindication to kidney transplantation.

Gastrointestinal Disease

A number of GI diseases can be a source of significant posttransplantation morbidity.

PEPTIC ULCER DISEASE.   Before the introduction of effective therapy in the form of histamine antagonists, posttransplantation upper GI bleeding was a common and feared complication, and all patients underwent pretransplantation upper GI evaluation. This precaution may now be reserved for patients with symptoms or a history of peptic ulcer disease. Active peptic ulcer disease is a contraindication to transplantation, and if the disease persists despite medical therapy, surgical intervention may be indicated.

PANCREATITIS.   A pretransplantation history of pancreatitis increases the risk for posttransplantation pancreatitis. Both prednisone and azathioprine have been implicated in the etiology of pancreatitis. Hyperparathyroidism should be excluded as a possible factor. Other possible contributing factors, such as lipid disturbances, cholelithiasis, and alcohol abuse, should be addressed before transplantation.

CHOLELITHIASIS.   Patients with a history of cholecystitis should undergo pretransplantation cholecystectomy. Patients with asymptomatic cholelithiasis do not necessarily need to undergo cholecystectomy. Some programs recommend cholecystectomy for diabetic patients with asymptomatic cholelithiasis because posttransplantation cholecystitis may be difficult to diagnose, and posttransplantation operative intervention may be complicated. Some transplantation programs routinely perform right upper quadrant ultrasonography to exclude cholelithiasis.

Liver Disease

Hepatic cirrhosis and clinically active hepatitis and chronic liver disease are contraindications to kidney transplantation; these dis-

eases may progress to end-stage liver disease after transplantation, usually as a consequence of immunosuppression. Patients with
advanced or end-stage kidney and liver disease may become candidates for combined liver–kidney transplantation (Table 6.4). The
decision to transplant patients with serologic evidence of prior
hepatitis B or C infection who are clinically quiescent is discussed
in Chapter 11.

Metabolic Bone Disease

Renal osteodystrophy is discussed in Chapter 1. Every attempt
should be made to minimize the effects of impaired vitamin D
metabolism, metabolic acidosis, and secondary hyperparathyroidism in the pretransplantation period. Patients with persistent hyperparathyroidism unresponsive to medical therapy may
need to undergo pretransplantation parathyroidectomy to prevent the development of severe posttransplantation hypercalcemia (see Chapter 9). Subsets of patients, particularly female
and diabetic patients, are at an exaggerated risk for osteopenia
and pathologic fractures. These patients may benefit from early
diagnosis of bone loss and therapy directed at prevention of bone
disease.

Seizure Disorders

The major antiepileptic agents all increase the rate of metabolism
of cyclosporine and tacrolimus. When patients who are being
treated for a seizure disorder are referred for transplantation,
note should be made of the anticonvulsant regimen, and a neurologic consultation should be obtained to determine which, if any,
of the anticonvulsants are mandatory. If patients need to continue anticonvulsant therapy, the immunosuppressive protocol
may need to be adjusted to take this into account (see Chapter 4).

Chronic Pulmonary Disease

Perioperative risks associated with severe lung disease include
ventilator dependency and infection. Patients with suppurative
bronchiectasis or chronic fungal disease are not candidates for
kidney transplantation. Pulmonary function testing may help
determine suitability for transplantation. Patients with evidence
of chronic lung disease who continue to smoke must stop before
transplantation; smoking cessation programs may be helpful.

Risk Factors Related to Individual Patient Characteristics

Age

Both very young and older patients are at increased risk for graft
loss and morbidity, although most centers no longer have an arbitrary upper age at which patients are no longer accepted for transplantation. Several studies have reported that patients between
the ages of 55 and 65 years are not at a significantly increased risk
for posttransplantation morbidity so long as they do not suffer from
significant vascular disease and their general medical evaluation
is unremarkable. It is wise to exclude covert coronary artery disease with stress testing before transplantation in older patients.
Experience with transplant recipients in their late 60s and 70s
is limited. Each case should be examined on its merits; patients
should not be arbitrarily excluded from transplantation because

of their age. Older patients, however, must have realistic expectations about the improvement in their quality of life after transplantation—the transplant will not make them younger! Their condition may also deteriorate in the years they may be required to wait for a cadaveric organ if a living donor is not available. There is some evidence that older patients may be immunologically less aggressive and that the metabolism of cyclosporine by the cytochrome P450 system in the liver (see Chapter 4) may be slowed. They may also be more susceptible to the infectious side effects of immunosuppression.

Transplantation in children is discussed in Chapter 15.

Obesity and Malnutrition

Severe malnutrition is less common now that patients with ESRD are starting dialysis earlier. Dialysis units should ensure that patients are adequately dialyzed and nourished because malnourished patients are at greater risk for infection and poor wound healing. Obese patients are also at greater risk in the perioperative period from wound complications and pulmonary infections. The long-term risks from cardiovascular disease secondary to hypercholesterolemia and from hypertension are compounded by obesity. Prednisone therapy may induce rapid weight gain, and these patients must be encouraged to lose as much excess weight as possible before transplantation. Severe morbid obesity may be a contraindication to transplantation. The nutritional assessment of transplantation candidates is discussed in Chapter 18.

Candidates Being Treated With Peritoneal Dialysis

In general, the form of dialysis has no bearing on suitability for transplantation. Peritonitis and exit-site infections must be adequately treated, and about 6 weeks should elapse after an episode of peritonitis before patients are put on the active cadaveric waiting list. Occasionally, the location of the exit site of the dialysis catheter may prevent the use of that side for transplantation.

Predialysis Transplantation

Five to 10% of kidney transplantations are now performed in patients with advanced chronic kidney disease who are not yet dependent on dialysis. Predialysis patients may begin to accrue waiting-time "points" for the purposes of distribution of cadaveric kidneys when their estimated glomerular filtration rate (GFR) is less than 20 mL/min (see Chapter 3). Because the waiting time for a cadaveric transplant is typically measured in years, most patients require dialysis before a kidney becomes available, unless there is a living donor.

Early referral to a transplantation center of patients with progressive renal disease permits timely evaluation of ESRD treatment modalities (see Chapter 1). This is particularly important for diabetic patients because their disease progression may be rapid and because it may require months to prepare a living donor. For other forms of chronic kidney disease in which disease progression may be slower (e.g., chronic interstitial nephritis, polycystic kidney disease), careful clinical judgment is required to time the transplantation. If a living donor is available, it may be possible not to place a dialysis access and either transplant the patient when the earliest uremic symptoms develop or wait until the estimated GFR is less than 10 to 15 mL/min. For potential cadaveric kidney recipients, it is wise to place a dialysis access (or plan for peritoneal dialysis) as ESRD approaches and the patient is placed on the waiting list. It must be emphasized to patients that preparation for transplantation and preparation for dialysis are not mutually exclusive but can be performed in parallel. It is unwise to get into a "race against time" to find a kidney for patients who are reluctant to start dialysis.

Patients seeking predialysis transplantation should clarify their health insurance status to ensure that the cost of their evaluation and preparation of living donors is covered. In the United States, Medicare ESRD benefits do not commence before dialysis and transplantation. Preemptive transplantation may offer improved patient and graft survival over conventional transplantation, probably because it eliminates the complications and increased cardiovascular risk associated with long-term dialysis, and the incidence of acute rejection may also be less. Patients who receive a transplant before the development of frank uremic symptoms or commencement of dialysis, however, may not feel the improved sense of well-being typically enjoyed by dialysis patients after transplantation. They should be warned of such.

Highly Sensitized Patients

About 40% of the national pool of patients awaiting cadaveric transplants have high levels of preformed cytotoxic antibodies that may prevent them from receiving a kidney or prolong their wait considerably (see Chapter 3). Cytotoxic antibodies result from failed prior transplantation, multiple pregnancies, and multiple blood transfusions. Attempts have been made to reduce the antibody levels by intravenous infusions of immunoglobulin, plasma exchange, cyclophosphamide, and immunoabsorption, but these techniques have not yet proved widely applicable. Patients with high levels of antibodies should be warned of the probability of a prolonged wait for a kidney.

Previously Transplanted Candidates

The fate of second and multiple transplants is dependent to a considerable extent on the rate and etiology of the prior transplant loss. Patients who lost kidneys because of surgical complications or have kidneys that functioned for more than a year have a prognosis that is not significantly different from patients with primary transplants. If the primary transplant is lost to early rejection, the prognosis for another transplant is impaired, and the patient will do best with a highly matched cadaveric transplant or a well-matched living-related transplant if a suitable donor is available. Recurrent disease is likely to re-recur. Patients must be made aware of their impaired prognosis.

The process of evaluating a patient for a repeat transplantation is the same as for a primary transplantation. For patients whose first transplant life was prolonged, special attention should be paid to the possibility of covert coronary artery disease or malignancy.

Candidates for Double Organ Transplants

Patients with end-stage liver disease who are candidates for orthotopic liver transplantation (OLT) frequently have impaired renal function as a result of hepatorenal syndrome, "prerenal" dysfunction, acute tubular necrosis, or nephrotoxicity. In most cases, renal function improves after successful OLT despite what is often a prolonged period of dialysis dependence. Concomitant renal transplantation is therefore not indicated when it is anticipated that native renal function will improve.

Irreversible renal dysfunction may accompany end-stage liver disease; in these cases, it is logical to consider a combined procedure (Table 6.4). The addition of a kidney transplant adds relatively little to the considerable morbidity of an OLT, but a well-functioning kidney may facilitate posttransplantation management. The immunosuppressive regimen does not need to be modified. Results of the combined procedure are similar to those of OLT alone.

Experience with combined heart–kidney transplantation is more limited. The same principles regarding reversibility of renal dysfunction apply. Combined pancreas–kidney transplantation is discussed in Chapter 14.

Waiting Period for a Cadaveric Transplant: Reevaluation of Patients on the Waiting List

The median waiting time on the cadaveric list continues to increase and is 4 to 5 years or more in many centers. During this time, the health status of potential transplantation candidates may change, and periodic reevaluation of patients on the list is warranted. Ischemic heart disease can progress rapidly in dialysis patients; thus, periodic screening of patients at the greatest risk (those with a history of ischemic heart disease, diabetes, or advanced age) is warranted. Studies defining the optimal timing of repeat screening are lacking.

During the waiting period, patients must remain adherent to their dialysis regime and attempt to improve their physical and emotional health and rehabilitation. Close liaison between the personnel of the dialysis unit and the transplantation program is essential, and the transplantation program must be kept updated regarding significant medical developments. The program should maintain contact with the patients either by routine visits or by telephone. This contact ensures that the program is updated with medical and demographic data and that the patient does not feel forgotten or disheartened by a prolonged wait.

SELECTED READINGS

Danovitch GM. The epidemic of cardiovascular disease in chronic renal failure: a challenge to the transplant physician. *Graft* 1999;2:5108.

Doyle SE, Matas AJ, Gillingham K, et al. Predicting clinical outcome in the elderly renal transplant recipient. *Kidney Int* 2000;57:2144.

Frazier P, Davis-Ali S, Dahl K. Correlates of noncompliance among renal transplant recipients. *Clin Transplant* 1994;8:550.

Ismail N, Hakim RM, Helderman JH. Renal replacement therapies in the elderly. Part II. Renal transplantation. *Am J Kidney Dis* 1994;23:1.

Jeyarajah DR, McBride M, Klintmalm GB, et al. Combined liver-kidney transplantation: what are the indications? *Transplantation* 1997;64: 1091–1096.

Kasiske BL, Ramos EL, Gaston RS, et al. The evaluation of renal transplant candidates: clinical practice guidelines. *J Am Soc Nephrol* 1995;6:1.

Katz SM, Kerman RH, Golden D, et al. Preemptive transplantation: an analysis of benefits and hazards in 85 cases. *Transplantation* 1991;51:351.

Le A, Wilson R, Douek K, et al. Prospective risk stratification in renal transplant candidates for cardiac death. *Am J Kidney Dis* 1994;24:65.

Lehlou A, Lang P, Charpentier B, et al. Hemolytic uremic syndrome; recurrence after renal transplantation. *Medicine* 2000;79:90.

Lochhead KM, Pirsch JD, D'Alessandro AM, et al. Risk factors for renal allograft loss in patients with systemic lupus erythematosus. *Kidney Int* 1996;49:512.

Parfrey PS, Harnett JD, Foley RN, et al. Impact of renal transplantation on uremic cardiomyopathy. *Transplantation* 1995; 60:908.

Penn I. The effects of transplantation on preexisting cancers. *Transplantation* 1993;55:742.

Ramos EL, Tisher CC. Recurrent disease in the kidney transplant. *Am J Kidney Dis* 1994;24:152.

Schaubel D, Desmeules M, Mao Y, et al. Survival experience among elderly end-stage renal disease patients. *Transplantation* 1995;60:1389.

Shandera K, Sago A, Angstadt J, et al. An assessment of the need for voiding cystourethrogram for urologic screening prior to renal transplantation. *Clin Transplant* 1993;7:299.

Spital A. Should all human immunodeficiency virus-infected patients with end-stage renal disease be excluded from transplantation? *Transplantation* 1998;65:1187.

Stone J, Amend W, Criswell L. Antiphospholipid antibody syndrome in renal transplantation. *Am J Kidney Dis* 1999;34:1040.

The Transplant Operation and Its Surgical Complications

H. Albin Gritsch and J. Thomas Rosenthal

Kidney transplantation is an elective or semielective surgical procedure performed in patients who have undergone careful preoperative assessment and preparation. Chronic dialysis allows patients to be maintained in optimal condition and provides time to address potentially complicating medical and surgical issues. Chapter 6 describes these preparations. In this respect, kidney transplantation differs from heart or liver transplantation, in which the condition of the patient is often deteriorating rapidly in the pretransplantation period.

TRANSPLANTATION OPERATION

Immediate Preoperative Preparations

Chapter 5 describes the process of kidney transplant donation and provides a standard preoperative checklist (see Chapter 5, Table 5.7). If transplantation candidates have been well prepared, it is rarely necessary to call off surgery because of last-minute findings. Occasionally, cancellation of surgery is required because of recent events, such as new onset of chest pain or cardiographic changes, diabetic foot ulcers, peritonitis, pneumonia, or gastrointestinal (GI) bleeding. If the patient is anticoagulated to maintain dialysis access or mechanical cardiac valve function, fresh-frozen plasma may need to be administered to correct the internal normalization ratio (INR) to less than 2.

The decision to dialyze a patient before transplantation depends on the timing of the previous dialysis, clinical assessment of volume status, and serum electrolyte levels, particularly potassium. Because of the danger of intraoperative or postoperative hyperkalemia in oliguric patients, it is wise to dialyze patients with a serum potassium level of more than 5.5 mEq/L. In well-dialyzed patients, preoperative dialysis for fluid removal is usually unnecessary. If fluid is removed, it should be done with care to maintain the patient at or somewhat above his or her dry weight to facilitate postoperative diuresis. If time constraints demand it, a brief preoperative dialysis lasting 1 to 2 hours may be all that is necessary to reduce potassium levels and optimize the hemodynamic status.

Operative Technique

Because all kidney transplant recipients receive immunosuppressive drugs and many are anemic or malnourished at the time of surgery, wound healing is potentially compromised. Meticulous surgical technique, attention to detail, strict aseptic technique, and perfect hemostasis are essential. Drains are best avoided, but if they are used, they should be closed systems and should be removed as quickly as possible.

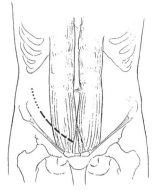

Fig. 7.1.   Standard incision for adult kidney transplantation. An oblique incision is made from the symphysis in the midline curving in a lateral and superior direction to the iliac crest.

Incision

An oblique incision is made from the symphysis in the midline curving in a lateral superior direction to the iliac crest (Fig. 7.1). It can be extended into the flank or as high as the tip of the 12th rib if more exposure is needed. In a first transplantation, the incision site may be in either lower quadrant. There are different approaches to the decision regarding which side to use. One approach has been to always use the right side, regardless of the side of origin of the donor kidney, because the accessibility of the iliac vein makes the operation easier than on the left side. Another approach is to use the side contralateral to the side of the donor kidney; that is, a right kidney is put on the left side, and *vice versa.* This technique was used when the hypogastric artery was routinely used for the anastomosis because the vessels lie in a convenient position and the renal pelvis is always anterior, making it accessible if ureteral repair is needed. The third approach has been to use the side ipsilateral to the donor kidney; that is, a right kidney is put on the right side, and vice versa. This choice is best when the external iliac artery is used for the arterial anastomosis. The vessels then lie without kinking when the kidney is placed in position. In repeat transplantations, the side opposite the original transplantation is generally used. In further transplantations, the decision regarding where to place the kidney is more complex; a transabdominal incision may be necessary, and more proximal vessels may be used.

   The retroperitoneal space is entered, and a pocket is made for the kidney. In patients with type 1 diabetes who may be eventual candidates for pancreas transplantation, the kidney is preferentially placed in the left iliac fossa to facilitate a possible pancreas transplantation on the right side (see Chapter 14).

Vascular Connections

Figure 7.2 shows the vascular connections for a kidney transplantation.

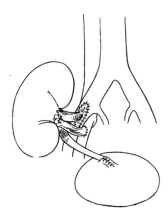

Fig. 7.2.   The standard hook-up. The donor renal artery is shown anastomosed end-to-end on a Carrel aortic patch to the recipient external iliac artery. The donor renal vein is anastomosed to the recipient external iliac vein. The donor ureter is anastomosed to the recipient bladder with an antireflux technique.

RENAL ARTERY.   The donor renal artery may be sewn to the external iliac artery in an end-to-side fashion or to the hypogastric artery in an end-to-end fashion. In a cadaveric kidney transplantation, the donor renal artery or arteries are usually kept in continuity with a patch of donor aorta called a *Carrel patch,* which makes the end-to-side anastomosis much easier and safer and facilitates the anastomosis of multiple renal arteries. In a living-related transplant, a Carrel patch is not available, and the renal artery itself is sewn to the recipient artery. If an end-to-side anastomosis is chosen, a 2.7-mm aortic punch is useful in creating the recipient arteriotomy. A fine nonabsorbent monofilament suture, such as 5-0 or 6-0 polypropylene, is usually chosen. In small children and in patients undergoing repeat transplantation on the same side, it may be necessary to use arteries other than the external iliac or hypogastric. The common iliac artery or even the aorta may sometimes be used. During the anastomosis time, the kidney is wrapped in a gauze pad with crushed ice saline to minimize warm ischemia.

MULTIPLE ARTERIES.   A variety of techniques have been proposed for handling multiple donor renal arteries. In cadaveric transplantations, it is best to keep them all on a single large Carrel patch, which minimizes the likelihood of damage to a small polar artery. In no case should polar arteries be sacrificed. Ligation of a lower-pole artery may lead to ureteral necrosis. There may be visible capsular vessels that supply a tiny part of the cortical surface of the kidney. These vessels may be ligated, and tiny superficial ischemic areas on the surface of the kidney may result. If there are multiple arteries in a live donor transplant or if a Carrel patch is not available, the donor arteries can be anastomosed individually or anastomosed to each other before being anastomosed to the recipient vessel. Occasionally, a small polar branch may be anastomosed end-to end to the inferior epigastric artery.

RENAL VEIN. The renal vein is sewn to the external iliac vein. Suture material similar to that used for the arterial anastomosis is usually chosen. If there are multiple renal veins, the largest may be used; the others can be ligated safely because of internal collateralization of the renal venous drainage. With cadaveric renal transplants, the donor vena cava may be used as an extension graft for the short right renal vein.

URETER. The ureter can be placed either into the recipient's bladder or into the ipsilateral native ureter as a ureterostomy. The native ureter may also be brought up to the allograft renal pelvis as a ureteropyelostomy. Most surgeons use the bladder whenever possible. Preferably, the recipient's bladder will have been shown to be functional before the transplantation; however, even small, contracted bladders that have not "seen" urine for prolonged periods can function well. If necessary, the ureter can be placed in a previously fashioned ileal or colonic conduit.

Establishing an antireflux mechanism is important to prevent posttransplantation pyelonephritis. In one method, the bladder is opened, the ureter is brought into the bladder by a separate opening posteriorly, and laterally, a submucosal tunnel is created. The ureter is sewn into the bladder from within, and the bladder is then closed. This technique is similar to a *Leadbetter-Politano reimplantation*.

The other approach is to make a single, small opening into the bladder and to sew the ureter in from the outside. Bladder muscle is then brought over the ureter to create the antireflux mechanism (Fig. 7.3). This technique is similar to a *Lich reimplantation*. Because of its simplicity, many surgeons have adopted this extravesical approach. Absorbable suture is used to prevent stone formation. Indwelling stents are not usually required but may be used if there is any question about the reimplantation. A 4.8-mm double-J stent is useful in this setting. Foley catheter drainage of the bladder is required for 3 to 5 days unless there are bladder abnormalities.

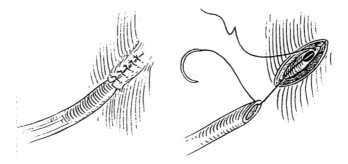

Fig. 7.3. A Lich reimplantation. A single, small opening is made in the bladder, and the ureter is sewn in from the outside. Bladder muscle is used to create an antireflux mechanism.

Drains

Drains may be placed through a separate small incision into the perirenal space to drain blood, urine, or lymph. Some surgeons routinely place drains, whereas others do not. Closed drains, such as the Jackson-Pratt type, are preferred over the open Penrose-type drains because of a lower risk for wound infection. When drains are used, they should be removed as soon as there is no longer significant drainage, typically 24 to 48 hours after transplantation.

Surgical Considerations in Young Children

Urologic disease is the cause of renal failure in nearly half of children with end-stage renal disease (see Chapter 15). It is therefore important to study bladder function in children with a history of urinary tract infections or voiding abnormalities. Reconstructive surgery must be coordinated with possible renal transplantation. The parents and child must be psychologically prepared for intermittent catheterization, which may be necessary postoperatively.

The transplantation procedure for children who weigh more than 20 to 25 kg is the same as the procedure for adults. In smaller children, comparatively large adult-sized kidneys are implanted because kidneys from equivalently sized infant donors are more prone to technical complications. A larger incision and more proximal blood vessels are used for implantation. The common iliac artery and vein or even the aorta and vena cava may be used. In children weighing more than 10 to 12 kg, an extraperitoneal approach may still be used. The right side is almost always preferable because of the easy exposure of the common iliac vein. In children weighing less than 10 to 12 kg, a midline transabdominal approach is necessary. The great vessels are approached by mobilizing the cecum, and the kidney is placed behind the cecum. To provide room for a large kidney in the right flank, a right native nephrectomy is sometimes necessary at the time of the transplantation to create room for the allograft. Careful intraoperative fluid management is crucial to prevent thrombosis of large kidneys in small children.

Intraoperative Fluid Management

Adequate perfusion of the newly transplanted kidney is critical for the establishment of an immediate postoperative diuresis and the avoidance of acute tubular necrosis (see Chapter 8). Volume contraction should be avoided and mild volume expansion maintained, conducive to the recipient's cardiac status. Central venous pressure should be maintained at about 10 mm Hg with the use of isotonic saline and albumin infusions, and systolic blood pressure should be kept above 120 mm Hg. If blood is required, cytomegalovirus-negative units should be used.

Immediately before the release of the vascular clamps, a large dose of methylprednisolone is usually given (up to 1 g in some programs; see Chapter 4). Mannitol (12.5 g) and furosemide (up to 200 mg) are also given, and fluid replacement is maintained accordingly. Direct injection of the calcium-channel blocker verapamil in a dose of 5 mg into the renal artery reduces capillary spasm and improves renal blood flow. This medication must be administered with caution in patients taking beta-blocker antihypertensive medications to avoid complete heart block. Postoperative management is discussed in Chapter 8.

Dual Kidney Transplantation

At the extremes of donor age, both donor kidneys are sometimes transplanted into a single recipient. The simultaneous use of both kidneys entails some additional risks to the recipients and is a reflection of the donor shortage.

For donors younger than 2 years of age, both kidneys are usually transplanted *en bloc* with the donor aorta and vena cava (Fig. 7.4); for donors between the ages of 2 and 5 years, the decision to transplant the kidneys separately or together is made by the transplant surgeon after assessing the size of the organs. For the *en bloc* procedure, the aorta and vena cava superior to the renal vessels must be of adequate length to allow closure without compromising the lumen of the renal vessels. All of the other branches of the great vessels are carefully ligated, the aorta is then anastomosed to the external iliac artery, and the vena cava is anastomosed to the external iliac vein. Both ureters are then anastomosed to the bladder. The kidneys must be carefully positioned to avoid kinking of the blood vessels and tension on the ureteral anastomoses. If the ureters are implanted into the bladder separately, the risk for injury to the second kidney in case of vascular thrombosis is reduced. The rate of technical complications, most typically urine leaks and vascular thrombosis, varies between 10% and 20% with young donor kidneys transplanted individually or *en bloc*. With greater experience and improved immunosuppressive agents, pediatric donors are being used more frequently because of the significant donor organ shortage.

Kidneys from older "marginal" donors are sometimes discarded for fear they will not provide adequate renal function for their recipients. To avoid this wastage, some centers now advocate the

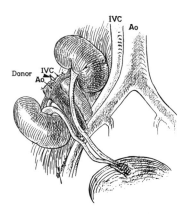

Fig. 7.4. Pediatric *en bloc* kidney transplantation. The donor aorta *(Ao)* and inferior vena cava *(IVC)* are anastomosed to the external iliac vessels. The ureters are anastomosed to the bladder using pediatric stents. (Reprinted with permission from Bretan PN, Koyle M, Singh K, et al. Improved survival of en bloc renal allografts from pediatric donors. *J Urol* 1997;157:1592.)

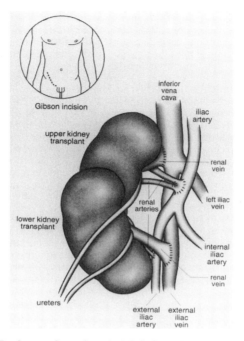

Fig. 7.5.   Dual transplantation of adult kidneys into a single recipient. (Reprinted with permission from Masson D, Hefty T. A technique for the transplantation of 2 adult cadaver kidney grafts into 1 recipient. *J Urol* 1998;160:1779.)

use of two kidneys from donors aged 60 years or older, if the calculated creatinine clearance is less that 90 mL/min at the time of admission or if there is evidence of significant histologic damage on the biopsy specimen taken at the time of organ retrieval. One kidney can be placed in each iliac fossa using a preperitoneal midline incision or separate lower abdominal incisions. Alternatively, both kidneys can be placed on one side, with anastomosis of the vessels of one kidney to the common iliac artery and the vena cava (Fig. 7.5). Early experience with double marginal kidneys suggests that results of graft survival and renal function are comparable to those achieved with single kidneys from older donors. Older recipients may do better with kidneys from older donors because their metabolic demands may be less.

SURGICAL COMPLICATIONS OF KIDNEY TRANSPLANTATION

The clinical presentation of surgical and nonsurgical complications of kidney transplantation may be similar. Graft dysfunction may reflect an acute rejection or a urine leak; fever and graft tenderness may reflect wound infection or rejection. Posttransplantation events have a broad differential diagnosis that must include technical complications of surgery as well as immunologic and other causes.

The fundamental algorithm in the management of posttransplantation graft dysfunction requires that vascular and urologic causes of graft dysfunction be ruled out before concluding that an event is due to a medical cause such as rejection or cyclosporine toxicity. The differential diagnosis of postoperative graft dysfunction is discussed in Chapter 8, and the radiologic diagnostic tools are discussed in Chapter 12. Doppler ultrasound is invaluable in the differentiation of medical and surgical postoperative complications.

Wound Infection

In the 1960s and 1970s, wound infection rates after kidney transplantation were as high as 25%. Wound infections should now occur in less than 1% of cases. This improvement is due to several factors: patients receiving transplants are healthier; lower steroid doses are used for both maintenance and treatment of rejection; and perioperative antibiotics are routinely used. In most cases, a first-generation cephalosporin is sufficient (see Chapter 10). Obviously, strict aseptic technique in the operating room is essential to prevent wound infection. If infections do occur, they should be treated with drainage and systemic antibiotics to avoid contamination of the vascular suture line and possible mycotic aneurysm formation. The risk of infection or other wound problems is significantly higher in obese patients.

Lymphocele

Presentation

Lymphoceles are collections of lymph caused by leakage from severed lymphatics that overlie the iliac vessels. They may develop and present within weeks after transplantation. The incidence of lymphoceles reported in the literature ranges from less than 1% to 10%. Some lymphoceles are small and asymptomatic. Others are large and produce symptoms. Usually, the larger the lymphocele, the more likely it is to produce symptoms and require treatment, although there are some cases of very small but strategically placed lymphoceles producing ureteral obstruction. Lymphoceles may present by producing ureteral obstruction; by compressing the iliac vein, leading to deep-vein thrombosis or leg swelling; or as an abdominal mass. Lymphoceles occasionally produce incontinence secondary to bladder compression, scrotal masses secondary to spontaneous drainage into the scrotum, or vena cava obstruction. Lymphoceles can be avoided by minimizing the dissection of the iliac vessels and by ligating all lymphatics. Electrocoagulation is not adequate.

Diagnosis

Lymphoceles are usually diagnosed by ultrasound (see Chapter 12). The characteristic ultrasound finding is a roundish, sonolucent, septated mass. Hydronephrosis may be present, and the ureter may be seen adjacent to and compressed by the lymphocele. More complex internal echoes may signal an infected lymphocele. Usually, the clinical situation and ultrasound appearance distinguish a lymphocele from other types of perirenal fluid collections, such as hematoma or urine leak. Simple needle aspiration of the fluid using sterile technique makes the diagnosis. The fluid obtained is clear and has a high protein content, and the creatinine concentration is equal to that of serum.

Treatment

No therapy is necessary for the common, small, asymptomatic lymphocele. Percutaneous aspiration should be performed if there is suspicion of a ureteral leak, obstruction, or infection. The most common indication for treatment is ureteral obstruction. If the cause of the obstruction is simple compression due to the mass effect of the lymphocele, drainage alone will resolve the problem. The ureter itself is often narrowed and may need to be reimplanted because of its involvement in the inflammatory reaction in the wall of the lymphocele. Repeated percutaneous aspirations are not advised because they seldom lead to dissolution of the lymphocele and often result in infection.

Infected or obstructing lymphoceles can be drained externally using either a closed or an open system. Closed systems are superior because they control the fluid and are less susceptible to infection. Sclerosing agents, such as povidone iodine (Betadine), tetracycline, or fibrin glue, can be instilled into the cavity with good results. Lymphoceles can also be drained internally by marsupialization into the peritoneal cavity, where the fluid is resorbed. Marsupialization can be done as an open surgical procedure or laparoscopically. It is important to ensure that the opening in the lymphocele is large enough to prevent peritoneal overgrowth, which can produce recurrence or bowel entrapment and incarceration. Omentum is often interposed in the opening to prevent closure. Care must be taken to avoid injury to the ureter, which may lie in the wall of the lymphocele. On rare occasions, the actual site of lymph leak can be identified and ligated.

Bleeding

The risk for postoperative bleeding can be minimized by close attention to pretransplantation coagulation parameters, which should be considered during the pretransplantation work-up (see Chapter 6). Aspirin and anticoagulant medications should be discontinued before transplantation, and well-dialyzed patients may have improvement of the platelet dysfunction and abnormal bleeding time associated with uremia. Postoperative bleeding seldom arises from the vascular anastomoses unless a mycotic aneurysm ruptures or the graft itself ruptures. These events are not likely to occur until a few days after transplantation and are associated with exsanguinating hemorrhage. Early postoperative bleeding can occur from small vessels in the renal hilum, which may not have been apparent before closure because of vasospasm. After surgery, when perfusion improves, these hilar vessels can then bleed. Meticulous preparation of the allograft and hemostasis during the operation minimizes this risk. Close observation of vital signs and serial hematocrits is necessary for the first several postoperative hours to recognize this type of bleeding. Ultrasound can confirm the presence of perigraft hematoma. Surgical exploration may be necessary. If bleeding occurs, coagulation parameters should be studied to ensure that there is no occult coagulopathy. Administration of blood, efficient dialysis, estrogen infusions, and vaso-pressin all improve platelet function and reduce bleeding time in uremic patients.

Late hemorrhage can result from the rupture of a mycotic aneurysm. The bleeding may be profound. Nephrectomy and repair of the artery are usually required. Rarely, the external iliac artery may have to be ligated and blood supply to the ipsilateral leg provided by extraanatomic bypass.

Graft Thrombosis

Arterial or venous thrombosis occurs most often within the first 2 to 3 days after transplantation, although it may occur as long as 2 months after transplantation. The reported incidence varies widely from 0.5% to as high as 8%. The incidence of thrombosis may be increased in patients with a prior thrombotic tendency, positive anticardiolipin antibodies, or high platelet counts (more than $350 \times 10^9/L$). The early variety of thrombosis is most often a reflection of surgical technique; the later is most often associated with acute rejection. If the kidney has been functioning well, thrombosis is heralded by a sudden cessation of urine output and rapid rise in serum creatinine, often with graft swelling and local pain. Platelets may be consumed, and thrombocytopenia and hyperkalemia may develop. Venous thrombosis may present with severe graft swelling, tenderness, and gross hematuria. If a patient's native kidneys were making large quantities of urine, however, the only sign of thrombosis may be the rising creatinine level; if the allograft had not been functioning, there may be no overt signs of thrombosis at all. For this reason, grafts that are not functioning are routinely imaged radiologically to ensure ongoing blood flow to the graft. Diagnosis of thrombosis is by a Doppler ultrasound or isotope flow scan (see Chapter 12). These techniques help distinguish thrombosis from other causes of acute anuria, such as rejection or obstruction. Confirmed thrombosis usually requires graft nephrectomy.

The transplanted kidney has no collateral blood supply, and its tolerance for warm ischemia is short. Unless the problem can be diagnosed quickly and repair carried out immediately, the kidney will be lost. Although there are a few case reports of kidney salvage after thrombosis, most grafts sustaining either arterial or venous thrombosis are lost. Streptokinase has not been reported to be useful for arterial thrombosis. It has been successfully used in a case of renal vein thrombosis that occurred late after transplantation and was associated with deep-vein thrombosis of the leg that extended up to the transplant vein.

Renal Artery Stenosis

Renal artery stenosis is a late complication and occurs in 2% to 12% of transplant recipients. Its presentation, diagnosis, and management are discussed in Chapters 9 and 12. Two major types of stenosis are seen. One is a discrete, suture line stenosis, which is most often seen after end-to-end anastomosis. The other type is a more diffuse, postanastomotic stenosis, which can occur after any type of arterial anastomosis. The term *pseudo–renal artery stenosis* has been used to describe the situation that may occur if an atherosclerotic plaque in the iliac vessels impairs blood flow to the transplant renal artery. Table 7.1 lists potential causes of stenosis. The

Table 7.1.   Potential causes of renal artery stenosis

1. Rejection of the donor artery
2. Atherosclerosis of the recipient vessel
3. Clamp injury to the recipient or donor vascular endothelium
4. Perfusion pump cannulation injury of the donor vessel
5. Faulty suture technique: pursestring effect, lumen encroachment by the suture, improper suture material, fibrotic inflammatory reaction to polypropylene in the setting of abnormal hemodynamics
6. End-to-end anastomosis with abnormal fluid dynamics
7. Angulation due to disproportionate length between graft artery and iliac artery
8. End-to-end anastomosis with vessel size disproportion
9. Pseudo renal artery stenosis by critical iliac atherosclerotic lesion
10. Kinking of the renal artery

postulate that rejection can cause renal artery stenosis has not been conclusively proved.

When technically feasible, percutaneous transluminal angioplasty, often with the placement of intraarterial stents, offers the safest mode of treatment with a high rate of success. In one series, more than 80% of patients were cured 2 years after treatment, although recurrence may occur in up to 20% of cases. If angioplasty is not technically feasible or fails as a primary form of therapy, surgical repair is necessary. Graft loss after surgical repair has been reported in up to 30% of cases and is a reflection of the difficulty in directly approaching the vascular anastomosis in a noncollateralized kidney.

Urine Leaks

Etiology and Diagnosis

Urine leaks may occur at the level of the bladder, ureter, or renal calyx. They typically occur within the first few days after transplantation or at the onset of posttransplantation diuresis in patients with delayed graft function. Urine leaks may be technical in etiology as a result of a nonwatertight ureteral reimplantation or bladder closure. They may also be due to ureteral slough secondary to disruption of ureteral blood supply; the blood supply to the distal donor ureter is the most endangered by the harvesting procedure. Leaks may also occur as a result of a tight ureteral stenosis that leads to forniceal rupture in the presence of a high urine volume.

If the transplantation incision is drained, a urine leak may present with copious drainage. Any excess fluid drainage from the incision should be sent urgently for creatinine estimation. Any significant elevation in concentration over that of plasma confirms that the fluid is urine (occasionally, at a time of a falling serum creatinine level serous fluid may be trapped at a slightly higher creatinine level than the current plasma level). If the wound is not drained, a urine leak may present with agonizing pain, rising plasma creatinine level due to the reabsorption of urine, and a fluid density mass on ultrasound. This clinical picture may be confused with rejection though the pain of a urine leak is typically much more severe than the aching pain of an acute rejection. Fluid leaking from the incision line may have a typical uriniferous odor. If ultrasound shows a fluid collection, the fluid should be tapped under sterile conditions and sent urgently for a creatinine estimation. A renal scan will often identify the leak by showing radioisotope outside the urinary tract. A cystogram may show leakage of contrast outside of the bladder (see Chapter 12).

Treatment

There should be no delay in instituting therapy. A Foley catheter reduces intravesical pressure and occasionally may reduce or stop leakage altogether. Percutaneous antegrade nephrostomy may be used to diagnose the leak and control the flow of urine. Some leaks can be managed definitively with external drainage and stent placement alone. It may be difficult, however, to access the collecting system percutaneously because there is often not enough hydronephrosis present. If the leak is due to a ureteral slough, percutaneous treatment will never work and only delays definitive treatment. For these reasons, when leaks occur, early surgical exploration and repair are usually required.

The type of surgical repair depends on the level of leak and the viability of the tissues. Bladder fistulas should be closed primarily. A calyceal leak that is the result of obstruction is treated by removal of the obstruction. If a ureteral leak is a simple anastomotic leak, resection of the distal ureter and reimplantation is the easiest solution. If the ureter is nonviable because of inadequate length of blood supply, ureteropyelostomy using the ipsilateral or contralateral native ureter is a good option. Cystopyelostomy has also been done to replace a sloughed ureter. Here, the bladder is mobilized and brought directly to the allograft renal pelvis without an intervening ureter. The advantage of using the native ureter over direct anastomosis of the bladder to the renal pelvis is that the native ureter is antirefluxing, which may result in a lower incidence of pyelonephritis.

An indwelling double-J stent is usually left in place after repair of a urine leak. Nephrostomy drainage is not essential, although if a prior percutaneous nephrostomy has been done, it is wise to leave it in place until several days after surgery. It should be removed only after a trial of nephrostomy occlusion to ensure continuity of distal drainage. The double-J stent can be removed cystoscopically several weeks later, followed by ultrasound to ensure that urine is not recollecting.

Ureteral Obstruction

Diagnosis

Ureteral obstruction is usually manifested by impairment of graft function. Obstruction may be painless because of the absence of innervation. Hydronephrosis may be seen on ultrasound; increasing hydronephrosis is good evidence of obstruction. Low-grade dilation of the collecting system secondary to edema at the implantation site is often seen on early posttransplantation ultrasound examinations and should not necessarily lead to the conclusion that there is obstruction present. Confirmation of the obstruction and identification of the site can be made by intravenous pyelogram, although often graft function is not adequate to allow good visualization. Obstruction can be confirmed by retrograde pyelogram, although the ureteral orifice may be difficult to catheterize. Renal scan with furosemide wash-out is a good screening test but does not provide clear anatomic detail. The most effective way to visualize the collecting system is by percutaneous antegrade pyelography.

Etiology and Treatment

Acute postoperative obstruction usually requires surgical repair. Blood clots, a technically poor reimplantation, and ureteral slough are the common causes of early acute obstruction after transplantation. Ureteral fibrosis secondary to either ischemia or rejection can cause an intrinsic obstruction, and obstruction associated with polyoma BK virus has also been described (see Chapters 10 and 13). Extrinsic obstruction can be caused by ureteral kinking or periureteral fibrosis from lymphoceles or graft rejection. Calculi are rare causes of transplant obstruction.

Intrinsic ureteral scars can be treated effectively by endourologic techniques in an antegrade (Fig. 7.6) or retrograde approach. If graft dysfunction is associated with significant or increasing hydronephrosis, obstruction is confirmed with a fine-needle percutaneous nephrostogram (step A in Fig. 7.6; see Chapter 12). If obstruction is confirmed, a guide wire is passed endoscopically through the stricture (step B in Fig. 7.6). If the stricture is short (i.e., less than 2 cm), balloon dilation allows a working element to be passed, and under direct vision, the stricture is incised with a cold knife (step C in Fig. 7.6). The stricture can also be approached retrograde through the bladder cystoscopically. A stent is left indwelling (step D in Fig. 7.6) and removed cystoscopically after 2 to 6 weeks. The nephrostomy is removed after an antegrade nephrostogram has confirmed that the urinary tract is unobstructed. Early reports suggest success rates of 70% to 80% with these techniques. Endourologic techniques can also be used to remove calculi, which can also be destroyed by extracorporeal shock-wave lithotripsy.

Extrinsic strictures or strictures that are longer than 2 cm are less likely to be amenable to percutaneous techniques and require surgical treatment, as do those strictures that fail endourologic incision. The same surgical options are used as for ureteral leaks: direct reimplantation of the ureter above the stricture or anastomosis of the native ureter or bladder to the renal pelvis if the stricture is high.

Gastrointestinal Complications

Gastrointestinal complications of renal transplantation are not uncommon. Nausea and vomiting may simply be related to the multiple medications these patients require, but more serious conditions, such as bowel obstruction, cholecystitis, infectious gastritis, pancreatitis, gastric ulceration, and colonic perforation, may occur. A high degree of suspicion is crucial because immunosuppressed patients may not present with typical symptoms of peritonitis.

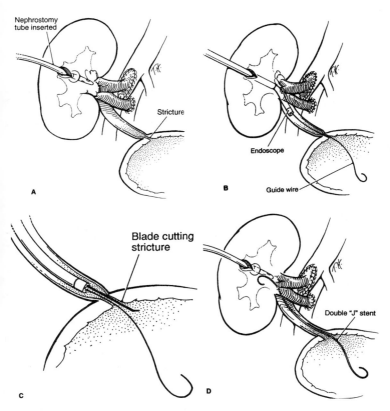

Fig. 7.6.   Stages in the endourologic treatment of ureteral structure. See text for description of steps.

Timely diagnosis and surgical treatment are essential to avoid significant mortality. Sodium polystyrene sulfonate (Kayexalate)–sorbitol enemas should not be administered to uremic patients because they have been associated with colonic necrosis. Constipation is a common postoperative problem; sodium phosphate (Fleet) enemas should be avoided in patients with poor renal function because of the high phosphate load.

ALLOGRAFT NEPHRECTOMY

Indications

Kidneys that have failed either for technical reasons or from rejection may need to be removed. Indications for allograft nephrectomy are symptoms and signs that typically occur when immunosuppression is withdrawn but may be delayed by weeks or months. These may include low-grade fever, graft tenderness and swelling, malaise, thrombocytopenia, and hematuria. It may be possible to lessen the symptoms and avoid nephrectomy by temporary re-institution of small doses of steroids. Avoidance of nephrectomy is preferred because the procedure may have an unfavorable effect on the prognosis of a future transplant and may cause a steep elevation in the percentage of preformed cytotoxic antibodies (see Chapter 3). If the graft loss is acute and occurs within 1 year of transplantation, nephrectomy may be necessary in up to 90% of cases. Graft loss from chronic rejection after 1 year results in nephrectomy in up to half of cases. The rejected graft that remains *in situ* typically becomes a small, fibrotic mass. Acquired cystic disease may develop as described in chronically diseased native kidneys.

Procedure

The removal of a failed allograft may be technically more difficult than the transplantation itself because of the inflammatory response and scarring due to rejection. Usually, the old incision is reopened. Care must be taken to avoid the peritoneum, which may have become draped across the surface of the kidney. If the nephrectomy is performed soon after transplantation, especially if there has not been a great amount of rejection, the kidney can be removed entirely because it is not very adherent to surrounding structures. If there has been recurrent rejection, the kidney usually adheres to surrounding structures and needs to be removed subcapsularly. The hilar vessels are friable and should be ligated and suture ligated. It is almost always safe to leave a small amount of donor vessel in the recipient so that repair of the recipient iliac vessels is not necessary.

Hemostasis should be meticulous. Some dead space is always left after nephrectomy. If this fills with blood, abscess formation is more likely. Although a closed drain may be used, it may inadequately drain the blood and create the potential for infection by its presence. Electrocoagulation of the entire raw surface of the capsule should be performed, and spraying thrombin topically may improve hemostasis. Topical and parenteral antibiotics are routinely used.

Complications

Although there are few series in the literature, the reported morbidity for allograft nephrectomy is high. The potential complications include acute bleeding during surgery secondary to injury to the iliac artery or vein; injury to other surrounding structures, such as the bowel; infection; and lymph leaks. Leaving small segments of the allograft renal artery or vein does not usually cause long-term problems, although rupture can occur if they become secondarily infected. Likewise, leaving a small amount of allograft ureter in place can result in some gross hematuria after the allograft nephrectomy; the hematuria is almost always limited and usually does not require reoperation.

NON–TRANSPLANTATION-RELATED SURGERY

Immunosuppressed transplant recipients may occasionally require significant surgical intervention not directly related to the transplantation, such as coronary artery bypass, cholecystectomy,

Table 7.2.   Precautions for kidney transplant recipients undergoing posttransplantation surgical procedures

1. Maintain hydration.
2. Use nonnephrotoxic prophylactic antibiotics.
3. Give calcineurin-inhibitor by mouth when possible.
4. Modify intravenous cyclosporine dose when necessary.
5. Provide perioperative steroid coverage.
6. Adjunctive immunosuppressants can be held for several days.
7. Avoid nephrotoxic antibiotics and analgesics.
8. Monitor graft function and plasma potassium and acid–base status.
9. Consider wound healing impairment.

or hip replacement. Nephrologists or members of the transplantation team are often requested to aid in the perioperative management of such patients, and certain precautions are required (Table 7.2).

The renal function of many transplant recipients is impaired to varying degrees, and the capacity to concentrate urine and lower urinary sodium concentration may be limited. Maintenance of hydration is, therefore, particularly important perioperatively to avoid further reduction in renal function. If a patient will be unable to take immunosuppressive medications orally for more than 24 hours, cyclosporine should be given intravenously in a dose that is about one third of the total daily oral dose (see Chapter 4) over 4 to 8 hours. Although functional adrenal suppression in patients taking 10 mg/day or less of prednisone is uncommon, 100 mg of hydrocortisone is typically given every 8 hours postoperatively until the patient can return to the preoperative oral prednisone dose. For patients receiving triple therapy (see Chapter 4), azathioprine can be safely withheld for 2 to 3 days, as can mycophenolate mofetil. Nonnephrotoxic antibiotics should be given prophylactically, and if intravenous contrast is required for radiologic studies, a saline diuresis should be maintained. In patients with markedly impaired graft function, careful monitoring of postoperative plasma potassium levels and acid–base status is mandatory.

SELECTED READINGS

Abouljoud MS, Deierhoi MH, Hudson SL, et al. Risk factors affecting second renal transplant outcome with special reference to primary allograft nephrectomy. *Transplantation* 1995;60:138.

Alfrey EJ, Lee CM, Scandling JD, et al. When should expanded criteria donor kidneys be used for single versus dual kidney transplants? *Transplantation* 1997;64:1142.

Churchill BM, Steckler RE, McKenna PH, et al. Renal transplantation and the abnormal urinary tract. *Transplant Rev* 1993;7:21.

Davidson I, Ar'Rajab A, Dickerman B, et al. Perioperative albumin and verapamil improve early outcome after cadaver renal transplantation. *Transplant Proc* 1994;26:3100.

Gruessner RW, Fasola C, Benedetti E, et al. Laparoscopic drainage of lymphocele after kidney transplantation, indications and limitations. *Surgery* 1995;117:288.

Hobart MG, Modlin CS, Kapoor A, et al. Transplantation of pediatric en bloc cadaver kidneys into adult recipients. *Transplantation* 1998; 66:1689.

Merkus JWS, Huysmans FTM, Hoitsma AJ, et al. Treatment of renal allograft artery stenosis. *Transplant Int* 1993;6:111.

Nargund VH, Cranston D. Urologic complications after renal transplantation. *Transplant Rev* 1996;10:24.

Pleass HC, Clark KR, Rigg KM, et al. Urologic complications after renal transplantation: a prospective randomized trial comparing different techniques of ureteric anastomosis and the use of prophylactic ureteric stents. *Transplant Proc* 1995;27:1091.

Remuzzi G, Grinyo J, Ruggenenti P, et al. Early experience with dual kidney transplantation in adults using expanded donor criteria. *Am Soc Nephrol* 1999;10:2591.

Rosenthal JT. Complications of renal transplantation and autotransplantation. In: Smith RB, Ehrlich RM, eds. Complications of urologic surgery. Philadelphia: WB Saunders, 1990:231–256.

Satterthwaite R, Aswad S, Sunga V, et al. Outcome of en bloc and single kidney transplantation from very young cadaver donors. *Transplantation* 1997;63:1405.

Wong W, Fynn SP, Higgins RM, et al. Transplant renal artery stenosis in 77 patients: does it have an immunologic cause? *Transplantation* 1996;61:215.

8

The First Two Posttransplantation Months

William J.C. Amend, Jr., Flavio Vincenti, and Stephen J. Tomlanovich

The "early" period after renal transplantation usually refers to the first 2 months after transplantation. It is useful to further divide this period to allow consideration of the different diagnostic and therapeutic issues that affect both routine and complicated transplant management and tend to change with time. It is a fair generalization to say that surgical issues predominate in the first days after transplantation, and medical and immunologic issues tend to predominate thereafter. A combined surgical and medical transplantation team should follow the patients during this period. In this chapter, patient management on the first day after transplantation, the next 2 to 8 days, and the next 9 to 60 days is considered separately. Although this separation is somewhat arbitrary, it is supported by the observation that most acute rejection episodes have been found to occur in the first 2 months. Patients who successfully navigate their way through these first 2 months can usually look forward to prolonged graft function. Immunosuppressive therapy during this period is discussed in Chapter 4.

THE FIRST POSTOPERATIVE DAY

Recovery Room Assessment

Patients should be evaluated by the transplantation team immediately on arrival from the operating room. This initial assessment should first address routine postsurgical issues such as hemodynamic and respiratory stability. Most patients are extubated and awake. The operative record should be reviewed to assess fluid and blood loss and replacement and to ensure that intraoperative immunosuppressive protocols have been followed (e.g., corticosteroids, OKT3; see Chapter 4). The surgeon should report any untoward intraoperative events and the appearance of the transplanted organ after completion of the anastomosis and release of vascular clamps. It is often possible to anticipate early graft function based on the intraoperative perfusion characteristics of the kidney, the firmness or turgidity of the allograft, and the intraoperative urine volume. Special situations, such as the use of pediatric *en bloc* kidneys (see Chapter 5), transplantation into a difficult vascular bed, or the use of ureteral stents, should be clearly noted.

Routine postoperative orders are reviewed in Table 8.1. The length of time a patient remains in recovery depends on both medical and logistic factors. The postoperative nursing environment must allow for close hemodynamic and fluid management. This environment can be in an intensive care unit or a surgical step-down unit, depending on the facilities available in a given institution. Special considerations for the postoperative management of diabetic patients are discussed in Chapter 14.

**Table 8.1.   Suggested postoperative orders on transfer
of kidney transplant recipient from the recovery room**

Postoperative Nursing Orders

1. Vital signs checked every hour for 24 hr, then every 4 hr when patient is stable
2. Intake and output every hour for 24 hr, then every 4 hr
3. Intravenous fluids per physician
4. Daily weight
5. Turn, cough, deep breathe every hour; encourage incentive spirometry every hour while awake
6. Out of bed first postoperative; ambulate daily thereafter
7. Head of bed at 30 degrees
8. Dressing changes every 4 hr for 24 hr, then every 8 hr and p.r.n.
9. Check dialysis access for function every 4 hr
10. No blood pressure; venipuncture in extremity with fistula or shunt
11. Foley catheter to bedside drainage, irrigate gently with 30 mL normal saline p.r.n. for clots
12. Catheter care every 8 hr
13. Notify physician if urine output drops to less than 50 mL/hr or if greater than 200 mL/hr
14. Notify physician if temperature is >180 mm Hg or <110 mm Hg
15. NPO until changed by surgical team
16. Chest radiograph in the morning
17. Electrocardiogram in the morning

Postoperative Laboratory Orders

1. Complete blood count with platelets, electrolyte, creatinine, glucose, and blood urea nitrogen every 6 hr for 24 hr, then every morning
2. Calcineurin-inhibitor level each morning
3. Chemistry panel, urine culture, and sensitivity twice a week

Hemodynamic Evaluation

Postoperative hemodynamic evaluation is crucial for several reasons: for routine postsurgical management, to optimize graft function, to assess the significance of the urine output (or lack thereof), and to undertake therapeutic intervention.

Hemodynamic evaluation may be somewhat difficult in patients with chronic renal failure with hemodialysis fistulas or shunts. Vascular sclerosis is common in uremic patients, especially in elderly and diabetic patients, and systolic hypertension in these patients is common. The clinician should be familiar with the patient's pre-transplantation blood pressure and antihypertensive medications. A review of the operative course with the transplantation surgeon may be useful for blood pressure management decisions because there is impaired intrinsic renal autoregulation and the initial blood flow to the allograft is primarily dependent on mean systemic arterial blood pressure. The surgeon can report the intraoperative level of mean arterial blood pressure that provided the best observed allograft turgor and urine output. Excessive postoperative arterial hypertension may increase the risk for anastomotic leak and cerebrovascular catastrophe. Reduced mean arterial pressures, on the other hand, increase the risk for both postoperative acute tubular necrosis (ATN) and irreversible vascular thrombosis at the fresh anastomotic sites. Sublingual nifedipine is effective and convenient for management of postoperative systolic hypertension. Intravenous labetalol, hydralazine, fenoldopam, esmolol, or nitroprusside can be used in resistant cases in which the systolic blood pressure is consistently more than 180 mm Hg.

Some kidney transplantation units use central venous pressure or pulmonary artery and pulmonary wedge pressure measurements in the first 24 to 48 hours after transplantation. These measurements can be useful especially when the clinical team is not sure of the need for and amount of fluid resuscitation. Because kidney transplant recipients may have varying degrees of heart failure (from uremic cardiomyopathy, hypertensive cardiomyopathy, and coronary artery disease), the more sophisticated preload monitoring techniques may be invaluable. Such patients ideally will have been identified in the pretransplantation period, and the results of the pretransplantation cardiac evaluation (see Chapter 6) should be available to aid in their postoperative assessment. Clinical judgment, however, should supersede slavish commitment to central venous pressure parameters. Thus, a normotensive patient with a good urine output may have a low recorded central venous pressure and yet not need fluid resuscitation.

Intravenous Fluid Replacement

Several factors need to be assessed to determine the rate and form of posttransplantation fluid replacement. In general, the patient should be kept euvolemic or mildly hypervolemic, and repeated hemodynamic assessment is required. Insensible fluid losses are typically 30 to 60 mL/hour. Vascular volume deficits can continue due to "third-spacing" over the first 12 to 24 postoperative hours and need to be replaced. Volume losses at the operative site must be considered, especially if there are concomitant changes in urine volume and hemodynamic status. Urine volume must be monitored hourly and replaced accordingly (see Urine Output).

Which Intravenous Fluid?

Insensible fluid loss is essentially water loss and is replaced by a 5% dextrose solution at about 30 mL/hour. If the patient is deemed hypervolemic, it may be wise not to replace this fluid and to allow the patient to reach the postoperative dry weight gradually over the ensuing days. Hourly urine output is replaced with half-normal saline on a milliliter-for-milliliter basis. Half-normal saline is used for urine replacement because the sodium concentration of the urine of a newly transplanted diuresing kidney is typically 60 to 80 mEq/L. Large nasogastric losses are replaced with normal saline. If the patient is hypovolemic or if an attempt is being made to increase urine volume (see Urine Output), isotonic saline boluses are given after bedside clinical and hemodynamic evaluation.

Potassium replacement is usually not required unless urine volumes are very high and should be given with great care in oliguric patients. Lactated Ringer solution and other premixed intravenous fluids are unnecessary. Their potassium and bicarbonate content is inadequate if replacement is required, and it is better to supplement saline infusions with potassium, bicarbonate, and calcium on an as-needed basis. The necessity for blood transfusion is discussed under Early Postoperative Bleeding.

Urine Output

The initial urine volume can range from anuria to oliguria, "nonoliguria," or polyuria and may shift from one to the other based on parenchymal, urologic, or perfusion factors. A background knowledge of the patient's native urine output is crucial to assess the origin of the early posttransplantation urine output. Information about the donor kidney itself is crucial. When the transplant is from a live donor, postoperative oliguria is rare because of the short ischemia time (see Chapter 5); if it occurs, it must raise immediate concern regarding the vascularization of the graft or other technical problems, such as obstruction. On the other hand, when a patient receives a cadaveric kidney with a prolonged ischemia time or preprocurement ATN, postoperative oliguria can be anticipated. The mate kidney from a cadaveric donor often performs in a similar manner (i.e., has ATN or not) in both recipients, and it can be informative to call the transplantation center receiving the other kidney to inquire about its performance.

Various techniques and protocol modifications have been made to encourage postoperative diuresis (see Chapter 4 and Patients With Delayed Graft Function). Some protocols do not permit the use of an intravenous calcineurin inhibitor in the early postoperative period. Dopamine infusions at "renal-dose" levels of 1 to 5 μg/kg/min are used routinely at some centers to promote renal blood flow and counteract calcineurin inhibitor–induced renal vasoconstriction, but their value has not been proved. Fenoldopam, a more selective D_1 agonist, is being tested in a randomized clinical trial. Perioperative calcium-channel blockers are also sometimes used.

The Anuric and Oliguric Patient

Anuria is easy to define; oliguria is relative and, in the posttransplantation situation, usually refers to urine outputs of less than about 50 mL/hour. Before addressing the low urine output therapeutically and diagnostically, the patient's volume status and fluid balance must be assessed, and the Foley catheter is irrigated to ensure patency. If there are clots and an associated ball-and-valve effect at the catheter's internal ostium, the catheter should be removed while applying gentle suction in an attempt to capture the offending clot. Thereafter, a larger-sized catheter may be required. If the Foley catheter is patent and the patient is clearly hypervolemic (i.e., edematous, with congested pulmonary vasculature on chest radiograph or with elevated venous or wedge pressures), up to 200 mg of furosemide should be given intravenously. If the patient is judged to be hypovolemic, isotonic saline should be given in boluses of 250 to 500 mL, the response assessed; and the intravenous infusion repeated if necessary. If the patient is judged to be euvolemic, or if a confident clinical assessment cannot be made, a judicious isotonic saline challenge should be given, followed by a high dose of furosemide.

If a diuresis follows these maneuvers, urine output is again replaced milliliter for milliliter with half-normal saline. The volume challenge and furosemide dose may be repeated if urine volume falls off, but only after careful hemodynamic assessment. A constant infusion of furosemide in a dose of 5 to 10 mg/hour is employed in some centers. An algorithmic approach to the management of postoperative oliguria is suggested in Fig. 8.1.

Diagnostic Studies in Persistent Oliguria or Anuria

If the volume challenge, furosemide use, and volume replacement have no significant effect on the posttransplantation urinary output, diagnostic studies should be carried out to determine the cause of the early posttransplantation oliguric state (see Chapter 12). The urgency of this work-up depends somewhat on the clinical circumstances. If diuresis is anticipated, such as after a live donor kidney transplantation, diagnostic studies should be performed immediately—in the recovery room if necessary. If oliguria is anticipated, studies can usually be safely delayed by several hours.

The purpose of diagnostic studies is to confirm the presence of blood flow to the graft and the absence of a urine leak or obstruction. Blood flow studies are performed scintigraphically or by Doppler ultrasound. If the flow study reveals no demonstrable

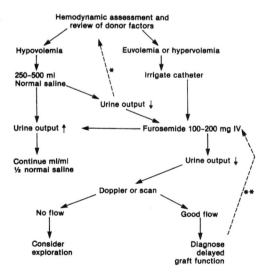

Fig. 8.1.   Algorithmic approach to posttransplantation oliguria. *The volume challenge can be repeated, but only after careful reassessment of the volume status and fluid balance; **Repeated doses of intravenous furosemide or furosemide "drips" may be valuable in patients whose urine output fluctuates. Persistent oliguria usually does not respond to a repeat dose.

blood flow, a prompt surgical reexploration is necessary to attempt to repair any vascular technical problem and diagnose hyperacute rejection. These kidneys are usually lost, however, and are removed during the second surgery.

If adequate blood flow is visible with the scintigraphic or Doppler studies, the possibility of ureteral obstruction or urinary leak needs to be considered and can be evaluated by the same imaging studies. In the first 24 hours after transplantation, as long as the Foley catheter has been providing good bladder drainage, the obstruction or leak is almost always at the ureterovesical junction and represents a technical problem that needs surgical correction. To avoid this complication, some surgeons place a ureteral stent at the time of transplantation. This can be attached to the Foley catheter and subsequently removed with the catheter when it is removed, or it can be removed cystoscopically several weeks after transplantation (see Chapter 7).

The Polyuric Patient

Occasionally, patients, usually recipients of live donor transplants, pass massive amounts of urine (more than 500 mL/hour) in the early posttransplantation period. Generally, these patients are hypervolemic, and urine replacement can be reduced stepwise to a less than milliliter-for-milliliter replacement. If a negative fluid balance is permitted, the volume status must be reassessed at frequent intervals and the fluid replacement returned to milliliter-for-milliliter replacement when the urine volume becomes more manageable or if the patient becomes relatively hypotensive. Potassium and calcium may need to be replaced in the polyuric patient.

Early Postoperative Bleeding

The possibility of surgical postoperative bleeding must be considered in any patient with a rapidly falling hematocrit and saline-resistant hypotension. If a drain is present, it may repeatedly fill with blood, and there may be a palpable or visible perinephric hematoma. Most hematomas spontaneously tamponade and do not require reoperation so long as the patient can be kept hemodynamically stable with crystalloid and colloid solutions and blood. The threshold for postoperative blood transfusion depends on the clinical circumstances. Older or diabetic patients who may have covert coronary artery disease should be transfused earlier rather than later. If possible, blood from cytomegalovirus (CMV)-negative donors should be given. At reoperation, an identifiable bleeding site is not uniformly discovered (see Chapter 7).

Postoperative Hemodialysis

If the patient is well dialyzed preoperatively and enters the operation normokalemic, early postoperative dialysis is usually not required. Oliguric patients, especially those with bleeding complications, may develop dangerous hyperkalemia and may require urgent therapy with intravenous calcium, bicarbonate, or insulin and glucose combinations. Sodium polystyrene sulfonate (Kayexalate) enemas should be avoided in the early postoperative period because they may cause colonic injury. Patients with persistent hyperkalemia should be dialyzed. A no-heparin protocol should be used, a bicarbonate bath is preferred, a biocompatible dialyzer should be used, and ultrafiltration should be avoided to prevent hypotension. A 2- or 3-hour dialysis treatment is usually adequate.

If the patient was receiving chronic ambulatory peritoneal dialysis before transplantation and the Tenckhoff catheter is in place, postoperative peritoneal dialysis may be possible. Generally, hemodialysis is preferred because of the possibility of a peritoneal leak or infection; a temporary hemodialysis catheter may be required for access.

THE FIRST POSTOPERATIVE WEEK

The first postoperative week is generally characterized by progressive improvement in the patient's overall condition in conjunction with steady improvement in kidney function. Most patients can leave the intensive care setting after 24 to 48 hours. Continued close observation of the urine output is still indicated, but fluid replacement need not be adjusted on an hourly basis and can be ordered on a 4- to 8-hour record of urine output. The urine volume is a useful indicator of kidney allograft function but may be misleading in patients who had appreciable urine output from their native kidneys. Mild fluctuation in urine volumes are acceptable, but a persistent drop in urine volume of greater than 50% or the sudden onset of oliguria or anuria must be promptly investigated (see Patients with Delayed Graft Function). The Foley catheter can usually be removed after 2 to 4 days, although a longer period may be wise for patients with a thin bladder wall or with prostatic hypertrophy. Patients should be observed to void frequently after catheter removal to avoid overdistention of the bladder. If there is concern regarding inadequate bladder emptying, the postvoid residual volume should be checked, and the Foley catheter may need to be replaced.

Patients should be ambulated within 24 hours of surgery and are usually started within 72 hours on a liquid diet and progress thereafter as tolerated. Abdominal distention and pain and the prolonged absence of bowel sounds require investigation by abdominal radiographs and consideration of the occasional occurrence of intraabdominal catastrophe. Incisional pain may persist throughout the first postoperative week but is usually mild. Severe pain or a change in the pain pattern should be thoroughly investigated to exclude rejection, perinephric hematoma, or a urine leak. Fever is not uncommon in the first week and is most commonly due to postoperative atelectasis. Opportunistic infections do not occur at this time, and extensive work-up of fever is usually not indicated. Persistent fever with no obvious infectious source may be a manifestation of unrecognized rejection.

The management of the transplant recipient in the first week is largely determined by the quality of function of the allograft. Patients typically exhibit one of three patterns of function: excellent graft function, slow graft function, or delayed graft function (DGF). At the end of the first week, the most powerful predictor of long-term graft function is the serum creatinine level.

Patients With Excellent Graft Function

In ideal circumstances, graft function and diuresis are excellent postoperatively, dialysis is not required, and the serum creatinine level declines rapidly so that patients achieve stable kidney function within the first posttransplantation week (the serum creatinine level may reach less than 2.5 mg/dL). Almost all the recipients of kidneys from live donors, as well as 30% to 50% of cadaveric kidney recipients, enjoy such a postoperative course. In patients with excellent early function, both the urine volume and serum creatinine levels are useful markers to monitor the occurrence of early rejection, calcineurin inhibitor toxicity, or other underlying pathologic events in the allograft.

If the course of these patients remains uneventful, it is not mandatory to perform routine imaging studies. Some transplantation centers elect to perform renal ultrasound and scintigraphic scans to provide baseline data.

Patients With Slow Graft Function

Patients with slow graft function or moderate graft dysfunction are nonoliguric and exhibit modest daily declines in serum creatinine levels. These patients do not usually require dialysis but do not have normal kidney function within the first postoperative week. In these patients, the urine volume and the daily serum creatinine concentration are useful markers to monitor the development of complications. Depending on the rate of decline in the serum creatinine concentration, it may be wise to obtain imaging studies to exclude the possibility that urine leak or partial obstruction is accounting for the slow improvement of function. Studies should certainly be performed if the serum creatinine concentration plateaus at a high level or begins to rise. Slow graft function is essentially a milder form of DGF, and its pathophysiology and clinical significance are similar.

Patients With Delayed Graft Function

Any newly transplanted kidney that does not function well can be said to be suffering from DGF. Most of these patients are oliguric, and in this regard, it is important to consider the patient's preoperative urine output, which, if large, can be a source of confusion because it cannot easily be differentiated from urine output from the transplant. Most patients with DGF require dialysis; using the need for dialysis alone to define DGF, however, may lead to underdiagnosis, particularly if there is some residual native kidney function. The frequency of DGF may be as low as 10% and as high as 50% in some programs. In recipients of transplants from living donors, this occurrence is exceptional and almost always portends a serious complication. Potential causes of DGF are listed in Table 8.2.

Posttransplantation Acute Tubular Necrosis

The terms DGF and ATN are often used interchangeably. It is wise to differentiate them. Not all DGF is due to ATN; covert accelerated acute rejection and technical complications such as vascular thrombosis account for some of the cases and cause permanent or so-called primary nonfunction. Posttransplantation ATN, as in ATN in the nontransplantation situation, is essentially a diagnosis of exclusion. When differentiated from other causes of DGF and when uncomplicated by the development of rejection, ATN appears, at least in the short term, to be a relatively benign condition that resolves spontaneously over days and sometimes

Table 8.2.   Differential diagnosis of delayed graft function

Acute tubular necrosis
Intravascular volume contraction
Arterial occlusion
Venous thrombosis
Ureteric obstruction
Catheter obstruction
Urine leak
Hyperacute rejection
Nephrotoxicity
Hemolytic-uremic syndrome

weeks. Recovery is usually first recognized by the patient and is heralded by a steady increase in urine output, diminution in intra-dialytic rise in creatinine concentration, and eventual steady improvement in kidney function.

The cadaveric kidney is subject to injury at every step along the path from donor death to organ procurement to surgical reanas-tomosis and the postoperative course (Table 8.3). Posttransplan-tation ATN is essentially an ischemic injury, which may be exag-gerated by synergistically acting immunologic and nephrotoxic insults. The transplanted kidney is particularly susceptible to *ischemia-reperfusion injury* as a result of the reintroduction of oxygen into tissues, with a high concentration of oxygen free rad-icals resulting from anaerobic metabolism. Superoxide anion and hydrogen peroxide are produced, which lead to lipid peroxidation of cell membranes. This process may be responsible for the com-monly occurring clinical sequence whereby an early posttrans-plantation diuresis is followed within hours by oliguria.

The oliguria of ATN is caused by a combination of diminished glomerular filtration rate (GFR), tubular obstruction with cellu-lar debris, back-leak of tubular fluid through damaged proximal tubular membranes, and increased interstitial pressure. Although blood flow to the renal cortex is reduced, there is a relatively greater reduction in GFR and tubular function that accounts for the com-monly encountered radiologic find of "good flow and poor excretion" on scintigraphic studies. The alterations in vascular resistance and increased intracapsular pressure produce the increased *resis-tive index* and reduced or reversed diastolic flow found on Doppler ultrasound (see Chapter 12).

ATN may have significant immunologic implications, which largely determine its effect on short-term and long-term graft prognosis (see Chapter 9). The ischemia reperfusion injury may cause up-regulation and exposure of histocompatability antigens, costimulatory molecules, and adhesion molecules (see Chapter 2). Nitric oxide, produced by the nitric oxide synthase enzymes, may provide the link between injury and immune activation. Activa-tion of inflammatory cytokines and growth factors (epidermal growth factor and transforming growth factor-beta) may facilitate the development of low-grade inflammation, which, in turn, facil-itates acute and chronic immune injury. The sequence is thus

Table 8.3.   Preoperative factors promoting ischemic injury in cadaveric renal transplantation

Premorbid factors
  Donor age
  Donor hypertension
  Donor cause of death
  Donor acute renal dysfunction
Preoperative donor management
  Brain-death stress
  Cardiac arrest
  Circulating catecholes
  Nephrotoxins
  Catabolic state
Procurement surgery
  Hypotension
  Traction on renal vessels
  Inadequate flushing and cooling
  Flushing solution
Kidney storage
  Prolonged cold storage
  Cold storage versus machine perfusion
  Prolonged anastomosis time
Recipient status
  Preoperative dialysis
  Recipient volume contraction
  Pelvic atherosclerosis
  Preformed antidonor antibodies
  Poor cardiac output

Modified from Shoskes DA, Halloran PF. Delayed graft function in renal transplantation. *J Urol* 1996;155:1831, with permission.

injury, inflammation, immune response, further injury. Immunologic factors may also make the kidney more susceptible to injury, as illustrated by the observation that patients receiving a second transplant with high levels of preformed antibodies are more likely to develop ATN.

The reported effect of DGF on long-term graft survival and function has been the subject of much controversy. Some studies report little or no effect, whereas others report a greater than 20% reduction in 1-year graft survival when early graft function is impaired. Much of the discrepancy can probably be accounted for by failure to differentiate between ATN and other causes of delayed function. There are also degrees of ATN severity, and patients who require prolonged posttransplantation dialysis are clearly at increased risk for early graft loss. Kidneys with ATN that do not develop rejection appear to do as well in the short term as kidneys without ATN that do not develop rejection. Hence, it is the immunologic consequences of ATN that appear to be responsible for its prognostic significance. Highly matched kidneys may be less susceptible to the harmful affects of DGF presumably because ATN exposes the mismatched kidney to a more aggressive immune attack.

In addition to any acute or chronic repercussions of ATN, it also complicates patient management, and every attempt should be made to minimize its frequency and severity.

Prevention and Management

The fact that ATN is unusual in recipients of live donor transplants emphasizes the factors that need to be addressed if ATN is to be prevented in recipients of cadaveric kidneys. Programs that avoid the use of "marginal" kidneys and insist on short cold ischemia times can reduce their incidence of ATN to less than 5%. Many programs accept a higher incidence as an unavoidable consequence of the pressure to provide kidneys to the growing population of patients in need (see Chapter 1). There are also important financial implications to the development of posttransplantation ATN because the hospital stay is often prolonged and the immunosuppressive protocol used may be more expensive.

Some transplantation programs modify their immunosuppressive protocols in the presence of ATN, usually on the premise that cyclosporine or tacrolimus administration should be avoided or minimized in this situation (see Chapter 4). Avoidance of cyclosporine or tacrolimus may reduce the length of the oliguric period, but the incidence of DGF is not clearly lower with alternative protocols. Some programs routinely use antibody induction in the presence of anticipated or established DGF, and there is evidence that commencing the antibody infusion before the graft reperfusion may be beneficial, presumably because of suppression of adhesion and costimulatory molecule expression. Clinical trials of oxygen free radical scavengers, prostaglandin E analogues, pentoxyfylline, and monoclonal antibodies against adhesion molecules have not shown benefit. Clinical trials of the dopamine agonist fenoldopam are in progress.

DGF complicates management because it masks clinical detection of posttransplantation events. Graft thrombosis and acute rejection are difficult to detect in an anuric or oliguric patient, and a urine leak will not manifest itself if the kidney does not make urine! Thus, in this situation, there must be greater reliance on noninvasive imaging studies to assess the status of the allograft. Doppler ultrasound or scintigraphic scans should be performed at regular intervals to ensure maintenance of blood flow and to exclude urine leak and obstruction (see Chapter 12). Where available, fine-needle aspiration biopsy is particularly useful in this setting (see Chapter 13) because it allows repeated, minimally invasive monitoring of intragraft events. Core biopsy is performed at intervals in some centers to ensure that the diagnosis is indeed ATN and not covert rejection. Criteria for dialysis and dietary management during this period are the same as for any patient with postoperative end-stage renal failure, although particular care should be taken to avoid hypotension during dialysis, which may serve to perpetuate ischemic injury.

Rejection

Accelerated Acute Rejection

Accelerated rejection is due to presensitization and is mediated by antibodies to donor human leukocyte antigens (HLAs). The rejection occurs after an anamnestic response, and a critical level of antibodies is produced that results in a potentially irreversible vascular rejection. Accelerated rejection can occur immediately after transplantation (*hyperacute rejection*), or it may be delayed by several days. Patients are usually anuric or oliguric and often have fever and graft tenderness. The renal scan shows little or no uptake, and there may be evidence of intravascular coagulation. The differential diagnosis in this setting includes both arterial and venous thrombosis; however, patients with these vascular complications frequently do not have symptoms. Surgical exploration of the allograft may be indicated, and when in doubt, an intraoperative biopsy is performed to determine its viability. Patients may sometimes respond to aggressive treatment with plasmapheresis, OKT3, and intravenous immunoglobulin (see Chapter 4).

The pathology of accelerated acute rejection is discussed in Chapter 13. Because of assiduous attention to the pretransplantation crossmatch (see Chapter 3), it occurs rarely. A form of anti–HLA class I–mediated rejection has been described in which the pretransplantation crossmatch is negative yet becomes positive after transplantation. These patients are oliguric but have persistent blood flow. Histologic studies show absence of typical cell-mediated rejection but evidence of glomerular endothelial injury.

Early Cell-Mediated Rejection

Classic cell-mediated rejection can be detected in the latter part of the first transplantation week, although it typically occurs somewhat later. Recipients of one-haplotype–matched live donor transplants and patients who have had recent blood transfusions, especially those who receive donor-specific blood transfusions, may develop a reversible, cell-mediated rejection early in the first posttransplantation week. These cell-mediated rejections can be differentiated from accelerated humoral rejection by a renal scan, which shows decreased but persistent perfusion. If in doubt, a kidney biopsy may be indicated. Treatment of acute rejection is discussed in Chapter 4, and pathology is discussed in Chapter 13.

Nonimmunologic Causes of Graft Dysfunction

There are a variety of nonimmunologic causes of graft dysfunction in the first posttransplantation week. Technical vascular complications, such as renal artery or renal vein thrombosis, may result in abrupt loss of function. Urologic complications, such as obstruction, urine leaks from the ureteroneocystostomy, or necrosis of the ureter, can present with deterioration in kidney function, increased pain over the allograft, or drainage of fluid through the wound. The combination of Doppler ultrasound and scintigraphic scan can be extremely useful in determining the diagnosis. In cases of obstruction, an antegrade pyelogram provides the most accurate localization of the obstruction (see Chapter 12). In patients with a suspected urine leak associated with wound drainage, a prompt diagnosis can be made if the creatinine concentration of the fluid is greater than the simultaneously measured plasma level. Any excessive drainage from the incision or a surgical drain should be sent for creatinine estimation. Indigo carmine can also be injected intravenously and the presence of a leak confirmed by the blue color of the drainage.

The use of a calcineurin inhibitor during the first week after transplantation may result in abnormalities in graft function (see Chapter 4). The recovery from ATN may be delayed, and even in patients with excellent graft function, cyclosporine and tacrolimus can cause an abrupt deterioration in function that needs to be differentiated from early rejection or graft thrombosis. This response is most likely due to renal vasoconstriction and can be reversed by decreasing the calcineurin inhibitor dose.

Both cyclosporine and tacrolimus may be associated with a *hemolytic-uremic syndrome* (HUS) or *thrombotic microangiopathy* (see Chapters 4 and 13), and occasional cases have been described in patients receiving OKT3. HUS may be evident clinically by virtue of the typical laboratory findings of intravascular coagulation (e.g., thrombocytopenia, distorted erythrocytes, elevated lactic dehydrogenase levels) accompanied by an arteriolopathy and intravascular thrombi on transplant biopsy. Development of calcineurin inhibitor–induced HUS may be covert, however, and the laboratory findings may be inconsistent. The syndrome may occur soon after the introduction of the calcineurin inhibitor, but it also may be delayed; blood levels of cyclosporine and tacrolimus are not necessarily elevated. The initial transplant biopsy may also be misleading; thus, a high level of clinical suspicion is required. It is crucial to make the diagnosis because improvement in transplant function may follow discontinuation or reduction of the calcineurin inhibitor and institution of plasmapheresis.

Medical Management

Cardiovascular and hemodynamic stability remain extremely important during the first week after transplantation to ensure adequate perfusion of the allograft. Drugs that can alter intrarenal hemodynamics, such as angiotensin-converting enzyme (ACE) inhibitors or nonsteroidal antiinflammatory agents, should be avoided. Although control of hypertension during the first week after transplantation is important, tight control should be avoided to prevent episodes of hypotension. Calcium-channel blockers are effective and well-tolerated antihypertensive agents, and they have some theoretical and practical advantages over other agents (see Chapters 4 and 9) in the early posttransplant course.

Changes in immunosuppressive strategy during the first week after transplantation should be based as much as possible on the results of diagnostic studies. Combined therapeutic and diagnostic maneuvers can be useful on a short-term basis; for example, decrease in graft function after introduction of cyclosporine or tacrolimus may be managed by withholding or reducing the dose for 1 or 2 days. More aggressive pursuit of a definitive diagnosis with core kidney biopsy or angiogram should be considered in patients with significant risk factors, including highly sensitized individuals; patients who have had a previous, rapidly rejected kidney transplant; and patients who have native kidney diseases with a high risk for early recurrence. Generally speaking, core kidney biopsies should be avoided in the first week because there may be a greater incidence of bleeding. Finally, particular attention should be paid to the nutritional support of these highly catabolic patients (see Chapter 18), and ambulation and physical activity should be encouraged in anticipation of discharge.

Care of the Surgical Incision

With modern surgical techniques and prophylactic perioperative antibiotics, significant wound infections and problems have become uncommon after transplantation. Obese patients are more susceptible to wound dehiscence and infection. A serosanguineous incisional ooze is not uncommon after transplantation, and if it is profuse enough that it can be collected into a syringe, its creatinine concentration should be measured to ensure that it is not a urine leak. Staples and sutures are usually removed after 12 to 14 days.

THE FIRST TWO POSTOPERATIVE MONTHS

The next 2-month period is characterized by the transition from inpatient to outpatient management. Most stable patients are discharged 4 to 14 days after surgery. Transplantation centers vary with respect to their enthusiasm for early discharge, and logistical issues, such as travel distance to the transplantation center, the availability of a helpmate, and the frequency of outpatient clinics, need to be considered. Before discharge, it is crucial to counsel the patient about his or her medications. The patient should be familiar with their names, doses, and purposes as well as their side effects and possible drug interactions, especially with calcineurin inhibitors. Diet, exercise, and wound care are discussed. The patient should be encouraged to ambulate and to begin light aerobic exercise, such as walking or biking. Premenopausal, sexually active women must receive contraceptive counseling because many women presume, often mistakenly, that they are still infertile. Patients must be taught to recognize the symptoms and signs of infection and rejection. It is wise to instruct patients to maintain a diary of their vital signs, urine output, and medications, although this can be discontinued after the first few weeks. Patients should be warned and prepared for the possibility of readmission to the hospital.

Discharge from the hospital often engenders anxious anticipation in both the patient and family, and empathic counseling should be available on an informal and formal level.

Clinical Course

By the second posttransplantation week, the graft function of most patients with DGF due to ATN begins to improve. Some patients remain oliguric for several weeks, and constant surveillance for covert rejection and urologic complications is required (see Patients With Delayed Graft Function). Patients who still require dialysis can receive it on an outpatient basis.

Because many of the patients are at home during this period, close attention to the development of allograft pain, fever, weight gain, or decreased urine output is important. If any of these signs or symptoms occur, patients are instructed to contact the transplantation team, whose representatives must be available on a 24-hour basis. Patients without complications should be seen as outpatients at least twice weekly for the first month and weekly for the next month. During each outpatient visit, a routine physical examination is required to assess the volume status, adjust blood pressure medications, and examine the allograft to detect enlargement, tenderness, or the presence of a new bruit. Routine laboratory work should include a urinalysis, complete blood count, plasma creatinine and blood urea nitrogen levels, and an electrolyte panel that includes phosphate and calcium levels. Hepatic enzyme levels should be checked regularly.

At each clinic visit, the medications should be carefully reviewed with the patient, and changes, particularly of critical immunosuppressive medications, should be explained with great care. At this stage, the patient is often taking a multitude of medications: immunosuppressives, antihypertensives, and infection prophylactic agents. Every attempt should be made to simplify the therapeutic regimen and reemphasize the importance of adherence. Meticulous attention to detail is crucial in this posttransplantation period, and early intervention is necessary to minimize morbidity and mortality.

Well patients should gradually return to normal activity, and some patients will wish to return to work after 4 to 6 weeks. A 3-month leave of absence from work is legitimate. Regular, graduated aerobic exercise should be encouraged, and normal social and family life should resume.

Differentiation of Infection, Rejection, and Cyclosporine Toxicity

The accurate recognition and treatment of infection, rejection, and cyclosporine toxicity and their differentiation from surgical posttransplantation complications is a constant concern in the early posttransplantation period. The treatment of common posttransplantation infections is discussed in Chapter 10 and the treatment of rejection in Chapter 4.

Fever

Fever may indicate either rejection or infection. Infection during the first month is rarely due to opportunistic organisms and usually results from bacterial pathogens in the wound, urinary tract, or respiratory tract. CMV infection may mimic acute rejection; it occurs in about 20% to 30% of patients 1 to 6 months after transplantation (see Chapter 10), and its possible presence needs to be constantly considered, particularly in recipients of kidneys from CMV-positive donors.

Posttransplantation fever must always be taken seriously. Acute rejection is often present with seemingly innocuous flu-like symptoms or upper respiratory tract infection. The fever and the symptoms consistently and rapidly resolve when the rejecting patient receives pulse steroids (see Chapter 4). Rejection in patients receiving calcineurin inhibitors is often not associated with fever because of impaired production of cytokines. Febrile patients should have a chest radiograph and be fully cultured. They usually require readmission to the hospital or close outpatient follow-up.

Elevated Creatinine Level

Measurement of the serum creatinine level is a simple, inexpensive diagnostic test that lies at the core of early posttransplantation management. Its significance is not lost on patients, who often wait in trepidation at each clinic visit for their creatinine "verdict." Large elevations in plasma creatinine concentration (i.e., greater than 25% from baseline) almost always indicate a significant, potentially graft-endangering event. Smaller elevations may represent laboratory variability, and recognition of their significance is sometimes more of an art form than a science! If there is any question regarding a small asymptomatic rise in the plasma creatinine concentration, the test should be repeated within 48 hours, and the directional change usually facilitates its clinical evaluation.

Anatomic or surgical problems must be excluded before "medical" diagnoses are made to explain deteriorating graft function. Doppler ultrasound is invaluable (see Chapter 12), and it should be performed before any major therapeutic intervention. Scintigraphic scans are nonspecific in the setting of ATN, rejection, or drug toxicity and are of limited diagnostic value at this stage.

The gold-standard diagnostic tool is either the kidney biopsy or fine-needle aspiration biopsy (see Chapter 13). The timing and frequency of kidney biopsies vary between centers. One clinical approach to graft dysfunction is to make a therapeutic intervention empirically based on the clinical presentation and laboratory values. A favorable response confirms the diagnosis, but a lack of a response likely requires a tissue diagnosis. A tissue diagnosis of rejection should always precede a course of OKT3 or polyclonal antibodies. This policy is wise because unanticipated diagnoses, such as nephrotoxicity, CMV infection, posttransplantation lymphoma, or polyomavirus infection, may be made, and such findings require reduction of immunosuppression rather than intensification.

A more precise and increasingly routine approach to graft dysfunction is to perform a kidney biopsy whenever the serum creatinine level increases over the baseline value.

A 25% increase is usually enough to trigger a response that recognizes the observation that clinical diagnosis of graft dysfunction is unreliable. Therapy is then based on the histologic findings. In each transplantation center, a protocol should be developed that logically incorporates both noninvasive and invasive techniques to evaluate allograft dysfunction during this time period.

Protocol Biopsies

Up to 30% of clinically stable patients may experience *subclinical rejection* episodes that do not produce overt renal dysfunction or elevation in serum creatinine values. Subclinical rejections are typically mild by pathologic criteria (Banff type 1; see Chapter 13). Recognition of subclinical rejection requires uniform performance of protocol biopsies at prespecified posttransplantation intervals. The approach to treatment and the long-term effect of these episodes are unresolved, although a prospective study has shown that treatment with corticosteroids may lead to a reduction in the incidence of clinical rejections and improvement in long-term function and histology. Protocol biopsies performed for clinical purposes have not yet become standard practice in most transplantation centers, although they represent a potentially valuable approach to management.

Calcineurin Inhibitor Levels

Despite nearly two decades of experience with cyclosporine and a decade of experience with tacrolimus, there remains a lack of uniformity regarding the use of trough blood levels in routine patient management. Guidelines for dosage are provided in Chapter 4. It is clear that high blood levels of these agents do not preclude a diagnosis of rejection and that nephrotoxicity may occur at apparently low levels. Nephrotoxicity and rejection may coexist. With these provisos, however, it is fair to presume initially that a patient with deteriorating graft function and a very high cyclosporine or tacrolimus level is probably suffering from nephrotoxicity and that a patient with deteriorating graft function and very low levels is probably undergoing acute rejection. If the appropriate clinical therapeutic response does not have a salutary effect on graft function, the clinical premise needs to be reconsidered. Acute calcineurin inhibitor toxicity usually resolves within 24 to 48 hours of a dose reduction. Progressive elevation of the plasma creatinine level, even in the face of persistently high drug levels, is highly suggestive of rejection. Acute rejection may present as dramatic deterioration of graft function, whereas it is unusual for calcineurin inhibitor toxicity to produce a greater than 50% elevation of the plasma creatinine level.

Graft Tenderness
Graft tenderness on palpation in the first few days after transplantation is usually an innocuous finding related to recent surgery. In a stable patient, it is important to palpate the graft regularly to provide a clinical baseline for future changes. The development of graft tenderness in a previously pain-free, stable patient is a significant symptom that needs to be evaluated. A tender, swollen graft in a patient with a rising creatinine concentration and fever usually indicates rejection, although the possibility of acute pyelonephritis must be considered. Calcineurin inhibitor toxicity and CMV infection do not produce graft tenderness. Excruciating localized perinephric pain is usually due to a urine leak.

Fluid Retention and Oliguria
Both rejection and cyclosporine toxicity may produce weight gain and edema due to impaired GFR and avid tubular sodium reabsorption. Mild peripheral edema is common in stable patients receiving cyclosporine and usually responds to oral furosemide. Both acute rejection and calcineurin inhibitor toxicity can produce graft dysfunction in the absence of oliguria. Oliguria is common in acute rejection but makes a diagnosis of drug toxicity unlikely.

Common Laboratory Abnormalities

Urinalysis
Examination of the urine for the presence of red and white blood cells, bacteria, and protein should be part of the routine outpatient visit. Pyuria can indicate either rejection or infection, and the urine should be cultured. The presence of proteinuria may herald the early recurrence of the primary kidney disease or chronic rejection; in the case of patients at risk for recurrent focal sclerosis, the finding of proteinuria is an indication for graft biopsy because plasmapheresis may be indicated (see Chapter 9). Trace or "one plus" proteinuria, amounting to less than 500 mg/day,

is usually not a morbid finding. Transient microscopic hematuria is common after transplantation but requires urologic evaluation if it is persistent.

Hyperkalemia

Elevated serum potassium levels are common in the first few posttransplantation months in patients receiving calcineurin inhibitors. The mechanism of the hyperkalemia is discussed in Chapter 4. So long as the patient is not oliguric and kidney function is good, the hyperkalemia is rarely dangerous and can usually be managed safely with dietary potassium restriction and diuretics. Care should be taken to avoid concomitant use of drugs that may further exaggerate hyperkalemia, such as ACE inhibitors, betablockers, and oral phosphate supplements.

Hypophosphatemia, Hypercalcemia, and Hypomagnesemia

The mechanisms of posttransplantation hypophosphatemia and abnormalities of divalent ion metabolism are discussed in Chapter 9. Profound hypophosphatemia may develop in the first few weeks after transplantation, particularly in patients with excellent graft function. Phosphate supplements, in a dose of 250 to 500 mg three times daily, should be given if the serum phosphate levels fall below 2 mg/dL (see Chapter 18). Phosphate supplementation is usually adequate to control mild posttransplantation hypercalcemia. Magnesium supplements should probably be given for cyclosporine- or tacrolimus-induced hypomagnesemia if the serum magnesium level falls below 1.5 mg/dL, although they are often ineffective.

Hyperchloremic Metabolic Acidosis

Proximal, distal, and type IV renal tubular acidosis have been described after transplantation, and mild hyperchloremia and hypobicarbonatemia are common. Renal tubular acidosis may be a manifestation of immune-mediated impairment of hydrogen ion secretion, of acute or chronic interstitial renal disease impairing tubular ammonia secretion, of parathyroid hormone-induced reduction in proximal tubular bicarbonate reabsorption, of cyclosporine-induced impairment in tubular aldosterone responsiveness, and of tacrolimus use. The ensuing metabolic acidosis is usually not severe enough that it requires therapeutic intervention, and the finding is too nonspecific to be of much diagnostic value.

Anemia, Leukopenia, and Thrombocytopenia

Profound anemia at the time of transplantation is much less common in the present erythropoietin era. Erythropoietin is usually discontinued at the time of transplantation, and the hematocrit level may fall after transplantation and then rise toward normal over weeks and months. Many patients are iron deficient after transplantation, and assessment of iron stores with repletion of iron intravenously, when necessary, may be more effective than prolonged oral iron repletion (see Chapter 18). Resistant anemia needs to be evaluated, with the possibility of gastrointestinal bleeding high on the differential diagnosis list. Patients receiving azathioprine often develop macrocytosis, and all the antiproliferative drugs (e.g., azathioprine, mycophenolate mofetil, sirolimus) may produce varying degrees of pancytopenia (see Chapter 4). A complete blood count should be performed at least weekly in the early posttransplantation period and less frequently with time. In the absence of clinical evidence of infection, thrombocytopenia and leukopenia are usually drug related. Because the calcineurin inhibitors generally do not cause hematologic abnormalities, it is usually safe to continue them and reduce the dose or discontinue other components of the immunosuppressive regimen for a short time, until the abnormality resolves. If leukopenia is severe, granulocyte-stimulating factor can be given and appears to be safe in the posttransplantation period. Posttransplantation polycythemia is discussed in Chapter 9.

Transaminitis

Elevation of the levels of the hepatic transaminases associated with discrete alterations in hepatic function is common after transplantation and is usually a transient and self-limiting manifestation of drug toxicity. More severe manifestations of liver disease may require further investigation and modification of the immunosuppressive regimen (see Chapter 11).

SELECTED READINGS

Al-Awwa IA, Hariharan S, First RM. Importance of allograft biopsy in renal transplant recipients: correlation between clinical and histological diagnosis. *Am J Kidney Dis* 1998;31:S15.

Danovitch GM, Nast CC. Diagnosis and therapy of graft dysfunction. In: Owen WF, Pereira BJ, Sayegh MH, eds. *Dialysis and transplantation.* Philadelphia: WB Saunders, 2000;31:568.

De Fijter JW, Bruijn JA. Acute nonoliguric renal failure after renal transplantation. *Am J Kidney Dis* 1999;33:166.

Jassem W, Roake J. The molecular and cellular basis of reperfusion injury following organ transplantation. *Transplant Rev* 1998;12:14.

Katznelson S, Wilkinson AW, Rosenthal TR, et al. Cyclosporine-induced hemolytic-uremic syndrome: factors that obscure its diagnosis. *Transplant Proc* 1994;26:2608–2609.

Meehan SM, Siegel CT, Aronson AJ, et al. The relationship of untreated borderline infiltrates by the Banff criteria to acute rejection in renal allografts biopsies. *J Am Soc Nephrol* 1999;10:1806.

Nickerson P, Jeffery J, Gough JJ, et al. Beneficial effects of treatment of early subclinical rejection: a randomized study. *J Am Soc Nephrol* 1999;10:1801.

Pascual M, Vallhonrat H, Cosimi B, et al. The clinical usefulness of the renal allograft biopsy in the cyclosporine era. *Transplantation* 1999;67:737.

Shoskes DA, Halloran PF. Delayed graft function in renal transplantation. *J Urol* 1996;155:1831.

9

Long-Term Posttransplantation Management and Complications

Bertram L. Kasiske

CURRENT SUCCESS AND FUTURE CHALLENGE

The care of renal transplant recipients can be roughly divided into early and late posttransplantation periods. This division, although somewhat arbitrary, is justified by the facts that episodes of acute allograft rejection are most common in the first few months after transplantation and that relatively large amounts of potent immunosuppressive medications, with their resultant complications, must be administered (see Chapter 4). For patients who survive the first few months with a functioning allograft, doses of immunosuppression can then usually be reduced. Most statistical analyses use 12 months to define the onset of the late posttransplantation period. For example, the *United Network for Organ Sharing (UNOS) Scientific Registry* usually reports short-term graft survival and graft survival beyond the first year (half-life) separately as major posttransplantation outcomes.

The incidence of acute rejection and early graft failure has declined dramatically as a result of new immunosuppressive medications (see Chapter 4). One-year graft survival is now 85% to 90% in most transplantation centers. This success has occurred despite the fact that the risk for graft failure has increased with the acceptance of transplantation candidates who are older and have more cardiovascular disease and other risk factors (see Chapter 6). In addition, the shortage of cadaveric organs has encouraged centers to accept older, "marginal" kidneys that also add to the risk for graft failure (see Chapters 3 and 5). It would appear, therefore, that the new immunosuppressive regimens have helped overcome this increased risk, reducing the rate of early graft failure.

Declines in early graft loss have, unfortunately, not been matched by equivalent declines in the rate of late renal allograft failure. The rate of late renal allograft failure is often measured by graft half-life. Allograft half-life is the time that one half of the patients who survive beyond the first posttransplantation year are still alive with a functioning kidney. Therefore, half-life is determined by both the rate of death and return to dialysis (or retransplantation). There has been an increase in renal allograft half-life in the past several years (see Chapter 3, Fig. 3.5). For patients receiving cadaveric renal transplants in 1988, the half-life was 7.6 years; whereas for those receiving cadaveric kidneys in 1995, the half-life had increased to 11.6 years. However, the half-life of two-haplotype–matched living-related kidney recipients over this same time period was 22.8 years. This suggests that we have a long way to go before the half-life for cadaveric renal transplants can be considered optimal.

This chapter is divided into two main sections. Part I reviews the causes of late renal allograft failure and explores the pathogenesis of some of the more common causes of late graft failure. Part II offers a practical guide to the prevention of graft failure and other major complications of the late posttransplantation period. Emphasis is placed on prevention. Posttransplantation liver disease is discussed in Chapter 11, and posttransplantation infectious diseases are discussed in Chapter 10.

PART I. CAUSES OF LATE ALLOGRAFT FAILURE

DEFINING THE CAUSE OF ALLOGRAFT FAILURE

It is more difficult to define the cause of allograft failure than it may seem. Allograft failure is usually defined either by the patient's death or by the patient's need to undertake new treatment for end-stage renal disease (i.e., chronic dialysis or retransplantation). Making a distinction between these two categories of allograft failure may have important implications for understanding how to prevent allograft failure. However, making the distinction may sometimes be difficult. For example, a patient with severe acute rejection may temporarily require dialysis support and may die of complications of immunosuppression before the rejection can be reversed. Did this patient die with a functioning graft, or was the graft lost because of acute rejection? Studies have shown, however, that most patients who die with a functioning kidney have good renal function. In these cases, attempts to understand the pathogenesis of allograft failure should focus on understanding the cause of death and its pathogenesis.

In the United States, *death with a functioning allograft* accounts for 42.5% of all graft loss. The goal of renal transplantation should be to have every patient die with a kidney that functions well. Unfortunately, most deaths that now occur with a functioning allograft are premature and are at least theoretically preventable. Most of the premature deaths that occur in the late posttransplantation period can be directly or indirectly attributed to the events that initially led to end-stage renal disease and the consequences thereof (see Chapter 1) and to allograft dysfunction or the immunosuppression used to prevent or treat allograft rejection. The three most common causes of death in the late posttransplantation period are cardiovascular disease (CVD), infection, and cancer (Fig. 9.1).

CAUSES OF DEATH AFTER TRANSPLANTATION

Cardiovascular Disease

Atherosclerotic CVD kills patients by causing myocardial infarction, congestive heart failure, stroke, ischemic colitis, and peripheral vascular disease. In the case of ischemic colitis and peripheral vascular disease, the terminal event may be infection (e.g., sepsis from a perforated cecum or cellulitis). To understand how to prevent posttransplantation CVD deaths and complications, it is crucial to define the etiologic risk factors (Table 9.1). Identifying risk factors is important for two reasons. Some risk factors can be modified, and for some of these, there is strong evidence from studies in the general population that intervention improves survival. It is also important, however, to identify risk factors that cannot be mod-

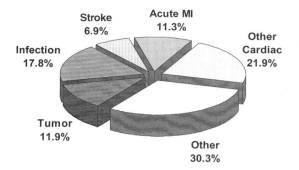

Fig. 9.1.   Causes of death after renal transplantation. Data are from the United States Renal Data System 1998 Annual Data Report from a cohort of all patients transplanted between 1994 and 1996.

ified because these risk factors help to identify high-risk patients who can be targeted for screening (and in some cases, intervention with revascularization) as well as for treatment of other modifiable risk factors.

Patients with pretransplantation CVD are at increased risk for posttransplantation CVD complications. Such patients should be targeted for aggressive management of modifiable CVD risk factors. Atherosclerosis is often diffuse; therefore, it should not be surprising that patients with a history of cerebral vascular disease (e.g., ischemic strokes) are at increased risk for ischemic heart dis-

Table 9.1.   Risk factors for posttransplantation cardiovascular disease

Risk Factor	Strength of Evidence
Pretransplantation cardiovascular disease	++++
Diabetes (including posttransplantation diabetes)	++++
Cigarette smoking	+++
Hyperlipidemia	+++
Hypertension	++
Platelet and coagulation abnormalities	++
Allograft dysfunction and rejection	++
Hypoalbuminemia	++
Erythrocytosis	+
Oxygen free radicals	+
Infections	+
Increased homocysteine	+

ease (e.g., myocardial infarctions) and *vice versa*. Although pre-transplantation CVD greatly increases the risk for posttransplantation CVD complications, much of the risk for CVD in the late posttransplantation period is acquired after transplantation. It is a mistake to adopt a nihilistic attitude and use the presence of pretransplantation CVD as an excuse to avoid aggressive risk factor management after transplantation. Rather, the opposite approach should be taken: to identify and intervene aggressively in high-risk patients.

Diabetes is the most common cause of end-stage renal disease leading to transplantation, and diabetes is arguably the most important risk factor for posttransplantation CVD. Both type 1 and type 2 diabetes greatly increase the risk for ischemic heart disease, cerebral vascular disease, and peripheral vascular disease. Diabetic control may become more difficult after transplantation, and patients with type 2 diabetes often become insulin requiring (see Chapter 6).

About 20% of non-diabetic patients develop hyperglycemia after transplantation, and 5% to 10% require therapy with oral hypoglycemic agents or insulin. Older patients, obese patients, blacks, and patients with a strong family history of diabetes are at higher risk for posttransplantation diabetes. Diabetes developed after transplantation has been shown to have a similar effect on morbidity and graft survival as pretransplantation diabetes. Corticosteroids, cyclosporine, and tacrolimus all contribute to glucose intolerance (see Chapter 4).

Numerous epidemiologic studies in the general population have shown that cigarette smoking is an important, modifiable risk factor for CVD. Studies have reported that smoking is as prevalent in renal transplant recipients as it is in the general population. These same studies have shown that cigarette smoking is linked to CVD in the late posttransplantation period.

Countless epidemiologic studies and numerous large, randomized, controlled trials in the general population have shown that hyperlipidemia causes CVD. The evidence is strongest that elevations in low-density lipoprotein cholesterol (LDL) contribute to the pathogenesis of atherosclerosis; however, evidence is also very strong that low levels of high-density lipoprotein cholesterol (HDL) contribute to CVD risk as well. In addition, there is growing evidence that hypertriglyceridemia is an independent risk factor for CVD in the general population. A number of studies have also found correlations between lipoprotein(a) [Lp(a)] and CVD, although there are not yet effective means to lower Lp(a). Several studies have found the same associations between lipoprotein elevations and CVD in renal transplant recipients that have been found in the general population. The most important cause of hyperlipidemia after renal transplantation is immunosuppressive medication. Corticosteroids, cyclosporine, and sirolimus all cause elevations in lipid levels to varying degrees (see Chapter 4). Other causes include diet, genetic predisposition, proteinuria, and possibly decreased renal function.

Data from several epidemiologic and interventional studies have shown that hypertension contributes to CVD in the general population, although it has proved difficult to demonstrate that hypertension specifically causes CVD in renal transplant recipients. This may be due in part to the fact that most transplantation physicians treat blood pressure aggressively. Certainly, there is no reason to believe that the relationship between hypertension and CVD is different in renal transplant recipients than in the general population. Corticosteroids, cyclosporine, and tacrolimus can all elevate blood pressure after renal transplantation. Graft dysfunction also contributes to hypertension. Occasionally, allograft renal artery stenosis causes hypertension and graft dysfunction (see Chapter 7). Several studies have also found that the presence of the native kidneys is associated with increased blood pressure after renal transplantation.

Studies in the general population have implicated various platelet and coagulation abnormalities in the pathogenesis of CVD events. Evidence from randomized controlled trials suggests that low-dose aspirin prevents recurrent CVD events in patients with known coronary artery disease. Less certain is the role of aspirin in primary prevention. Several studies have shown that renal transplant recipients have a hypercoagulable state, and some studies have linked coagulation abnormalities to CVD in transplant recipients. Not surprisingly, many of these coagulation abnormalities have been attributed to immunosuppressive agents.

Observational studies have found that allograft dysfunction is also associated with subsequent CVD complications. Decreased renal function and proteinuria can contribute to other risk factors, such as hyperlipidemia, hypertension, and hyperhomocysteinemia. Allograft dysfunction is also more common in patients who have had acute rejection and have been treated with higher doses of immunosuppressive medications known to affect several CVD risk factors adversely. In some studies, however, allograft dysfunction has been an independent risk factor for CVD. It has been speculated that allograft rejection may be associated with a systemic, inflammatory response that may contribute to the pathogenesis of CVD; at least one study has shown that hypoalbuminemia is an independent risk factor for posttransplantation CVD, and chronic inflammation may reduce serum albumin levels. Atherosclerosis could be both a cause and an effect of chronic inflammation.

Erythrocytosis is common after renal transplantation, and hematocrit has been associated with CVD events in at least one study. Although atherosclerosis could theoretically contribute to hematocrit elevations, it is at least equally plausible that a high hematocrit could contribute to changes in blood viscosity and thereby lead to vascular thrombosis.

Although epidemiologic studies have often reported an association between antioxidant vitamin usage and CVD, more convincing clinical data supporting a role for oxygen free radicals in the pathogenesis of CVD have been elusive. In particular, most large, randomized, controlled trials in the general population have failed to show that antioxidant vitamins protect against CVD events. Some evidence suggests that oxygen free radicals may be more prevalent, and antioxidant defenses may more often be compromised in renal transplant recipients than in the general population.

A number of epidemiologic studies in the general population have implicated various infections, including cytomegalovirus (CMV) infection, in the pathogenesis of CVD. In addition, some studies have found evidence for the presence of infectious agents in atherosclerotic lesions. It is certainly plausible, however, that individuals with CVD may be more susceptible to infection, and infectious agents may be playing an "innocent bystander" role in systemic atherosclerosis. One study found that heart transplant recipients treated with CMV prophylaxis had less coronary artery disease. On the other hand, few studies have found an association between CMV or other infections and CVD in renal transplant recipients, despite the fact that the prevalence of such infections is very high. Thus, this interesting hypothesis remains unproved.

A number of observational studies have found a strong association between increased levels of plasma homocysteine and CVD in the general population. It has been suggested that homocysteine may cause vascular endothelial damage and thereby lead to atherosclerosis. Large, multicenter, controlled trials are being conducted to determine whether lowering homocysteine will reduce the incidence of CVD events in the general population. The results of these trials will be particularly important for renal transplant recipients because elevated levels of homocysteine are more common in transplant recipients than in the general population. This is no doubt largely a result of the fact that renal dysfunction itself, which is common in allograft recipients, elevates plasma homocysteine.

Infection

Infection is an inevitable consequence of immunosuppression (see Chapter 10). Unlike CVD that is linked to immunosuppressive medications through the adverse (nonimmunosuppressive) consequences of specific agents, infection is directly attributable to the overall level of immunosuppression. Figure 10.1 in Chapter 10 provides a timeline for the major types of posttransplantation infection. CMV infection is arguably the most common infection after renal transplantation. Infection occurs most often in the early posttransplantation period when patients are most immunosuppressed. Fortunately, the availability of effective antiviral therapy with ganciclovir has greatly reduced its lethal potential. Occasionally, patients will develop chronic retinitis from CMV infection, but this is rarely life-threatening. Chronic liver disease, usually due to viral hepatitis, is an important cause of posttransplantation mortality (see Chapter 11). The hepatitis C virus has now replaced the hepatitis B virus as the most common cause of chronic hepatitis after renal transplantation. Influenza is an important cause of preventable morbidity and mortality after transplantation. A number of other viral infections are associated with malignancies in the late posttransplantation period (Table 9.2).

Bacterial infections are common in the late posttransplantation period because of underlying risk factors and immunosuppression. As previously discussed, the high prevalence of peripheral vascular disease among diabetic patients and other transplant recipients greatly increases the risk for cellulitis and life-threatening bacterial sepsis. Ischemic bowel disease can also lead to septic shock and death. Bladder dysfunction, caused by diabetes and other anatomic urologic abnormalities, combine with immunosuppression to increase the risk for urinary tract infections and gram-negative

Table 9.2.   Infections in the late posttransplantation period

Viral

Chronic hepatitis (hepatitis B and C viruses)
Influenza (influenza A and B viruses)
Lymphoproliferative disorders (Epstein-Barr virus)
Kaposi's sarcoma (herpesvirus 8)
Squamous cell carcinomas (papillomaviruses)

Bacterial

Urinary tract infections (gram-negative organisms)
Intraabdominal sepsis (gram-negative organisms)
Cellulitis (gram-positive organisms)
Pneumonia (gram-positive organisms)
Tuberculosis (*Mycobacterium tuberculosis*)

Opportunistic

Pneumocystis pneumonia (*Pneumocystis carinii*)
Toxoplasmosis (*Toxoplasma gondii*)
Nocardiosis (*Nocardia* sp.)
Aspergillosis (*Aspergillus* sp.)
Listeriosis (*Listeria monocytogenes*)
Candidiasis (*Candida* sp.)
Cryptococcosis (*Cryptococcus neoformans*)
Histoplasmosis (*Histoplasma capsulatum*)
Coccidiomycosis (*Coccidiodes immitis*)
Blastomycosis (*Blastomyces dermatitidis*)

---

bacterial sepsis. Tuberculosis is common in the late posttransplantation period, especially among high-risk populations.

Several other, potentially life-threatening, opportunistic infections occur sporadically but are nevertheless relatively common in the late posttransplantation period. Examples include infection with *Pneumocystis carinii, Toxoplasma gondii, Nocardia* species, *Aspergillus* species, *Listeria monocytogenes, Candida* species, *Cryptococcus neoformans, Histoplasma capsulatum, Coccidioides immitis,* and *Blastomyces dermatitidis.* Infection with opportunistic organisms can present as pneumonia, meningitis, cellulitis, osteomyelitis, or generalized sepsis. Diagnosis requires a high index of suspicion and an aggressive diagnostic approach.

Malignancy

Malignancies are common after renal transplantation; they are also more common in chronic dialysis patients. Much of our knowledge of the malignancy–transplantation association has come from large registries, such as the *Cincinnati Transplant Tumor Registry* under the leadership of the late Dr. Israel Penn and the *Australia–New Zealand Dialysis and Transplantation Registry.* These data indicate that the incidence of nonskin malignancies in renal transplant recipients is 3.5-fold higher than that of age-matched controls. This increase can be attributed to an increased incidence of most tumors (Table 9.3). However, the observed-to-expected incidence is not uniform among different types of tumors. Some tumors, such as breast cancer in women and prostate cancer in men, do not appear to be more common among renal transplant recipients than among the general population. The differences in the observed-to-expected incidence of different malignancies are consistent with the notion that more than one mechanism may explain the increased incidence of cancer after renal transplantation.

Some malignancies are undoubtedly caused by viral infections. Viruses that may otherwise reside in the host without untoward complications may cause potentially lethal malignant transformations in immunocompromised renal transplant recipients. Some of the tumors that occur with the highest incidence compared with the general population have possible viral causes. For example, the posttransplantation lymphoproliferative disorders (PTLD) have been linked to infection with the Epstein-Barr virus (EBV; see later). The human herpesvirus-8 has been implicated in the high incidence of Kaposi's sarcoma after renal transplantation. Human papillomaviruses have been implicated in the pathogenesis of squamous cell cancer of skin, vulva, vagina, and possibly uterine cervix. Liver cancer may be caused by chronic infection with hepatitis B and C viruses.

Urinary malignancies may occur more frequently among renal transplant recipients because renal disease may sometimes be associated with malignant and premalignant conditions. Similarly, an increased risk for the rarely occurring parathyroid cancer may be attributable to long-standing renal disease and events occurring before transplantation. Other mechanisms are undoubtedly at play. Immunosuppressive agents may damage DNA and lead to malignant transformation of cells and may also inhibit normal immune surveillance and thereby allow cells that have undergone malignant transformation to grow and divide unchecked. In an animal model, cyclosporine has been shown to promote cancer progression by a direct transforming growth factor-beta (TGF-beta)–related cellular effect that is independent of the host's immune cells.

Malignancies may occur at any time after transplantation. However, some are more than likely than others to occur early after transplantation. These include PTLD (relatively common) and Kaposi's sarcoma (relatively rare). Most other tumors tend to occur later. In the Australia–New Zealand Dialysis and Transplantation Registry, the mean time to the diagnosis of nonHodgkin's lymphomas (PTLD) was 8 to 10 years after transplantation. Moreover, the incidence of malignant tumors continues to increase throughout the late posttransplantation period. The cumulative incidence of nonskin malignancies is about 33% by 30 years after transplantation. The cumulative incidence of skin cancer is much higher, but few patients die of skin cancer after renal transplantation.

Few studies have systematically examined risk factors for post-transplantation malignancies. Most investigators believe that the cumulative effects of immunosuppression *per se,* rather than any particular agent or agents, is principally responsible for the

Table 9.3.   **Malignancies after renal transplantation**[a]

Type of Malignancy (No. Reported)	Risk Ratio (95% CI)[b]
Non-Hodgkin's lymphoma (83)	7.40 (5.90–9.18)[c]
Central nervous system lymphoma (17)	>1000 (939–>10,000)[c]
Hodgkin's disease (2)	1.23 (1.38–4.43)[c]
Leukemia (27)	3.60 (2.37–5.23)[c]
Multiple myeloma (6)	1.92 (0.70–4.17)
Kaposi's sarcoma (18)	85.7 (50.8–135.5)[c]
Buccal cavity (30)	2.52 (1.70–3.60)[c]
Pharynx (3)	1.45 (0.30–4.24)
Esophagus (14)	5.04 (2.49–8.00)[c]
Stomach (9)	1.39 (1.18–3.64)[c]
Small intestine (1)	1.56 (0.04–8.71)
Colon (50)	2.26 (1.68–2.98)[c]
Rectum and anus (22)	1.43 (0.90–2.16)
Liver (8)	5.67 (2.45–11.18)[c]
Gallbladder and bile ducts (4)	2.11 (0.57–5.39)
Pancreas (13)	2.77 (1.47–4.73)[c]
Larynx (7)	2.77 (1.11–5.70)[c]
Trachea, bronchus, lung (60)	2.10 (1.61–2.71)[c]
Pleura (4)	3.15 (0.86–8.06)
Bone (2)	3.23 (0.39–11.65)
Breast (44)	1.00 (0.73–1.14)
Cervix—in situ (50)	13.51 (10.03–17.82)[c]
Cervix—invasive (15)	3.78 (2.11–6.23)[c]
Uterus (11)	1.63 (0.81–2.92)
Ovary (2)	0.43 (0.05–1.55)
Vulva or vagina (40)	43.5 (30.1–58.0)[c]
Prostate (21)	0.66 (0.41–1.01)
Testis (5)	1.76 (0.57–4.11)
Penis (7)	24.1 (9.70–49.7)[c]
Bladder (54)	7.19 (5.40–9.39)[c]
Kidney (54)	6.90 (5.18–9.00)[c]
Ureter (10)	250 (120–460)[c]
Central nervous system (nonlymphoma) (6)	0.91 (0.31–1.98)
Thyroid (11)	3.42 (1.71–6.13)[c]
Parathyroid (2)	200 (24–722)[c]
Other endocrine (1)	100 (2.5–557)[c]
Miscellaneous (72)	6.98 (5.46–8.79)[c]
TOTAL (785)	3.50 (2.64–3.04)[c]

[a] Data of the Australia–New Zealand Dialysis and Transplant Registry are from 8618 recipients of cadaveric donor kidneys transplanted between 1965 and 1997. Disney APS, et al. ANZ DATA Registry Report 1998.
[b] Values are observed-to-expected (compared with age-matched controls) with 95% confidence intervals (CI).
[c] Failure of the confidence intervals to include one indicates the risk difference is statistically significant.

increased incidence of nonskin malignancies after renal transplantation. Age has been shown to increase the risk for posttransplantation tumors, and it may be wise to minimize the amount of immunosuppression used in transplant recipients older than 60 to 65 years of age. Cigarette smoking is also associated with a higher risk for posttransplantation malignancies.

CHRONIC ALLOGRAFT NEPHROPATHY

Chronic allograft nephropathy is second only to death with a functioning kidney as the most common cause of late graft failure. The term *chronic allograft nephropathy* is preferred to the frequently used "chronic rejection" because the etiology includes factors that can be considered both immune, or *alloantigen dependent,* and nonimmune, or *alloantigen independent* (Table 9.4). The distinction between alloantigen-dependent and alloantigen-independent factors is a convenient one, but multiple factors often coexist, and early events may program later events. For example, ischemic injury may make the graft more susceptible to acute rejection (see Chapter 8), and graft survival after acute rejection is impaired in the presence of hypertension.

In 1953, in one of the first reports of successful human cadaveric renal transplantation, the transplantation pioneer David Humes and coworkers described pathologic findings from a patient who died almost 6 months after cadaveric renal transplantation:

> The tubular degeneration, casts, focal cellular infiltration, and interstitial edema were felt to be consistent with the picture of ischemic nephrosis. There were striking changes in the intrinsic

Table 9.4.   Putative risk factors for chronic allograft nephropathy

Alloantigen-Dependent Risk Factors

Acute rejection
Histocompatibility mismatch
Prior sensitization
Suboptimal immunosuppression
Medication noncompliance

Alloantigen-Independent Risk Factors

Ischemic injury and delayed graft function
Older donor age
Donor and recipient size mismatching
Calcineurin-inhibitor nephrotoxicity
Hyperlipidemia
Hypertension
Cigarette smoking
Hyperhomocysteinemia
Oxygen free radicals
Infection (e.g., cytomegalovirus)
Proteinuria

blood vessels. A severe degree of arteriosclerosis had developed. There was marked thickening of the intima with narrowing of the lumen, in some vessels almost to the point of occlusion. The inner portion of the intima showed dense sclerosis, and the outer portion, just within the inner elastic lamina, contained numerous lipid-laden macrophages.

This description fits well with what we now call chronic allograft nephropathy, the histologic features of which are described in detail in Chapter 13.

Clinically, chronic allograft nephropathy usually presents in one of two ways: (1) as a finding in patients undergoing biopsy for an acute rise in serum creatinine or proteinuria, or (2) as a finding in patients undergoing biopsy for gradually declining renal function or proteinuria. Chronic allograft nephropathy is the most common cause of posttransplantation nephrotic syndrome. Studies have also shown that protocol biopsies obtained in patients with no obvious clinical or laboratory abnormalities may also reveal chronic allograft nephropathy. Thus, it should be no surprise that the biopsy findings of chronic allograft nephropathy are often poor predictors of the subsequent clinical course, particularly if the histologic findings are mild. Patients with transplant glomerulopathy or severe arterial lesions on biopsy often have progressive declines in renal function. The causes of chronic allograft nephropathy are poorly understood.

Alloantigen-dependent Risk Factors

The most convincing evidence that alloantigen-dependent factors are important in the pathogenesis of chronic allograft nephropathy comes from several epidemiologic studies demonstrating an association between acute and chronic rejection. There is now little doubt that patients who have acute rejection episodes are more likely than patients with no acute rejection to develop chronic allograft nephropathy; an episode of acute rejection in the first 6 months after transplantation increases the risk for late graft loss by up to 50%. Not all acute rejection episodes, however, lead to chronic allograft nephropathy, and it is difficult in individual patients with acute rejection to predict the likelihood of developing chronic allograft nephropathy. Acute rejections that occur late (after the first 3 months) appear to be more predictive of chronic allograft nephropathy than those that occur during the first 3 months. It is unclear, however, whether acute rejection episodes that occur late because of attempts to withdraw immunosuppressive agents are as predictive of chronic allograft nephropathy as those that occur late on full doses of immunosuppression. It is clear that acute rejections that are more severe, either by histology or by the degree of increase in serum creatinine, are also more likely than less acute severe rejections to herald chronic allograft nephropathy. Finally, multiple acute rejections also appear to be more predictive of chronic allograft nephropathy.

The number of major histocompatibility complex (MHC) antigens that are mismatched between the recipient and donor is associated with chronic allograft nephropathy and late allograft failure (see Chapter 3, Fig. 3.6). Clearly, cadaveric kidney transplants that have zero MHC mismatches have the best long-term allograft survival. Less marked, but nevertheless statistically significant, are differences in late allograft survival between kidneys that have one through six MHC mismatches. The effect of MHC mismatches on graft half-life (reflecting the rate of allograft failure among those who have survived with a functioning kidney for at least 1 year) is further evidence that alloantigen-dependent factors are important in the pathogenesis of chronic allograft nephropathy.

Similarly, some studies have also found an association between the number of preformed antibodies present in recipients at the time of transplantation and subsequent chronic allograft nephropathy. This is usually measured as the percentage of panel-reactive antibodies (PRA), or the percentage of a panel of random donor lymphocytes to which the prospective recipient's plasma reacts. In some studies, PRA has correlated with long-term allograft survival.

If it could be shown that higher doses of immunosuppression prevent chronic allograft nephropathy, this too would be evidence that alloantigen-dependent factors are important. Data showing that higher doses or more potent immunosuppression reduces the incidence of chronic allograft nephropathy, however, are equivocal. It is noteworthy that the introduction of cyclosporine in the 1980s led to dramatic (25% to 30%) reductions in the rate of acute rejection early after transplantation and greatly improved 1-year graft survival in most programs. During this era, however, there was little improvement in graft half-life, suggesting that cyclosporine had little effect on chronic allograft nephropathy. The nephrotoxicity of cyclosporine may cancel any benefit that a reduced incidence of acute rejection from cyclosporine may have on chronic allograft nephropathy.

Several studies have shown that poor adherence to medications increases the likelihood of late graft failure, presumably from chronic allograft nephropathy. This too has been cited as evidence supporting the hypothesis that chronic allograft nephropathy is caused by alloantigen-dependent factors. These same patients are likely to be noncompliant with follow-up visits and thus inhibit the ability to detect treatable acute rejection episodes and thereby increase the risk for chronic allograft nephropathy. Patients who are noncompliant with immunosuppression, however, may also be noncompliant with antihypertensive agents as well as other medications, and this could also increase the risk for chronic allograft nephropathy. Thus, it is difficult to attribute the adverse consequences of noncompliance entirely to alloantigen-dependent mechanisms causing chronic allograft nephropathy.

Alloantigen-independent Risk Factors

Patients with delayed, or "slow," graft function have a higher rate of late allograft failure (see Chapter 8). The serum creatinine level at the time of discharge from hospital has been shown to be a determinant of late graft loss. One theory holds that ischemic injury and delayed graft function result in a reduced number of functioning nephrons and that inadequate "nephron dosing" causes chronic allograft nephropathy and late allograft failure. However, delayed graft function is also associated with an increased incidence of acute rejection that could also explain its adverse effects on late graft survival. If true, this might suggest that closer surveillance of patients for acute rejection during and after periods of delayed graft function could reduce the rate of late allograft failure.

With the current organ shortage and long waiting times for cadaveric kidneys, many centers now accept kidneys from older donors. Donor age is clearly associated with a higher rate of late allograft failure (see Chapter 3, Fig. 3.7). Many of the histologic characteristics of chronic allograft nephropathy are similar to those seen in normal aging. It is unclear exactly how age of the kidney increases the risk for late allograft failure. The inadequate number of nephrons in older kidneys may create a physiologic response that sets in motion mechanisms ultimately leading to graft failure. The *accelerated senescence theory* proposes that the intrinsic age of the kidney (genetically determined in every cell and expressed in telomere length) limits its longevity in the recipient; the aging process is further accelerated by the repeated injury and stress represented by the alloantigen-dependent and alloantigen-independent factors discussed previously. By whatever mechanisms, the use of older kidneys appears to be a major cause of chronic allograft nephropathy.

The most direct test of the hypothesis that inadequate nephron dosing may lead to chronic allograft nephropathy is to determine whether the size of the kidney affects long-term outcomes. Clearly, larger kidneys have a proportionally greater filtration capacity (although not necessarily a greater number of nephrons) than smaller kidneys. It has been theorized that placing a small kidney into a large recipient may create a situation of inadequate nephron dosing for that recipient and thereby precipitate chronic allograft nephropathy. A number of studies, however, have failed to demonstrate that this donor-to-recipient size mismatching increases the risk for chronic allograft nephropathy or late allograft failure.

The calcineurin inhibitors are nephrotoxic (see Chapter 4). The histologic changes of chronic calcineurin inhibitor toxicity are nonspecific and can resemble those of chronic allograft nephropathy. The extent of interstitial fibrosis that is a feature of chronic allograft nephropathy and calcineurin inhibitor toxicity has been correlated to the expression of TGF beta mRNA, which may, in turn, be stimulated by cyclosporine (see Chapter 4, Fig. 4.3). Therefore, chronic calcineurin inhibitor toxicity could be yet another alloantigen-independent mechanism contributing to the pathogenesis of chronic allograft nephropathy. The fact that graft survival has not been reduced by the increased incidence of acute rejections after cyclosporine withdrawal in randomized, controlled trials may be due to the offsetting effects of nephrotoxicity in the controls continuing to take cyclosporine in these studies. Withdrawing cyclosporine may produce a trade-off between the adverse effects of acute rejection and the beneficial effects of reduced nephrotoxicity, the net result being no difference in allograft survival. Additional studies with long-term follow-up are needed to confirm this hypothesis.

The most distinctive histologic characteristic of chronic allograft nephropathy is the fibrointimal proliferation seen in arteries. In some ways, this vasculopathy resembles accelerated atherosclerosis, prompting investigators to consider whether alloantigen-independent risk factors for atherosclerotic vascular disease may also be risk factors for chronic allograft nephropathy. Observational studies in some transplantation centers have found that recipients with hypercholesterolemia are at increased risk for developing chronic allograft nephropathy. In randomized controlled trials in heart transplant recipients, 3-hydroxy-3-methylglutaryl coenzyme A (HMG-CoA) reductase inhibitors reduced graft vasculopathy. As yet, there are no studies in renal transplant recipients demonstrating that lipid-lowering agents reduce chronic allograft nephropathy.

Registry data have shown that elevated blood pressure is also associated with graft failure. Of course, it is plausible that graft dysfunction causes hypertension, rather than hypertension causing graft dysfunction and chronic allograft nephropathy. Unfortunately, there are no randomized trial results to determine whether aggressive blood pressure lowering will reduce the rate of late graft failure. Similarly, cigarette smoking is another risk factor that could have a negative effect on graft vasculopathy and contribute to chronic allograft nephropathy. Unfortunately, there are few studies examining the effects of cigarette smoking on allograft function in renal transplant recipients. Likewise, homocysteine may be injurious to vascular endothelial cells, and transplant recipients have increased levels of plasma homocysteine compared with controls. In addition, homocysteine levels correlate with renal allograft function. However, reduced renal function is known to cause higher levels of homocysteine, and there are no data suggesting that reducing homocysteine improves graft survival. Similarly, oxygen free radicals are of theoretical importance in the pathogenesis of systemic atherosclerosis and could also play a role in endothelial injury and the vasculopathy of chronic allograft nephropathy. There are few data, however, suggesting that oxygen free radicals cause chronic allograft nephropathy in humans. Finally, infections have long been considered a possible mechanism in the pathogenesis of systemic atherosclerosis. If true, the increased incidence of CMV and other infections could also contribute to the vasculopathy of chronic allograft nephropathy. To date, the evidence that infections contribute to chronic allograft nephropathy is largely circumstantial.

Most epidemiologic studies suggest that the incidence of persistent proteinuria after transplantation (e.g., more than 1 to 2 g per 24 hours for longer than 6 months) is about 20%. Of course, the incidence of proteinuria in these studies is greater with longer duration of follow-up. Cross-sectional studies suggest that about two thirds of patients with persistent proteinuria have chronic allograft nephropathy on biopsy. Although it is clear that chronic allograft nephropathy can cause proteinuria, proteinuria may also have toxic effects on the allograft that contribute to chronic allograft nephropathy. Indeed, a number of studies have identified proteinuria as an important risk factor for graft loss to chronic allograft nephropathy. Proteinuria has been shown to cause interstitial nephritis in experimental animals. In addition, studies in humans with renal disease have consistently reported that the amount of urine protein excretion predicts renal disease progression. Thus, it is possible that proteinuria could cause tubulointerstitial damage and contribute to renal injury in chronic allograft nephropathy.

In summary, chronic allograft nephropathy is an important cause of graft failure in the late posttransplantation period. The pathogenesis of chronic allograft nephropathy is poorly understood. Epidemiologic studies, however, have identified both alloantigen-independent and alloantigen-dependent risk factors that correlate with chronic allograft nephropathy and graft failure. Intervention studies are needed to determine whether these risk factors have a pathogenic role and to define safe and effective therapies for chronic allograft nephropathy.

ACUTE REJECTION IN THE LATE POSTTRANSPLANTATION PERIOD

A small proportion of renal allografts are lost to acute rejection in the late posttransplantation period. Noncompliance with immunosuppressive medications may play an important role in some, if not most, late acute rejections and should always be considered when they occur. Because most patients do not admit to missing doses of medications, it is difficult to know how often noncompliance causes acute rejection and graft failure. Transplant centers frequently attempt to reduce doses of immunosuppression, replace drugs with less toxic or less expensive alternatives, or withdraw an agent to convert stable patients from triple to double immunosuppressive therapy. Such changes in immunosuppression are always associated with some risk for acute rejection. If patients are monitored closely, acute rejection can be detected early and can usually be treated successfully. On the other hand, if acute rejection goes undetected, as is often the case with noncompliant patients, it can cause or accelerate graft failure.

RECURRENT AND *DE NOVO* RENAL DISEASE

The reported incidence of recurrence of the original renal disease in the allograft is variable (Table 9.5). This is likely because of differences in the duration of follow-up and differences in the frequency with which patients undergo biopsies. It is probable that as graft failures from death and rejection decline, the incidence of graft failure from recurrent disease will increase. It is also frequently difficult to establish whether some diseases represent recurrences or *de novo* glomerular disease.

The incidence of recurrent and *de novo* disease among a large cohort (4,913 subjects), with 22% receiving living-related donor transplants) in the *Renal Allograft Disease Registry* was 3.4% over a mean follow-up period of 5.4 years. Diagnoses were focal segmental glomerulosclerosis (FSGS; 34.1% of the total), immunoglobulin A (IgA) nephropathy (13.2%), diabetes (11.4%), membranoproliferative glomerulonephritis (MPGN; 10.8%), membranous nephropathy (9.6%), hemolytic-uremic syndrome or thrombotic thrombocytopenia purpura (4.8%), and other (16.1%). There was a significant increase in graft failures among the recurrent and *de novo* disease groups (55%) compared with the others (25%; $p < 0.001$). In contrast, in a small cohort (60 subjects) of two-haplotype–matched living-related donor transplants followed for a mean of 8.3 years, the incidence of recurrent disease was 15% (9 of 60) and was 27% (9 of 33) in patients with glomerulonephritis as the original kidney disease. The higher incidence of disease recur-

Table 9.5.   Recurrent renal disease: range of reported incidence

Underlying Disease	Rate of Recurrence (%)	Graft Failure if Recurrence (%)
Focal segmental glomerulosclerosis	25–50	10–65
Membranoproliferative GN type I	20–30	6–66
Membranoproliferative GN type II (DDD)	90–100	19–50
Membranous nephropathy	5–10	1–44
IgA nephropathy	40–50	2–41
Henoch-Schönlein purpura	75–90	20–40
Anti-GBM nephritis	10–25	<1
Hemolytic-uremic syndrome, TTP	10–28	40–63
Diabetes	100	5–10

GN, glomerulonephritis; DDD, dense deposit disease; GBM, glomerular basement membrane; IgA, immunoglobulin A; TTP, thrombotic thrombocytopenic purpura.

rence in the latter study may reflect the lack of competing graft loss to rejection in well-matched recipients exposed to relatively long follow-up.

In data from large registries, it is more difficult to discern the incidence of disease recurrence than to define the outcome of patients after recurrent disease has been diagnosed. In data from the *European Dialysis and Transplant Association,* the percentage of patients with graft failure for FSGS was 24%; for MPGN type II, 19%; MPGN type I, 6%; for IgA nephropathy, 6%; and for other types of glomerular diseases, 4%.

The overall rate of recurrence for FSGS is 24% to 50%; however, patients who have lost a prior transplant because of recurrent FSGS are at much higher risk. Early recognition of recurrent FSGS is particularly important because it may respond to plasmapheresis (see Chapter 15). MPGN type II (dense deposit disease) recurs in almost 100% of patients and often leads to graft failure. MPGN type I recurs in about 20% to 30% of patients and leads to graft failure in about 50%. Membranous glomerulonephritis can present as *de novo* disease but probably recurs in 5% to 10% of patients. About 25% of patients may ultimately lose their grafts from recurrent membranous nephropathy. Histologic recurrence of IgA nephropathy is common. Allograft failure to IgA nephropathy is higher than once reported and is now probably about 25%. Henoch-Schönlein purpura recurs in a high proportion of patients and leads to graft failure in about 25%. Antiglomerular basement membrane disease recurs in 10% to 25% but rarely causes graft failure. Diabetes recurs histologically in 100% of patients after a few years. Graft failure due to diabetes occurs in about 5% to 10%

patients, but this percentage may increase as graft failure due to rejection declines.

ROLE OF NONCOMPLIANCE IN LATE ALLOGRAFT FAILURE

It is difficult to assess how frequently patients are noncompliant with immunosuppressive medications, but it is probably more frequent than generally appreciated. As a group, transplant recipients may be especially reluctant to admit to noncompliance if they believe that doing so may jeopardize their chances of ever receiving another transplant. Investigators at the University of Alabama carefully reviewed the records of 184 patients who had lost their grafts more than 6 months after transplantation and found that about 50% had chronic rejection as a primary or contributing cause of graft failure. Most of these patients had a significant history of noncompliance. This was defined by having at least two of the following: (1) admission of noncompliance by the patient, (2) failure to keep scheduled appointments, or (3) undetectable cyclosporine blood levels on more than one occasion. Chronic rejection in compliant patients accounted for only 19% of late graft losses. When acute and chronic rejection were combined, 35% of all graft losses after the first 6 months were thought to be due to noncompliance. Thus, noncompliance was suspected to be a major cause of late graft failure.

At Hennepin County Medical Center in Minneapolis, patients were asked to have their serum creatinine checked monthly and to make sure that results were reported to the transplantation center. It was found that patients who failed to have these measurements performed regularly were significantly more likely to have late graft failure. This effect did not become manifest until several years after transplantation, consistent with the notion that, with time, some patients may become complacent.

Patients may become noncompliant with medications for a number or reasons. They may harbor the false belief that taking medication regularly is unnecessary. This belief may be reinforced by several years of an uneventful posttransplantation course. Many patients believe that the effects of immunosuppression continue indefinitely, even when doses of medication are missed. Such patients are more likely to be noncompliant than those who have a better understanding of the duration of action of immunosuppressive medications. Some patients may become noncompliant because they fear the adverse effects of medication more than they fear graft rejection. This is particularly true of adolescents, who abhor the social stigma of the body habitus changes caused by corticosteroids and, to a lesser extent, cyclosporine. Financial disincentives for medication noncompliance are discussed in Chapter 19.

Patients may simply forget to take doses of medications. In a recent survey of 100 members of the *Transplant Recipient International Organization* (TRIO), less than 30% were taking fewer than 5 medications, and 35% reported taking 10 to 20 different medications each day. Only 2% of the medications required a single daily dose. (In general, studies have shown that the number of times a day that patients must take medications is a stronger predictor of noncompliance than the total number of medications.) There were 25% who admitted missing doses of medications, and

55% of these gave forgetfulness as the reason. It is likely that the members of the TRIO represent a highly motivated population of transplant recipients. Only 35% of the participants were kidney transplant recipients, and recipients of other, nonrenal organs may suffer lethal consequences if their grafts fail.

Noncompliance can lead to graft failure through several different mechanisms. Patients who receive inadequate immunosuppression because of noncompliance may develop acute or chronic rejection that leads to graft failure. Noncompliance with clinic visits and laboratory follow-up can also contribute to late graft failure. Acute rejection in the late posttransplantation period rarely presents with signs and symptoms until it is far advanced. Thus, to be successfully treated, acute rejection must be detected early, and this can only be done by detecting increases in serum creatinine levels soon after they occur. It follows that patients who do not see physicians and who do not have frequent measurements of serum creatinine levels are less likely to have rejection detected at an early stage when it is treatable.

PART II. MANAGEMENT OF RECIPIENTS IN THE LATE POSTTRANSPLANTATION PERIOD

THE 10 MOST IMPORTANT THINGS TO DO!

Caregivers often feel impotent when it comes to treating and preventing diseases that cause morbidity and mortality. There is much that we do not know. This is particularly true in a relatively new field, such as renal transplantation. For example, we do not know how to treat chronic allograft nephropathy. We do not even know precisely what chronic allograft nephropathy is, yet we know that it is a major cause of graft failure in the late posttransplantation period. The dilemma is similar to that which caregivers face when they have patients suffering from inoperable, three-vessel coronary artery disease, inoperable cancer that responds poorly to chemotherapy, or other diseases and complications for which there may not be effective therapies.

On the other hand, there is a substantial amount of evidence to suggest ways to prevent at least some major disease complications that are common after renal transplantation. Studies have shown, however, that despite good evidence that a particular therapy or preventive strategy is beneficial, that therapy or preventive strategy may not be applied. Hypertension, for example, is a known risk factor for stroke and ischemic heart disease, and numerous studies have documented the safety and efficacy of antihypertensive medications. Nevertheless, many studies have also shown that hypertension is poorly controlled, even among patients who are seen regularly in hospitals and clinics. Attention to atherosclerotic risk factors may be the most important way to improve the longevity of transplant recipients, yet these risk factors are often not addressed nor adequately emphasized. Part of the responsibility no doubt falls on the patients themselves; much also falls on physicians and other caregivers.

Resources are limited; there is only so much that can be done. It seems prudent, therefore, to adopt a priority system for delivering health care. Such a system should emphasize measures that are known to be effective, that is, strategies that are evidence based. In the case of renal transplantation, we know the major causes of

Table 9.6.   The 10 most important things
to do in the late posttransplantation period

1. Reduce immunosuppression whenever possible.
2. Adopt a strategy to prevent noncompliance.
3. Monitor renal function closely.
4. Perform biopsy early and often to detect late acute rejection.
5. Aggressively treat hyperlipidemia.
6. Aggressively treat hypertension.
7. Do everything possible to encourage patients to quit smoking.
8. Screen for breast, cervical, prostate, colorectal, and skin cancer.
9. Immunize against influenza and pneumococcal pneumonia.
10. Consider prophylaxis with aspirin, calcium, and hormone-replacement therapy.

morbidity and mortality in the late posttransplantation period. In many cases, we have a substantial amount of evidence to suggest effective measures to prevent many of the common posttransplantation complications. This evidence, if not available from studies in renal transplant recipients, can often be extrapolated from studies in the general population. The challenge is to make the most of what we have. This section outlines 10 strategies for the management of renal transplant recipients in the late posttransplantation period. The emphasis is on specific complications for which we have evidence that the problem is common and the intervention is effective (Table 9.6).

Strategy 1: Reduce Immunosuppression Whenever Possible
Death is a common cause of renal allograft failure in the late posttransplantation period. The ultimate goal is to have all of our patients die with a functioning graft, but not prematurely, as is now too often the case. Cardiovascular disease, cancer, and infection are the leading causes of death in the late posttransplantation period, and immunosuppression plays a major role in the pathogenesis of each of these complications. Each immunosuppressive agent has both immune and nonimmune toxicity. Immune toxicity is usually nonspecific; that is, immune toxicity is the result of the total amount of all immunosuppression over a given period of time. Immune toxicity can only be avoided if patients become tolerant to their transplanted kidney. Unfortunately, most patients will reject their kidney if immunosuppression is completely withdrawn, and the best we can do is to select the minimal amount of immunosuppression that prevents rejection. This minimal amount should ideally be tailored to the needs of specific patients, but we are able to do that only in a very crude way.

The principal obstacle to reducing the overall amount of immunosuppression is acute rejection. A number of risk factors for acute rejection have been identified (Table 9.7). These risk factors can be taken into account when determining the amount of immunosuppression that may be appropriate for individual patients in the late posttransplantation period. In general, outcomes are better for live donor kidneys. This is especially true for haploidentical,

Table 9.7.   Tailoring the *amount* of immunosuppression to the individual patient

Risk Factor	Patients Who May Need *More* Immunosuppression	Patients Who May Need *Less* Immunosuppression
Donor source	Cadaveric	Living
Major histo-compatibility	>0 Mismatches	0 Mismatches
Prior trans-plantation experience	>1, Rejected quickly	0 or 1, Prolonged survival
Age	<18 years old	>60 years old
Race	Black	White
Timing of acute rejection	Late	Early
Severity of acute rejection	Severe, vascular	Mild, cellular
Number of acute rejections	>1	0 or 1

living-related transplants. For cadaveric kidney recipients, the number of major histocompatibility mismatches has been shown to be associated with the rate of late allograft failure (see Chapter 3, Fig. 3.6). In particular, patients with zero mismatches are at significantly lower risk for late graft failure when compared with patients with as few as one mismatch, and at least one study has shown that the number of HLA-DR mismatches predicts acute rejection after elective withdrawal of cyclosporine. Patients who have had more than one previous transplant have a higher risk for graft failure. In addition, the chances of such a patient receiving yet another kidney are reduced, making the risk associated with reducing immunosuppression higher. Young patients (younger than 18 years of age) have a higher incidence of acute rejection and need more immunosuppression than patients 30 to 50 years of age. On the other hand, elderly patients are more likely to die of complications of immunosuppression than to lose their kidneys to acute rejection, and many transplantation centers attempt to use less immunosuppression in elderly transplant recipients.

Blacks are at increased risk for late allograft failure. The reasons for this are probably multiple but include possible differences in immunoreactivity to the graft and poor bioavailability of calcineurin inhibitors. Acute rejection is a strong predictor of outcome, particularly from chronic allograft nephropathy. However, not all acute rejections lead to graft failure. Characteristics of acute rejection that correlate to increased risk for graft failure and, by inference, an increased need for long-term immunosuppression include late rejections, severe rejections, and multiple acute rejections. All of the above factors can be used to judge the amount of immunosuppression that may be best for individual patients in the late posttransplantation period.

A number of randomized controlled trials have studied the feasibility of electively withdrawing immunosuppressive agents in the late posttransplantation period. Withdrawal of both prednisone and cyclosporine has been studied extensively, yet withdrawal of these agents remains controversial (see Chapter 4, Part IV). Elective cyclosporine withdrawal is associated with about a 10% risk for acute rejection in the months following withdrawal. Most of these rejection episodes can be successfully treated and reversed. Despite this increased risk for rejection, there appears to be no increased risk for graft failure in several randomized, controlled trials. Even controlled trials with long-term follow-up (e.g., greater than 4 years) have been unable to demonstrate an increased risk for graft failure after cyclosporine withdrawal. In contrast, acute rejection after prednisone withdrawal appears to increase the risk for late allograft failure in randomized controlled trials. Additional studies are warranted to define better the circumstances under which immunosuppression withdrawal is advisable.

In addition to deciding on the minimum amount of immunosuppression needed to prevent acute rejection, physicians and patients must also choose among the most effective, but least toxic, of several different agents. In general, it is prudent to tailor the choice of agents to the risk profile or adverse effects that are most troubling to the individual (Table 9.8). In patients who have severe hyperlipidemia, especially those who are at high risk for cardiovascular disease, it may be wise to minimize the use of cyclosporine, prednisone, and sirolimus. Each of these drugs causes hyperlipidemia. Switching a patient from cyclosporine to tacrolimus, for example,

Table 9.8.   Tailoring the _type_ of immunosuppression to the individual patient

Risk Factor or Complication	Agents to Reduce or Withdraw
Severe hyperlipidemia	Cyclosporine, prednisone, sirolimus
Severe hypertension	Cyclosporine, prednisone
Severe tremor	Tacrolimus, cyclosporine
Difficult-to-control diabetes	Prednisone
New (posttransplantation) diabetes	Tacrolimus, cyclosporine, prednisone
Anemia, neutropenia, thrombocytopenia	Azathioprine, MMF, sirolimus
Very low renal function	Cyclosporine, tacrolimus
Severe liver disease	Azathioprine, cyclosporine, sirolimus
Gout requiring allopurinol	Azathioprine
Inability to pay for medications	Cyclosporine, tacrolimus, sirolimus, MMF

MMF, mycophenolate mofetil.

may reduce low-density lipoprotein cholesterol by the same amount as therapy with an HMG-CoA reductase inhibitor. Similarly, reducing cyclosporine or prednisone may help to control blood pressure. Patients with severe tremor will be especially eager to reduce or withdraw tacrolimus or cyclosporine in the late posttransplantation period if this is possible. Similarly, patients with difficult-to-control diabetes may be good candidates for minimizing doses of prednisone. New-onset, posttransplantation diabetes may sometimes resolve by reducing doses or discontinuing tacrolimus, cyclosporine, or occasionally prednisone. Bone marrow suppression may be an indication for reducing doses of azathioprine, mycophenolate mofetil, or sirolimus. Patients with marginal renal function may sometimes delay starting dialysis by decreasing or stopping calcineurin inhibitors. Patients with severe liver disease may benefit from lowering or discontinuing azathioprine. Allopurinol can dramatically increase blood levels of azathioprine; hence, azathioprine may need to be reduced or discontinued in patients with gout. Finally, many patients cannot afford to pay the high cost of immunosuppression. The use of expensive medications for patients who cannot afford them increases the risk for noncompliance and graft failure. Prednisone and azathioprine are a fraction of the cost of newer immunosuppressive agents and yet may provide adequate immunosuppression for many patients.

Strategy 2: Adopt Strategies to Prevent Noncompliance
There are few randomized, controlled trials to suggest how to prevent noncompliance with immunosuppressive medications. On the other hand, a number of observational studies have demonstrated that noncompliance is an important, preventable cause of allograft failure. These same studies have provided clues to preventative measures that are most likely to be effective.

1. Minimize the number of daily doses of medication. Whenever possible, use medications that can be dosed once daily.
2. Educate patients. In particular, dispel the common misconception that the immunosuppressive effects of medications extend beyond the dosing interval. Patients need to be constantly reminded that failure to take medications regularly will eventually result in graft failure.
3. Help patients establish a system to remind them to take their medications. Enlist the help of friends, family, and public health aides. Use egg-carton style pill containers or other mnemonic devices.
4. Maintain close contact with patients throughout the late posttransplantation period. Insist that patients need to have frequent follow-up with the transplantation center, and make every effort to locate patients who are lost to follow-up. Clinic visits and laboratory checks are a valuable reminder to patients of the importance of taking medications. When negotiating contracts with providers, insist that patients be allowed to follow-up with the transplantation center at regular intervals.
5. Know whether your patients have trouble paying for their medications. If this is the case, assign someone to help them. Most transplantation programs have found that it is often

necessary to have a dedicated social worker or pharmacist available to help patients find ways to cover the cost of their immunosuppressive medications.

6. Identify patients who are at high risk for noncompliance. Adolescent patients are at increased risk, often because they are fearful of the cosmetic effects of prednisone and cyclosporine. Patients who are poorly educated are also at increased risk for noncompliance. Similarly, low family income is associated with noncompliance. Socioeconomic factors place members of racial minorities at increased risk for noncompliance. Studies have shown that patients who were noncompliant with medication, diet, and dialysis therapy before transplantation are more likely to be noncompliant after renal transplantation.

7. Patients who are at high risk for noncompliance should be targeted with risk factor intervention in much the same way that we target patients who are at high risk for cardiovascular disease with intensive risk factor management. In both instances, the benefit is likely to be the greatest when the risk is the highest.

Strategy 3: Monitor Renal Function Closely

Frequent monitoring of renal function in the late posttransplantation period helps to enforce compliance with immunosuppressive medications and provides the only reliable means to detect acute rejection when it may still respond to treatment. A program requiring patients to make certain that serum creatinine is measured regularly and reported to the transplantation center also provides an indirect means for the center to monitor compliance. Patients who fail to have their serum creatinine level checked regularly should be contacted and reminded of the importance of close, ongoing follow-up to prevent graft failure. Patients and caregivers should be constantly reminded that acute rejection rarely presents with signs and symptoms in the late posttransplantation period. Serum creatinine levels can be measured in most laboratories relatively inexpensively. This test is the only practical tool that can be used to screen for acute rejection in the late posttransplantation period. It is not too much to ask patients to have their serum creatinine level measured regularly in the late posttransplantation period.

At least once a year, and preferably more often, urine should be checked for protein excretion. Persistent proteinuria (i.e., more than 1 g in 24 hours for at least 6 months) is associated with an increased risk for graft failure. Proteinuria can be most reliably detected by either a timed urine collection (which is cumbersome) or a protein-to-creatinine ratio measured in a random "spot" urine sample (which is convenient). Dipstick screening is less reliable because the protein concentration is also dependent on the state of diuresis. There are two reasons why it is important to detect proteinuria:

1. Reducing high levels of proteinuria with angiotensin-converting enzyme (ACE) inhibitors or receptor antagonists may help reduce levels of serum cholesterol and alleviate coagulation and other metabolic abnormalities associated with nephrotic-range proteinuria.

2. There is growing circumstantial evidence that proteinuria may itself be injurious to the kidney and may contribute to the pathogenesis of chronic allograft nephropathy.

Strategy 4: Perform Biopsy to Detect Late Acute Rejection

There is evidence to suggest that even low-grade tubulitis, or *borderline acute rejection,* may increase the risk for chronic allograft nephropathy. A small, randomized, controlled trial has demonstrated that treating acute rejection on protocol biopsies during the first few months after transplantation resulted in a lower serum creatinine level at 2 years, as compared with controls who underwent less frequent biopsies and relied instead on increased serum creatinine levels to prompt biopsy and treatment (see Chapter 8). Few centers perform protocol biopsies, that is, biopsies on all patients at predetermined intervals, in the late posttransplantation period. However, the message is clear. It is important to have a high level of suspicion for acute rejection and a low threshold for obtaining a renal allograft biopsy. An acute, sustained rise in serum creatinine should prompt immediate evaluation. The strategy of routinely monitoring serum creatinine levels (described previously) will only be successful if biopsies are obtained quickly and acute rejection is treated. Such a strategy will also avoid unnecessary intensification of immunosuppression when rejection is not present. After chronic allograft nephropathy is established, repeated biopsies may be unnecessary because repeated treatment may be unwise (see Chapter 4).

Strategy 5: Treat Hyperlipidemia Aggressively

Hyperlipidemia is common after renal transplantation. Elevations in total cholesterol are almost invariably accompanied by elevations in LDL cholesterol. Triglycerides are also frequently elevated. Several studies have found correlations between hyperlipidemia and cardiovascular disease after renal transplantation. Studies in the general population have provided incontrovertible evidence that treatment of elevated LDL reduces the risk for ischemic heart disease events and decreases mortality. Because an increased LDL level is the most common lipid abnormality after renal transplantation, it is reasonable to follow the National Cholesterol Education Program (NCEP) guidelines for treatment (Table 9.9). A National Kidney Foundation task force on CVD reached the same conclusion, but went further to suggest that transplant recipients should be considered in the highest risk category when applying the NCEP guidelines. Accordingly, transplant recipients with LDL cholesterol levels of more than 130 mg/dL should be considered for pharmacologic treatment, especially if they have preexisting CVD, diabetes, or other risk factors.

Reduction of the urine protein excretion with an ACE inhibitor or receptor antagonist may help to reduce lipid levels for patients with nephrotic-range proteinuria. Reduction or discontinuation of cyclosporine, sirolimus, or prednisone may also help lower lipid levels. Diet is effective in reducing cholesterol and LDL, but the effect is usually modest. A number of studies have shown that HMG-CoA reductase inhibitors are safe and effective in lowering LDL cholesterol after renal transplantation. Plasma levels of

**Table 9.9.   National Cholesterol
Education Program guidelines**

Risk Factors for Ischemic Heart Disease

Male: age 45 years
Female: age 55 years (or premature menopause without estrogen-
   replacement therapy)
Diabetes
Hypertension (blood pressure 140/90 mm Hg on several occasions or
   taking antihypertensive medication)
Current cigarette smoking
Family history (definite myocardial infarction or sudden death
      before 55 years in father or other male first-degree relative, or
      before 65 years in mother or other female first-degree relative)
HDL cholesterol <35 mg/dL
For HDL cholesterol 60 mg/dL, subtract one risk factor

Threshold and Target LDL Cholesterol Levels

Risk category	Drug treatment threshold LDL	Drug treatment target LDL
0–1 Risk factor	190 mg/dL	<160 mg/dL
2 Risk factors	160 mg/dL	<130 mg/dL
Ischemic heart disease	130 mg/dL	100 mg/dL

HDL, high-density lipoprotein; LDL, low-density lipoprotein.
From the Expert Panel on Detection Evaluation and Treatment of High Blood
Cholesterol in Adults. Summary of the Second Report of the National Cholesterol Education Program (NCEP) (Adult Treatment Panel II). *JAMA* 1993;269:
3015–3023, with permission.

HMG-CoA reductase inhibitors are increased in cyclosporine-
treated renal transplant recipients, and it is generally prudent to
use about half the usually prescribed dose. Patients who still have
high LDL cholesterol levels may be candidates for combination
therapy. Low-dose bile acid sequestrants can be combined with
an HMG-CoA reductase inhibitor. Bile acid sequestrants should
probably not be taken at the same time as cyclosporine and should
not be used in patients with very high triglyceride levels. Fibric
acid analogues, such as gemfibrozil, can also be used in combination with HMG-CoA reductase inhibitors. Some fibric acid analogues (not gemfibrozil), however, have been reported to increase
the serum creatinine level. Combination therapy should be used
with caution because it increases the risk for myositis and rhabdomyolysis.

Strategy 6: Treat Hypertension Aggressively
Hypertension occurs in 60% to 80% of renal transplant recipients.
It is associated with an increased risk for graft failure. Studies in
the general population have shown that treatment with antihypertensive agents reduces the risk for cardiovascular disease.
There is no reason to believe that treating blood pressure elevations would not be beneficial in renal transplant recipients.

All classes of antihypertensive agents can be used to lower blood pressure in renal transplant recipients, and each has its advantages and disadvantages (Table 9.10). Although there are limited data on the effects of reduced dietary sodium chloride intake on blood pressure in renal transplant recipients, this is a reasonable first step. A low dose of a thiazide diuretic is also reasonable for patients with creatinine clearance estimated to be greater than 25 to 30 mL/min. Low doses of thiazides (e.g., 12.5 to 25 mg/day) are effective and do not generally perturb lipid or glucose metabolism. Both a low-salt diet and thiazide diuretics may help with edema, which is a common problem after transplantation. A thiazide diuretic may also help in the management of the hyperkalemia that is common in cyclosporine-treated transplant recipients. Transplant recipients may be sensitive to volume contraction; therefore, diuretics may cause a reversible increase in serum creatinine levels. Thiazides often potentiate the antihypertensive effects of other agents, especially ACE inhibitors. Thiazides are inexpensive. Beta-blockers are also relatively inexpensive and are especially attractive for patients with ischemic heart disease, which is common after renal transplantation. Relative contraindications to beta-blocker therapy (e.g., peripheral vascular disease, reactive airways disease, and hypoglycemic reactions) are rarely a reason to forego the use of this important class of medication.

Physicians are sometimes reluctant to use angiotensin converting enzyme (ACE) inhibitors and angiotensin II antagonists in transplant patients for fear of inducing hemodynamic impairment of allograft function. Several studies however, have shown that

Table 9.10. **Some advantages and disadvantages of antihypertensive agent classes**

Class	Advantages	Disadvantages
Low-dose thiazide	↓Cost, ↓edema, ↓hyperkalemia	↑Creatinine
Beta-blockers	↓Cost, ↑survival in patients with ischemic heart disease	↑Lipids
ACEI	↓Proteinuria, ↓erythrocytosis, ↑Cough	↓Creatinine, anemia, ↑Potassium
AII-RA	↓Proteinuria, ↓erythrocytosis ↓ACEI-cough, ↓ACEI-hyperkalemia	↑Cost, ↑creatinine, Anemia
Calcium blockers	↑Cyclosporine levels, ↑renal blood flow	↑Edema
Vasodilators	↓Afterload in patients with congestive heart failure	↑Heart rate

ACEI, angiotensin-converting enzyme inhibitors; AII-RA, angiotensin II receptor antagonists.

these drugs are generally safe, effective, and well-tolerated. They may reduce proteinuria and stabilize the deterioration in renal function in chronic allograft failure, possibly by reducing the production of TGF beta. They may also have additional benefit in reducing the incidence of cardiovascular events in high risk patients. Occasionally, ACE inhibitors may increase serum creatinine, but this is usually a transient and reversible effect. Hyperkalemia can often be managed by adding a thiazide diuretic or a loop diuretic. ACE inhibitors may cause anemia in transplant recipients; This side effect can be exploited for the treatment of posttransplantation erythrocytosis. Cough occurs in about 15% of patients on ACE inhibitors but is much less frequent with angiotensin II receptor antagonists. Otherwise, angiotensin II receptor antagonists appear to have all of the advantages and disadvantages of ACE inhibitors (Table 9.10).

Calcium antagonists are also effective in renal transplant recipients. They can contribute to edema, which is already prevalent among transplant patients. Calcium antagonists appear to improve the preglomerular, arterial vasoconstriction that mediates cyclosporine-induced declines in renal blood flow. They may help to alleviate the propensity of the calcineurin inhibitors to exacerbate delayed graft function immediately after cadaveric transplantation. Nondihydropyridine calcium antagonists, e.g. diltiazem and verapamil, increase calcineurin inhibitor blood levels and can thereby be used to help reduce the cost of cyclosporine. Dihydropyridine calcium antagonists have less effect on cyclosporine blood levels (see Chapter 4, Part I). Finally, vasodilators and alpha-blockers are also effective in treating hypertension. They can cause reflex tachycardia and may need to be used in combination with beta-blockers. The most potent vasodilator, minoxidil, is very effective in treating severe hypertension, especially in combination with a beta-blocker and a diuretic. Hair growth with minoxidil limits its long-term usefulness in women. Other agents that are useful include sympatholytics, central and peripheral alpha-antagonists, and combined alpha/beta blockers.

Most patients require combination therapy. Some require several agents. Useful combinations include the following:

- A diuretic with an ACE inhibitor or receptor antagonist. A calcium antagonist can also be added.
- Calcium antagonists, beta-blockers, and diuretics can also be combined effectively. Recent concerns about the reflex sympathetic response to calcium antagonists may be mitigated by the concomitant use of a beta-blocker.
- The combination of a vasodilator, a beta-blocker, and a diuretic is also very effective.

When hypertension cannot be controlled, particularly if attempts to reduce blood result in decreased allograft function, the possibility of renal allograft artery stenosis should be considered (see Chapter 7). Color-flow Doppler examination of the renal artery may aid in the diagnosis, but interpretation of this test is difficult, and false-positive results are common. Radionuclide scanning is usually not helpful. Magnetic resonance angiography or renal arteriography should be used for diagnosis when suspicion of renal allograft artery stenosis is high (see Chapter 12). Percutaneous transluminal angioplasty may improve renal function and reduce the need for antihypertensive medications in 60% to 85% of cases. Restenosis may occur in up to 30%. Surgery should probably be reserved for critical stenoses that threaten the integrity of the graft.

The native kidneys often contribute to hypertension after renal transplantation. Studies to determine the role of the native kidneys in causing hypertension, however, are probably not useful. In particular, renal vein renins do not reliably predict blood pressure reduction after native kidney nephrectomy. Therefore, in difficult-to-control hypertension, consideration should be given to empirical removal of the native kidneys. Laparoscopic surgery may reduce the morbidity of posttransplantation native kidney nephrectomy.

Strategy 7: Do Everything Possible to Encourage Patients to Quit Smoking

Cigarette smoking appears to be just as prevalent among renal transplant recipients as it is in the general population. Cigarette smoking has been shown to contribute to cardiovascular disease and to increase the already high risk for cancer after renal transplantation. Studies in nontransplanted populations have also shown smoking to be detrimental to renal function. Thus, every effort should be made to encourage transplant recipients to quit smoking. Smoking cessation programs that make use of nicotine replacement therapies have been shown in clinical trials to be effective. Guidelines for smoking cessation have been developed by the American Psychiatric Society and the Agency for Health Care Policy and Research.

Strategy 8: Screen for Breast, Cervical, Prostate, Colorectal, and Skin Cancer

Knowledge that many posttransplantation cancers are caused by viruses has not yet produced effective prophylactic strategies. Successful treatment of cancer after renal transplantation relies on surveillance and early detection. Guidelines for cancer screening developed for the general population are applicable to renal transplant recipients. Although breast cancer is not more prevalent after transplantation than in the general population, it is still prudent for women older than 50 years of age to undergo screening mammography with or without breast self-examination every 1 to 2 years. Women who are younger than 50 years of age who are at high risk (due to a family history of premenopausal breast cancer in a first-degree relative or a prior history of breast cancer) should also undergo screening mammography every 1 to 2 years with or without clinical breast examination. Cervical carcinoma is more prevalent in transplant recipients, and women older than 18 years of age should have an annual pelvic examination and Papanicolaou smear.

Prostate cancer does not appear to be more common among renal transplant recipients than in the general population, but screening with digital rectal examination is recommended. The sensitivity of the digital rectal examination is low and is operator dependent. Serum prostate-specific antigen, on the other hand, has a sensitivity of about 70% for the detection of prostate cancer in men. Prostatitis and benign prostatic hypertrophy can cause false-positive elevations, and the positive predictive value is only 25% to 50%. Nevertheless, the prostate-specific antigen test is probably useful for screening. Anogenital carcinoma is common after renal transplantation. Yearly physical examination and pelvic examination in women are useful to screen for anogenital lesions. Transplant recipients 50 years or older should undergo screening for colorectal cancer with annual fecal occult blood testing. Flexible sigmoidoscopy or colonoscopy should be performed every 5 years.

Skin cancers are common after renal transplantation. Annual self-examination and examination by a physician are warranted to screen for squamous cell carcinoma and malignant melanoma. Suspicious lesions should undergo biopsy. Patients should be instructed to avoid sun exposure and to use sun block, although the effectiveness of this strategy in adults is uncertain. Patients with multiple lesions should undergo formal dermatologic surveillance on a regular basis. In addition to local measures, oral isotretinoin may be beneficial and appears to be safe in transplant recipients.

The management of immunosuppression in patients who have developed cancer is difficult, and each case should be considered individually. There is clinical evidence that higher cyclosporine levels are associated with an increased incidence of cancer and experimental evidence that cyclosporine may accelerate the growth of metastatic cancer. It is unlikely that this finding is specific for cyclosporine; therefore, it is wise to minimize the immunosuppressive protocol, and in some cases, discontinuation of immunosuppression may be appropriate. The potential for graft loss needs to be weighed against the natural history and the staging of the malignancy. It is the patient who must ultimately decide on his or her priorities after receiving consultation from his or her oncologic and transplantation physicians. Posttransplantation lymphoproliferative disease is discussed later.

Strategy 9: Immunize Against Influenza and Pneumococcal Pneumonia

Infections are common in the late posttransplantation period (see Chapter 10). These infections are sporadic, and few specific measures are effective in reducing the risk for infection. Routine prophylaxis for *P. carinii* and *T. gondii* infections with trimethoprim-sulfamethoxazole is probably not warranted late after transplantation. The exception may be in patients who are receiving high doses of immunosuppression to treat rejection. The same is true for CMV infection prophylaxis. Although recurrent urinary tract infections are common, there is no evidence that routine prophylactic antibiotic therapy is effective.

Influenza types A and B are likely to be at least as common, and probably more severe, in renal transplant patients as in the general population. Therefore, transplant recipients should receive annual influenza vaccination. Although the vaccines are safe, they may be somewhat less effective in transplant recipients than in the general population because of the limitation in antibody response by immunosuppressant drugs. Nevertheless, the response to vaccination is high enough (50% to 100%) to warrant their use. During the influenza season, chemoprophylaxis with amantadine or rimantadine (effective only against influenza A) or one of the newer neuraminidase inhibitors (effective against influenza A and

B) should be considered for patients who have not yet been vaccinated. Consideration should also be given to the early diagnosis of influenza. If begun early, therapy can shorten the course of influenza infection and is probably warranted in immunosuppressed transplant recipients. Infections from *Streptococcus pneumoniae* are also common after renal transplantation and can cause considerable morbidity and mortality. The polyvalent pneumococcal vaccine should probably be administered every 2 years.

Strategy 10: Consider Prophylaxis With Aspirin, Calcium, and Hormone Replacement Therapy; Encourage Regular Exercise

Few therapies have been proved to be effective for disease prevention in the general population. Aspirin has been shown to prevent CVD events for patients with known CVD. The role of aspirin prophylaxis in primary prevention is less clear. Aspirin should be considered for renal transplant recipients with CVD, and possibly for patients who are at high risk for CVD events.

Regular aerobic exercise should be part of the therapeutic regimen of all patients at high CVD risk and may be particularly beneficial in counteracting the effects of corticosteroids on muscle and bone. Near-normal levels of physical functioning are possible after transplantation, particularly for those patients who engage in regular physical activity.

Corticosteroid-induced osteopenia and its consequences are a common cause of morbidity in the late posttransplantation period. Cross-sectional studies have consistently shown that bone mass is lower in transplant recipients than in age- and sex-matched controls. Vertebral bone loss is highest in the first posttransplantation year (3% to 9%) but continues thereafter at a rate of about 2% per year. A fracture rate of 7% to 11% has been described in nondiabetic kidney transplant recipients and in diabetic recipients of kidney and pancreas transplants, the fracture incidence has been reported to be up to 45%. It is reasonable to screen for decreased bone mineral density at baseline and 6 months after transplantation with dual x-ray absorptiometry of the lumbar spine and hip. Patients with decreased bone mineral density may be candidates for oral calcium and vitamin D supplementation. Postmenopausal women may also benefit from hormone replacement therapy. Patients with abnormal bone mineral density 6 months after transplantation should be considered for additional follow-up examinations to measure the effectiveness of therapy. Bisphosphonates, which inhibit osteoclast activity, may be effective in treating posttransplantation osteopenia. However, bisphosphonates may be contraindicated in patients with bone disease characterized by low turnover. Low bone turnover can be diagnosed only with a bone biopsy. The role of bisphosphonates in preventing posttransplantation osteopenia is still being investigated, but preliminary studies are encouraging. It is difficult to prove a direct relationship between corticosteroid dose and bone loss, but it is reasonable to minimize steroid dose or consider discontinuation in the patients at highest risk.

Corticosteroids may also cause avascular necrosis, or osteonecrosis. The most common site for posttransplantation avascular necrosis is the femoral head, but other locations are occasionally

encountered. Up to 15% of transplant recipients may develop osteonecrosis in the first few years after transplantation, although the
incidence may be declining. The pathogenesis of osteonecrosis
is poorly understood, but corticosteroids can be implicated in most
cases. Osteonecrosis usually presents as hip or groin pain exacerbated by weight bearing. Magnetic resonance imaging is the most
sensitive method for diagnosis. Core decompression before the
femoral head collapses may relieve pain, but most often, patients
with avascular necrosis eventually require total hip arthroplasty.

Hypophosphatemia is common early after transplantation but
is less common in the late posttransplantation period. When
hypophosphatemia is encountered in the late posttransplantation period, it is often due to tertiary hyperparathyroidism, and
serum parathyroid hormone levels should be measured in all patients with late posttransplantation hypophosphatemia. On the
other hand, hyperphosphatemia may also be encountered, usually
in transplant recipients with renal insufficiency. Attempts should
be made to suppress elevated parathyroid hormone levels by increasing serum calcium to high-normal levels. Calcium can usually
be increased by reducing elevated serum phosphorous levels
(with dietary phosphorous restriction and phosphorous binders)
or by administering oral calcium and vitamin D supplements. If
increased parathyroid hormone levels cannot be suppressed, particularly if hypercalcemia becomes problematic, then parathyroidectomy may be required.

Hypomagnesemia is seen in about 10% of renal transplant
recipients treated with calcineurin inhibitors. Hypomagnesemia
may play a role in posttransplantation hyperlipidemia and hypertension. Treatment is usually by oral magnesium replacement.

OTHER MANAGEMENT ISSUES IN THE LATE
POSTTRANSPLANTATION PERIOD

Posttransplantation Lymphoproliferative Disease

The reported incidence of PTLD in the recipients of solid-organ
transplants ranges from 0.8% to as high as 20% and varies with
the type of transplantation, the patient's age, and the immunosuppressive regimen employed. In kidney transplant recipients,
the incidence is typically 1% to 2%.

PTLDs have several unusual features that distinguish them
from lymphomas found in the general population:

1. Most (96%) are non-Hodgkin's lymphomas (Hodgkin's disease
   is the most common lymphoma in age-matched controls) and
   are of B-cell origin.
2. Extranodal involvement (central nervous system, liver, lungs,
   kidneys, intestines) is common, and multiple sites are often
   involved.
3. There is a high rate of association with EBV infection. Seronegative recipients of an organ from a seropositive donor are
   at highest risk for PTLD.
4. The mortality rate is much greater for PTLD than for lymphomas in the general population. The course may be extremely fulminant, with progression to death within a few
   months of transplantation.

5. PTLD often presents as dysfunction of the transplanted organ and may be confused histologically with severe rejection.
6. The prolonged or repeated administration of antilymphocytic antibody preparations is a significant risk factor for the development of PTLD.
7. PTLD may respond to withdrawal or drastic reduction of immunosuppressive therapy. Standard chemotherapy and irradiation are not generally helpful and may exaggerate the degree of immune compromise.
8. Viral infection, particularly with CMV, may be a trigger for the development of PTLD. Prophylactic antiviral therapy, usually targeted against CMV infection (see Chapter 10), may serendipitously reduce EBV replication and the incidence of PTLD.

Role of Epstein-Barr Virus

EBV is a human DNA-transforming herpesvirus that primarily targets B lymphocytes. It is associated with an array of disorders ranging from infectious mononucleosis to nasopharyngeal carcinoma, Burkitt's lymphoma, and B-cell lymphomas in immunocompromised patients.

Transmission of EBV in transplant recipients is most commonly through the transplanted organ. EBV undergoes lytic replication because of inadequate EBV immune surveillance. The resultant increased burden of EBV in the naive recipient then infects the recipient's B cells. EBV has the innate capability of transforming and immortalizing host B lymphocytes, producing *lymphoblastoid cells*. An extrachromosomal particle of EBV genome can be found within the B-cell nucleus. In an immunocompetent host, a latent carrier state is established when the proliferation of the transformed B cells is contained by a normal immune response with intact cell-mediated immunity. About 95% of adults have serologic evidence of previous EBV infection. The presence of reactive T lymphocytes inhibits infected cell proliferation in a process termed *regression*. Immunosuppressive agents, particularly the antilymphocytic antibody preparations (see Chapter 4), prevent regression, and EBV-transformed cells may proliferate uncontrollably.

EBV-associated PTLD appears to progress through stages of transformation to a malignant state. The first stage resembles an infectious mononucleosis syndrome, with the development of polymorphic diffuse B-cell hyperplasias without cytogenic abnormalities or gene rearrangements. The second stage produces a subpopulation of cells with cellular and nuclear atypia and cytogenic abnormalities. In the third stage, a malignant monoclonal B-cell lymphoma develops. A form of fulminant PTLD has been described, often following multiple courses of OKT3. The disease may initially resemble a severe infectious mononucleosis-like illness but may progress rapidly, with death occurring within a few months of transplantation. At a later stage, the patient may present with localized lymphoproliferative tumor masses in the brain, lung, or gastrointestinal tract.

Clonality

The issue of the clonality of posttransplantation lymphomas has been a source of dispute. It has been suggested that polyclonal B-cell lesions are more likely to be benign and to respond to withdrawal of immunosuppression and acyclovir, whereas monoclonal lesions are believed to be frankly malignant. In fact, polyclonal lymphoproliferative disorders may represent an early stage in a spectrum that progresses from polyclonal activation of B cells by EBV to latently infected, malignantly transformed, monoclonal B-cell lymphomas.

Treatment

Restoration of host immunity is probably the most important therapy for the control of lymphoid proliferation. Patients with evidence of polyclonality are most likely to respond to reduction of immunosuppression. Acyclovir, which acts by inhibiting the EBV-associated DNA polymerase, is often used but is not of proven benefit. For patients with monoclonal tumors, immunosuppression should be drastically reduced or discontinued altogether. Acyclovir is less likely to be effective in monoclonal disorders, but conventional cytotoxic therapy and radiotherapy have also had disappointing responses, with mortality rates remaining at greater than 80%. There is limited experience using treatment with recombinant interferon-alpha. Anti–B-cell antibodies targeted against CD21, CD24, and CD20 (rituximab) have been used, and a response rate of 50% to 80% has been reported. Most patients in whom immunosuppression is stopped lose their grafts to inexorable rejection. Occasionally, tumors regress, and the patients and their grafts can be maintained on very-low-dose immunosuppression.

Hematologic Disorders

Anemia is common after renal transplantation. Iron deficiency is a frequent cause, and gastrointestinal bleeding should be excluded. Anemia from folate or vitamin B_{12} deficiency is unusual. Hemolysis is rare. In the late posttransplantation period, anemia is most commonly caused by immunosuppression or decreased renal function. Azathioprine, mycophenolate mofetil, and sirolimus can cause anemia, thrombocytopenia, and leukopenia, and the doses of these medications may need to be reduced. ACE inhibitors or receptor antagonists may also cause anemia. Parvovirus infection has been described to cause refractory anemia in patients receiving tacrolimus. When no underlying cause can be found, treatment with subcutaneous erythropoietin may be effective, particularly when renal function is impaired and iron stores are adequate. The efficacy of therapy can be monitored by observing changes in the reticulocyte count that precede an increase in the hemoglobin level.

Erythrocytosis is encountered in up to 20% of patients in the late posttransplantation period. It is most common during the first 2 years after transplantation. The cause of erythrocytosis appears to be related to defective feedback regulation of erythropoietin metabolism; it is not directly related to erythropoietin levels, and erythrocytosis rarely occurs in the absence of the native kidneys. Abnormalities in insulin-like growth factor-1 have been found in posttransplantation erythrocytosis and in polycythemia rubra vera. Hematocrit levels higher than 60% are associated with increased viscosity and thrombosis, and treatment should commence at a hematocrit level of greater than 55%. Low doses of ACE inhibitors or receptor antagonists are generally effective in reducing elevated hematocrit levels, but phlebotomy may be required.

Posttransplantation Reproductive Function

Male

After successful transplantation, about two thirds of male patients observe improved libido and increased sexual activity to predialysis levels. In some patients, there is no improvement, and occasionally sexual function deteriorates. Fertility, as assessed by sperm counts, improves in half of patients. The sex hormone profile tends to normalize; plasma testosterone and follicle-stimulating hormone levels increase; and luteinizing hormone levels, which may be high in dialysis patients, decrease to normal or low levels. Cyclosporine may impair testosterone biosynthesis through direct damage to Leydig cells and germinal cells, and a direct impairment of the hypothalamic-pituitary-gonadal axis has been suggested. There is no increased incidence of neonatal malformations in pregnancies fathered by transplant recipients.

Additional factors may account for failure of male sexual function to improve after transplantation. Antihypertensive medications may be responsible in some patients, autonomic neuropathy may impair erectile function, and interruption of both hypogastric arteries may occasionally impair vascular supply. Male patients should be asked about their sexual function and referred for urologic evaluation when necessary. There is no specific contraindication to the use of sildenafil (Viagra) in transplant recipients so long as standard precautions are taken regarding concomitant coronary artery disease.

Female

Women with chronic renal failure demonstrate loss of libido, anovulatory vaginal bleeding or amenorrhea, and high prolactin levels. Maintenance dialysis therapy results in improvement in sexual function in only a small percentage of women, and pregnancy is rare. Within a year of successful transplantation, menstrual function and ovulation typically return, and prolactin levels fall to normal.

Family Planning

All women of childbearing age should be counseled concerning the possibility and risks of pregnancy after kidney transplantation. Psychosocial issues should be discussed, genetic counseling should be provided for those with hereditary kidney disease, and consideration should be given to the long-term prognosis of the patient and the graft. Patients can be assured that birth defects are not increased with the use of azathioprine, cyclosporine, and tacrolimus during pregnancy, although intrauterine growth retardation and prematurity are common. Data regarding the stability of graft function during and after pregnancy should be discussed. All pregnancies should be planned and prepared for. Conception should be delayed 18 to 24 months after kidney transplantation and contraception practiced until then.

Contraceptive counseling should begin immediately after transplantation because ovulatory cycles may begin within 1 to 2 months of transplantation in women with well-functioning grafts. Low-dose estrogen-progesterone oral contraceptive preparations are advised. They should be used with caution because they may cause or aggravate hypertension or precipitate thromboembolism, especially in the context of cyclosporine immunosuppression. Calcineurin inhibitor levels should also be monitored soon after the contraceptive is started. The long-acting, subcutaneously placed hormone preparations are highly effective and well-tolerated. They have not yet been formally tried in the transplant situation and should be used only under careful supervision. The risk for infection may be increased with the use of an intrauterine device in immunocompromised patients, and their efficacy may be compromised by the antiinflammatory properties of the immunosuppressive agents. Barrier contraception is the safest modality but depends on user compliance for efficacy.

Pregnancy

Women with end-stage renal disease sometimes seek transplantation with the knowledge that a well-functioning graft will give them the only real chance for natural motherhood. It has been estimated that 2% of women of childbearing age conceive after transplantation. The incidence of spontaneous abortion has been reported to be 13% and that of ectopic pregnancy 0.5%. These frequencies are not different from those seen in the normal population. About one third of pregnant transplant recipients seek therapeutic abortion, a number that likely reflects inadequate family planning in women who have not previously considered themselves to be fertile. More than 90% of conceptions that continue beyond the first trimester end successfully.

Table 9.11 lists the criteria that should ideally be met before conception. A 90% incidence of successful pregnancies has been reported for women with a baseline serum creatinine of 1.5 mg/dL or less. Failure to meet all the listed criteria places the patient in a higher risk category but is not necessarily a contraindication to pregnancy. The *U.S. National Transplantation Pregnancy Registry* has been developed to provide current information concerning transplant recipient pregnancy for the benefit of patients and their physicians.

**Table 9.11. Criteria for the reduction
of posttransplantation pregnancy risk**

1. At least 1 year posttransplantation
2. Serum creatinine <2.0 mg/dL, preferably <1.5 mg/dL
3. No recent episodes of acute rejection
4. Normotensive or minimal antihypertensive regimen
5. Minimal or no proteinuria
6. Normal allograft ultrasound
7. Pregnancy-safe drug regimen (see text)

Antenatal Care

Pregnancy in a patient with a kidney transplant should be considered a high-risk condition and should be monitored in a tertiary care center with consultation by a transplantation nephrologist, obstetrician, and pediatrician. The pregnancy should be diagnosed as early as possible and accurate dating obtained by fetal ultrasound. In patients with good allograft function before conception, the glomerular filtration rate (GFR) remains stable or increases, as it does during a normal pregnancy. The GFR may decline to prepregnancy values during the third trimester. Most studies suggest that pregnancy itself does not have an unfavorable effect on long-term graft function as long as baseline function is excellent. Proteinuria may increase to abnormal levels in the third trimester but usually resolves postpartum and is of no prognostic significance unless it is associated with hypertension. About 30% of pregnant patients with kidney transplants develop pregnancy-induced hypertension, a figure that is four-fold greater than in uncomplicated pregnancies. The use of cyclosporine in pregnancy tends to increase the incidence of hypertension, which lowers birth weight.

Urinary tract infections are the most common bacterial infections and occur in up to 40% of pregnant transplant recipients. Pyelonephritis may develop despite adequate antibiotic treatment. Urinary tract infections are particularly common in patients who develop end-stage renal disease due to pyelonephritis.

Viral infections are of special concern because viruses are capable of crossing the placenta and infecting the fetus. An infant born to an HBsAg-positive mother should be given hepatitis B immunoglobulin within 12 hours of birth and HBV vaccine at another site within 48 hours (followed by a booster injection at 1 to 6 months). The combination of immunoglobulin and vaccine offers protection for more than 90% of infants. CMV surveillance buffy coat cultures and serology should be obtained routinely because virus reactivation is possible even with substantial existing antibody titers. If viral reactivation occurs, the pediatrician should be alerted to the necessity of screening the neonate for congenital CMV infection. Herpes simplex virus (HSV) infection before 20 weeks' gestation is associated with an increased rate of abortion. HSV is not thought to be a cause of intrauterine infection so long as the membranes are intact. A positive HSV cervical culture at term is an indication for cesarean section.

Immunosuppression in Pregnancy

PREDNISONE. Prednisone crosses the placenta, but a large proportion is converted to prednisolone, which allegedly does not suppress fetal corticotropin. Adrenal insufficiency in the neonate has been reported with maternal prednisone ingestion. Very large doses of corticosteroids administered to animals have resulted in congenital anomalies (cleft lip and palate), but no consistent abnormalities have been noted in the offspring of women treated with corticosteroids during pregnancy for rheumatologic disease or kidney transplantation. Overall, prednisone is considered to be relatively safe for use in pregnancy.

AZATHIOPRINE. At doses of 2 mg/kg or less, no anomalies attributable to azathioprine have been noted in human offspring. There are minimal data, however, on the long-term effects of azathioprine on first- or second-generation offspring. Azathioprine can cause transient gaps or breaks in lymphocyte chromosomes. Germ cells and other tissues have not been studied. It is not known whether the eventual sequelae could be the development of malignancies in affected offspring or other abnormalities in the next generation.

CALCINEURIN INHIBITORS. There are no animal or human data showing teratogenicity or mutagenicity of cyclosporine or tacrolimus, which appear to be safe during pregnancy. Intrauterine growth retardation and small-for-gestational-age neonates have been reported with cyclosporine use and may reflect chronic vasoconstriction. Cyclosporine is present in the fetal circulation at the same concentration found in the mother. The increased volume of distribution may produce low maternal blood levels, and dose elevations may be required.

OTHER IMMUNOSUPPRESSANTS. Few data are available concerning the safety of pregnancy for patients receiving the newer immunosuppressive agents (see Chapter 4); for the present, they should be avoided during pregnancy. Mycophenolate mofetil should be discontinued 6 weeks before conception is attempted. At present, there is insufficient information about the biologic effect of even small amounts of immunosuppressive agents on the neonate, and breastfeeding should be discouraged.

Labor and Delivery

Vaginal delivery is recommended because the transplanted kidney is placed in the false pelvis and there is little risk for obstruction of the birth canal or mechanical injury to the allograft. Cesarean section is usually performed only for standard obstetric reasons. Great care should be taken to identify and protect the transplanted ureter. Preterm delivery occurs in about half of pregnancies in transplant recipients because of the frequent occurrence of declining kidney function, pregnancy-induced hypertension, fetal distress, premature rupture of membranes, and premature labor. The incidence of small-for-gestational-age neonates is 20%. There is no increase in fetal abnormalities.

In the perinatal period, the steroid dose should be augmented to cover the stress of labor and to prevent postpartum rejection. Hydrocortisone, 100 mg every 6 hours, should be given during labor and delivery. Maternal hypertension and fluid balance should be monitored carefully. Graft function and the immunosuppressive regimen should be monitored with particular care in the first 3 months postpartum. Occasional cases of postpartum acute renal failure resembling hemolytic-uremic syndrome have been described.

SELECTED READINGS

Part I

Cosio FG, Peletier RP, Sedmak DD, et al. Renal allograft survival following acute rejection correlates with blood pressure levels and histopathology. *Kidney Int* 1999;56:1912.

Fishmann JA, Rubin RH. Infection in organ-transplant recipients. *N Engl J Med* 1998;338:1741.

Halloran PF, Melk A, Barth C. Rethinking chronic allograft nephropathy: the concept of accelerated senescence. *J Am Soc Nephrol* 1999; 10:167.

Hariharan S, Adams MB, Brennan DC, et al. Recurrent and de novo glomerular disease after renal transplantation: a report from renal allograft disease registry. *Transplant Proc* 1999;31:223.

Jain S, Furness PN, Nicholson ML. The role of transforming growth factor beta in chronic renal allograft nephropathy. *Transportation* 2000;69:1759.

Kasiske BL, Guijarro C, Massy ZA, et al. Cardiovascular disease after renal transplantation. *J Am Soc Nephrol* 1996;7:158.

Massy ZA, Guijarro C, Wiederkehr MR, et al. Chronic renal allograft rejection: immunologic and nonimmunologic risk factors. *Kidney Int* 1996;49:518.

Ojo AO, Hanson JA, Wolfe RA, et al. Longterm survival in renal transplant recipients with graft function. *Kidney Int* 2000;57:307.

Opelz G, Wujciak T, Ritz E, for the Collaborative Transplant Study. Association of chronic kidney graft failure with recipient blood pressure. *Kidney Int* 1998;53:217–222.

Penn I. De novo cancers in organ allograft recipients. *Curr Opin Org Transplant* 1998;3:188–196.

Perez FM, Rodriguez-Carmona A, Garcia FT, et al. Early immunologic and nonimmunologic predictors of arterial hypertension after renal transplantation. *Am J Kidney Dis* 1999;33:21.

Prommool S, Thangri GS, Cockfield SM, et al. Time dependency of factors affecting renal allograft survival. *J Am Soc Nephrol* 2000; 11:565.

Sheil AGR. Cancer report. In: Disney APS, ed. *Australia and New Zealand dialysis and transplant registry 1997.* Adelaide, South Australia, 1998:138–146.

West M, Sutherland DER, Matas AJ. Kidney transplant recipients who die with functioning grafts: serum creatinine level and cause of death. *Transplantation* 1996;62:1029.

Part II

Cueto-Manzano AM, Konel S, Hutchinson A. Bone loss in long-term renal transplantation: histopathology and densitometry analysis. *Kidney Int* 1999;55:2021.

Danovitch GM, Jamgotchian NJ, Eggena PH, et al. Angiotensin-converting enzyme inhibition in the treatment of renal transplant erythrocytosis: clinical experience and observation of mechanism. *Transplantation* 1995;60:132.

Gaston RS, Hudson SL, Ward M, et al. Late renal allograft loss: non-compliance masquerading as chronic rejection. *Transplant Proc* 1999;31:21S.

Ghandour FZ, Knauss TC, Hricik DE. Immunosuppressive drugs in pregnancy. *Adv Ren Rep Ther* 1998;5:31.

Hojo M, Morimoto T, Maluccio M, et al. Cyclosporine induces cancer progression by a cell-autonomous mechanism. *Nature* 1999;397:530.

Kasiske BL, Heim-Duthoy K, Ma JZ. Elective cyclosporine withdrawal after renal transplantation: a meta-analysis. *JAMA* 1993; 269:395.

Massari PU. Disorders of bone and mineral metabolism after renal transplantation. *Kidney Int* 1997;52:1412.

Massy ZA, Kasiske BL. Post-transplant hyperlipidemia: mechanisms and management. *J Am Soc Nephrol* 1996;7:971.

Miles AM, Sumrani N, Horowitz R. Diabetes mellitus after renal transplantation. *Transplantation* 1998;65:380.

Paya CV, Fung JJ, Nalesnik MA, et al. Epstein-Barr virus-induced posttransplant lymphoproliferative disorders. *Transplantation* 1999; 68:1517.

Stigant CE, Cohen J, Vivera M, et al. ACE inhibition and angiotensin II antagonists in renal transplantation: an analysis of safety and efficacy. *Am J Kidney Dis* 1999;35:58.

Weber TJ, Quarles D. Preventing bone loss after renal transplantation with bisphosphonates: We can . . . but should we? *Kidney Int* 2000; 57:735.

Wilkinson A. Use of angiotensin-converting enzyme inhibitors and angiotensin II antagonists in renal transplantation: Delaying the progression of chronic allograft nephropathy. *Transplant Rev* 2000;14:1.

10

Infectious Complications of Kidney Transplantation and Their Management

Bernard M. Kubak, David A. Pegues, and Curtis D. Holt

Of the solid organ transplantations, kidney transplantation is associated with the lowest rates of infection. In contrast to liver, heart, or lung allograft recipients, whose clinical and nutritional status often deteriorates before transplantation, the elective or semielective nature of kidney transplantation lowers the risk for infection. Despite these considerations, infections related to the transplantation procedure or to opportunistic pathogens can affect graft function and transplant outcome. This chapter highlights the infectious disease considerations in transplant candidates, posttransplantation infection prophylaxis, and the recognition and treatment of infectious syndromes with appropriate agents and dosages to minimize allograft toxicity.

GENERAL GUIDELINES FOR INFECTION RECOGNITION

Recognition of the following factors may assist in the identification of the causative pathogen and the initiation of appropriate therapy before laboratory confirmation:

1. The temporal occurrence of a presumed infectious episode relative to the date of transplantation (Fig. 10.1)
2. The infectious history of the donor, specifically, any infectious agent that can be directly transmitted with the donor graft
3. Preoperative recipient infectious history or exposures (e.g., exposure to tuberculosis, hepatitis viruses, human immunodeficiency virus [HIV], varicella zoster virus [VZV], cytomegalovirus [CMV], or Epstein-Barr virus [EBV]), immunizations, immune-altering conditions (e.g., surgical or functional asplenia, pretransplantation medical conditions requiring immunosuppressive agents, diabetes mellitus), substance or intravenous drug abuse, liver dysfunction, malnutrition, and geographic exposures (e.g., endemic mycoses, toxoplasmosis, *Strongyloides* species infection, intestinal parasites)
4. Acquisition of community and hospital-acquired organisms (e.g., *Streptococcus pneumoniae,* Enterobacteriaceae, and *Pseudomonas* species, methicillin-resistant *Staphylococcus aureus,* vancomycin-resistant enterococci)
5. The *net state of immunosuppression,* which is a qualitative expression reflecting the interaction of the following factors:

    A. The prophylactic immunosuppressive protocol employed Augmentation of immunosuppression during episodes of rejection
    B. Neutropenia

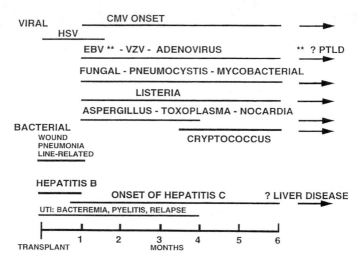

Fig. 10.1.   Timetable for occurrence of infection after transplantation.
CMV, cytomegalovirus; HSV, herpes simplex virus; EBV, Epstein-Barr
virus; VZV, varicella zoster virus; PTLD, posttransplantation lymphoproliferative disease; **, indicates possible relationship of EBV to
PTLD; UTI, urinary tract infection. Arrows indicate infections or
other manifestations that may present more than 6 months to years
after transplantation. (Modified from Rubin RH. Infection in the organ
transplant patient. In: Rubin RH, Young LS, eds. *Clinical approach
to infection in the compromised host.* New York: Plenum, 1994, with
permission.)

C. Open wounds, foreign bodies (e.g. catheters, stents), fluid
    collections, and devitalized tissues
D. Metabolic abnormalities (e.g. malnutrition, uremia, hyper-
    glycemia)
E. Infection with immunomodulatory viruses (e.g., CMV, EBV).
    Viruses such as CMV and HHV can exert an immunomodu-
    lating effect that has been implicated in allograft rejection,
    obliterative transplant arteriopathy, opportunistic infec-
    tions, and posttransplantation lymphoproliferative disorder
    (PTLD).

Table 10.1 summarizes the clinical risk factors for infection in
the pretransplantation and posttransplantation settings.

PRETRANSPLANTATION SCREENING:
RECIPIENT AND DONOR

Pretransplantation latent infections or infectious exposures can
lead to a reappraisal of transplant candidacy or, subsequently,
alterations in standard posttransplantation management. Untreated or unrecognized infections in the recipient can become
apparent in the posttransplantation period. Any infections, such
as vascular or urinary catheter–associated infection, pneumonia,
cellulitis, periodontal abscess, or smoldering intraabdominal, hepa-

Table 10.1.   Risk factors for infection in renal transplant recipients

Pretransplantation (Recipient)	Perioperative	Posttransplantation
Medical condition	**Surgery**	**Postoperative management**
Immunosuppression for chronic conditions (corticosteroids, cyclophosphamide)	Prolonged procedure or anesthesia	Catheters, stents, intubation
Diabetes mellitus	Graft injury or prolonged ischemia	Anastomotic breakdown or leak
Suboptimal nutritional status	Bleeding or multiple blood transfusions	Fluid collections or devitalized tissue
Unrecognized or inadequately treated infection		Early reexploration or retransplantation Leukopenia
Altered bacterial colonization	**Graft (donor)**	**Hospital flora acquisition**
Preoperative antibiotic exposures	Bacteremia or sepsis	Prolonged antibiotic therapy
Duration of hospitalization	Unrecognized infection in allograft Microbial contamination of preservation fluid	Increased antibiotic resistance
		Immunosuppression Multiple agents Antibody induction and rejection treatment Steroids—maintenance dose and pulses

tobiliary, or genitourinary tract infection, can reactivate or exacerbate in the immediate postoperative period during induction immunosuppression or subsequently, depending on the overall net state of immunosuppression.

General Screening
Pretransplantation evaluation is discussed in detail in Chapter 6. Evaluation of the patient for infectious disease should include a history of antibiotic allergies and cardiac valvular repairs, a dental assessment, a preoperative urine culture, and a chest radiograph to exclude active pneumonic processes and to identify evi-

dence of prior granulomatous or infectious disorders (Table 10.2). Patients from geographic areas with endemic mycoses should be identified and evaluated for disease. Of note, old "healed" granulomatous lesions representing prior tuberculosis, histoplasmosis, or coccidioidomycosis can reactivate in the posttransplantation setting under conditions of routine immunosuppression or after treatment of rejection. A purified protein derivative (PPD) skin test with appropriate controls (i.e., mumps, candidiasis, tetanus) should be applied; however, suboptimal reactivity of skin testing in renal failure patients can lead to false-negative results. Isoniazid prophylaxis may be indicated with an abnormal chest radiograph representing old tuberculosis despite a negative skin test. Guidelines should adhere to the American Thoracic Society recommendations on isoniazid prophylaxis for indications and duration of therapy; prophylactic isoniazid after transplantation is usually not required in patients who have previously completed a full curative course for active tuberculosis. Patients with polycystic kidney disease who have been treated for infected polycystic kidneys should have repeatedly negative urine cultures. Pretransplantation polycystic nephrectomy is occasionally required (see Chapter 6).

Serologic Testing

Preoperative serologic testing can help identify at-risk candidates and should include HIV (by enzymeimmunoassay [EIA] with Western blot analysis confirmation), EBV, hepatitis B virus (HBV; hepatitis B surface antibody, surface antigen, and core immunoglobulin G [IgG] and IgM antibody), hepatitis C virus (HCV; by antibody screening or with an RNA-detection assay as warranted; see Chapter 11), VZV, CMV, and specific endemic-mycosis antibody tests when applicable (e.g., anticoccidioidal antibody detection in any patient with endemic exposure no matter the duration).

Human Immunodeficiency Virus

All potential kidney transplant recipients should be tested for HIV regardless of the recognition of risk factors. HIV positivity has

Table 10.2.   Pretransplantation screening

Underlying medical conditions
Antibiotic and medication allergies or adverse reactions
Chest radiograph (e.g., prior granulomatous lesions, scarring)
Dental assessment
Immunizations (hepatitis, Pneumovax, tetanus, influenza)
History of sexually transmitted diseases
PPD skin test with adequate controls; history of tuberculous risk
    factors and exposure
Preoperative urine culture
Valvular repairs or replacements
Serologies: HIV, HBV/HCV, CMV, EBV, VZV, coccidioides,
    histoplasma, toxoplasma

PPD, purified protein derivative; HIV, human immunodeficiency virus;
HBV, hepatitis B virus; HCV, hepatitis C virus; CMV, cytomegalovirus;
EBV, Epstein-Barr virus; VZV, varicella-zoster virus

been regarded as a contraindication to kidney transplantation because of the enhanced progression of the disease with immuno-suppression and the relatively improved survival with hemodialy-sis. This policy is being reconsidered in some centers in certain well-defined circumstances (see Chapter 6). All potential trans-plant donors, both live and cadaveric, should be tested for HIV regardless of risk factors. Many centers reject kidneys from high-risk donors for fear of failure to detect antibody during the "win-dow" after infection (see Chapter 5). Although transmission of HIV by infected organs has been described, these precautions have reduced the risk for infection to an almost negligible degree.

Epstein-Barr Virus
EBV-seronegative recipients of grafts from EBV-seropositive donors or EBV-seropositive recipients may be at increased risk for PTLD, particularly if they receive prolonged or repeated courses of antilymphocytic therapy (see Chapter 9). The EBV-DNA titer can be assayed when increasing the overall net state of immuno-suppression, and surveillance by EBV polymerase chain reaction (PCR) can be performed, although for most kidney transplant recipients, this is unnecessary.

Hepatitis B and C
The finding of positive pretransplantation HBV and HCV serore-activity in both transplant donors and recipients has become more common with the availability of improved laboratory methods to detect viral-specific antibody, antigens, and nucleic acids. The effects of these findings on transplant candidacy and on the use of donor kidneys are discussed in Chapter 11.

Cytomegalovirus
CMV is the most common viral infection after kidney transplan-tation and may vary in severity from asymptomatic infection to multiorgan involvement and death. The incidence of CMV posi-tivity increases with age, and most adult dialysis patients have detectable IgG antibody to CMV. The clinical significance of the CMV antibody status of the donor and recipient is discussed later and shown in Table 10.3.

Coccidioidomycosis and Histoplasmosis
The pretransplantation identification of *Coccidioides immitis* com-plement fixation and immunodiffusion serologies or *Histoplasma capsulatum* serologies should alert the clinician to the possibility of reactivation disease after transplantation. Reactivation can occur during routine immunosuppression or after augmented immuno-suppression for rejection. Patients who have resided in geographic areas with endemic mycoses should be screened before transplan-tation and, if found to have prior infection, considered candidates for prophylactic antifungal agents (e.g., an azole agent in a patient with healed old granulomatous disease due to coccidioidomycosis or histoplasmosis).

Immunizations
When possible, incomplete immunizations in the recipient should be corrected before transplantation. The immune response to

Table 10.3. Relationship of incidence of cytomegalovirus infection and disease to seropositivity of donor and recipient

Donor	Recipient	Terminology	Cytomegalovirus Status		
			Infection (%)	Disease (%)	Pneumonitis (%)
Positive	Negative	Primary infection	70–88	56–80	30
Negative	Positive	Reactivation	0–20	0–27	Rare
Positive	Positive[a]	Reinfection or superinfection	70	27–39	3–14
		Reactivation	15–30		

[a] The source of infection and disease may be a new virus strain from the donor or latent virus in the recipient. The prevention of cytomegalovirus disease in renal transplantation. Am. J. Kidney Dis, *16*:175, 1990.

Data from Davis, C.L.:

vaccinations may vary among patients with long-standing renal failure. Pretransplantation candidates lacking standard pediatric or adult immunizations, splenectomized patients, and hemodialysis patients may benefit from pretransplantation vaccinations with influenza, pneumococcal, hepatitis B, and varicella vaccines as well as diphtheria-pertussis-tetanus (DPT), inactivated polio, and measles-mumps-rubella (MMR) vaccines. However, reduced efficacy of vaccinations in patients with renal failure must be recognized. Live vaccines should be avoided in immunocompromised patients (e.g., a renal transplant candidate with an underlying condition requiring immunosuppressive medications) and in patients who have undergone solid organ transplantation.

Of particular concern are pediatric renal failure patients with incomplete primary immunizations of live viral vaccines, such as MMR or varicella. The general recommendation of avoiding live attenuated viral vaccines in allograft recipients precludes the completion of the immunization series, thereby exposing the child to the risk for measles. Consequently, pretransplantation immunization offers the opportunity to prevent the posttransplantation risks of live, attenuated viral vaccines. In this respect, measles, MMR, and varicella vaccines could be administered several months before transplantation. Of note, vaccinated patients should be reminded that they may be capable of transmitting the vaccine virus to close contacts or susceptible high-risk individuals. Successful vaccination against CMV has not been achieved.

Donor- and Allograft-Transmitted Infections

It may be difficult to differentiate between a true donor allograft source of infection, exogenous infection, and reactivation of latent disease. The following agents have been implicated with reasonable certainty as being transmissible with the donor allograft: HIV, CMV, HBV, HCV, tuberculosis, and certain fungi, including *H. capsulatum, C. immitis, Cryptococcus neoformans, Candida albicans,* and *Monisporium apiospermum.* Probable transmission has been reported with HSV; aerobic gram-positive and gram-negative bacteria; anaerobes; *Candida* species, *Toxoplasma,* and *Strongyloides* species; atypical mycobacterium; and EBV. The consequences of such transmission include infectious disruption of the vascular anastomoses, formation of mycotic aneurysms, infective endocarditis, and donor-derived sepsis. The incidence of true donor-transmitted infection can be reduced by scrupulous screening and epidemiologic evaluation (see Chapter 5).

PATHOGENESIS OF INFECTION IN KIDNEY ALLOGRAFT RECIPIENTS

Several host-related, epidemiologic, and iatrogenic factors predispose renal allograft recipients to infection (Table 10.1). Prior medical conditions other than those pertaining to renal disease may confer increased susceptibility to infections. Furthermore, any exposure to broad-spectrum antibiotics or to the hospital environment before transplantation can result in nosocomial colonization, often with organisms displaying increased antimicrobial resistance. Organisms include Enterobacteriaceae or *Pseudomonas* species, methicillin-resistant *S. aureus,* vancomycin-resistant enterococci, and fungal pathogens. Preexisting latent infections, such as herpesviruses, CMV, tuberculosis, and toxoplasmosis, may reactivate and cause morbidity.

About 80% of infections in kidney transplant recipients are bacterial. Table 10.4a and 10.4b summarize the syndromes and microbial pathogens commonly encountered in kidney transplant recipients. Most bacterial infectious syndromes occurring after solid organ transplantation are comparable to infections occurring after nontransplantation genitourinary surgery in immunocompetent patients. Within the first month after transplantation, the risk for infection follows the surgical complexity of the transplantation procedure. Common infectious syndromes in kidney recipients include genitourinary tract infection, pneumonia with or without bacteremia, primary bacteremia, intraabdominal infections, superficial or deep wound infections, urinary tract infections (UTIs), vascular catheter and site infections, and suprainfections, or fluid collections or devitalized tissues.

Pulmonary bacterial infections constitute most of the life-threatening infections in kidney transplant recipients. Pneumonia is more likely to occur in the event of prolonged intubation, underlying lung disease, increased incidence of aspiration or atelectasis, diminished cough reflex, and impaired diaphragmatic function. The particular level of nosocomial exposure to certain pathogens may determine the development of pneumonia, especially with *Legionella* and *Pseudomonas* species as well as other gram-negative bacteria. *Legionella* and *Pseudomonas* species may be present in hospital water supplies.

Distinct clinical patterns of bacteremia are found in transplant recipients; the urinary tract is the most common portal for kidney recipients. Patients with gram-negative bacterial sepsis fare poorer among all transplant recipients. Some studies suggest that bacterial sepsis predisposes to CMV infection as a result of either high levels of tumor necrosis factor-alpha or poor immune response to CMV in the context of serious bacterial infections.

Historically, UTIs were the most common infectious complication of renal transplantation. Fortunately, antimicrobial prophylaxis with trimethoprim-sulfamethoxazole (TMP/SMX) or ciprofloxacin decreases the frequency of UTIs to less than 10% and essentially eliminates urosepsis unless urine flow is obstructed. TMP/SMX can also reduce the incidence of *Nocardia asteroides* infection and sepsis related to *Listeria monocytogenes*. Genitourinary infectious risks are directly related to complications of the surgical procedure, such as the incidence of urine leaks, wound hematomas, and lymphoceles. Genitourinary tract manipulation during transplantation, urinary catheters, anatomic abnormalities (e.g., ureterovesicular stenosis, ureteral stricture, vesicoureteric reflux), and neurogenic bladder all predispose to posttransplantation UTI. Bacterial suprainfection of urine leaks and fistulas, wound hematomas, and lymphoceles can occur. Early catheter removal decreased the incidence of UTIs in renal allograft recipients. Perinephric abscesses are rarely seen after transplantation, with lymphoceles predisposing to abscess formation by means of repeated percutaneous drainage. Fever, graft tenderness, and a characteristic ultrasound appearance assist in diagnosis. Common organisms include staphylococci, enteric gram-negative bacteria, enterococci, and rarely anaerobic bacteria or *Candida* species.

Table 10.4a.   Commonly encountered bacterial pathogens in renal transplant recipients listed by site of infection

Intra-abdominal	Septicemia	Urinary Tract	Pneumonia	Wound	Dermatologic (Cellulitis)
Enterobacteriaceae	Enterobacteriaceae	Enterobacteriaceae	Enterobacteriaceae	Mixed infection	*Staphylococcus* sp.
Enterococcus species	*Pseudomas aeruginosa*	*P. aeruginosa*	*P. aeruginosa*	Enterobacteriaceae	*Streptococcus* sp.
Anaerobes (*Bacteroides* sp.)	*S. aureus*	*Enterococcus* sp.	*S. aureus*	*Pseudomas* sp.	Enterobacteriaceae
Staphylococcus aureus	*Enterococcus* sp.		*Streptococcus pneumoniae*	*Enterococcus* species	*Pseudomonas* sp. (ecthyma)
Mixed infection	Anaerobes (*Bacteroides* sp.)		*Nocardia* sp.	*S. aereus*	*Nocardia,*
			Legionella sp.	Anaerobes (*Bacteroides* sp.)	*Mycobacteria* sp. (nodules)
			Mycobacteria sp.		
			Rhodococcus sp. (rare)		

Table 10.4b.   Commonly encountered nonbacterial pathogens in renal transplant recipients listed by site of infection

Pneumonia	Urinary Tract	Gastrointestinal	Central Nervous System	Dermatologic
Aspergillus, Candida, Cryptococcus sp.	*Candida* sp.	CMV, HHV	*Cryptococcus neoformans*	Candida
Pneumocystis	CMV	*Candida,*	*Aspergillus* sp.	HHV
CMV, HHV, respiratory viruses, EBV	Adenovirus	*Aspergillus sp.*	CMV, HHV, VZV,	Dermatophytes
Zygomycoses (*Mucor*)		Adenovirus	(EBV, polyoma)	(*Trichophyton*, other sp.)
Coccidioides, Histoplasma, other sp.				*Aspergillus, Cryptococcus* sp.; endemic mycoses, *Fusarium, Scedosporium* sp.

HHV, human herpes virus; CMV, cytomegalovirus; EBV, Epstein-Barr virus; VZV, varicella zoster virus.

The incidence of surgical wound infections in kidney transplant recipients ranges from 2% to 25%; wound infections typically occur within 3 weeks after transplantation and are usually related to technical complications and recipient factors, such as obesity. The process can involve the perinephric space or cause mycotic aneurysms at the site of the vascular anastomosis. Rarely, allograft nephrectomy is required.

Preexisting medical conditions unrelated to the specific end-organ failure, such as diverticular disease or biliary disease, can manifest in the posttransplantation period. Posttransplantation colonic perforation may occur from preexisting diverticular disease in the setting of intensified immunosuppression. Corticosteroid use may facilitate gastrointestinal perforation by decreasing surveillance of bacterial invasion in the gastrointestinal tract, mucosal integrity, and fibroblastic activity. A hypoperfused mucosa, possibly secondary to use of vasopressor agents, provides a less effective barrier to the extension of diverticular inflammation and infection.

Less common bacterial infections in kidney transplant recipients include sinusitis after nasogastric or endotracheal tube placements, cannulation-site abscess, tracheostomy site cellulitis, meningitis after a primary bacteremia, prostatitis, and prostatic abscess after urinary catheter misapplication. Catheters and instrumentation disrupt physical barriers and produce portals of entry for endogenous and nosocomial flora. The transplanted organ may also be or become a focus of infection as a result of ischemia and acute rejection after transplantation. Transfusion-associated infections (CMV, hepatitis viruses, HIV) may also develop in patients receiving large amounts of blood products.

Diagnosis

Infections in kidney transplant recipients can be difficult to diagnose. The concomitant immunosuppression and alterations in the immune response attenuate the usual clinical signs and symptoms of infection. Moreover, infection may be difficult to differentiate from other causes of graft dysfunction, and diagnosis can be delayed. Rapid clinical discrimination of overlapping clinical symptoms and the early institution of antimicrobial therapy are essential for effective treatment and prevention of septic complications. The presence of more than one causative pathogen within an infectious syndrome must be considered in an immunocompromised patient. For example, the immunomodulating effect of CMV infection can facilitate concomitant infection with bacterial or fungal pathogens, simultaneously or in succession (e.g., *Pseudomonas* or *Aspergillus* pneumonia and CMV viremia or pneumonitis).

Bacteremia and Fungemia

For the detection of bacterial or fungal septicemia, blood cultures should ideally be drawn before initiation of antimicrobial therapy. Fungal isolator tubes should be routinely included in a "sepsis" evaluation, especially if the patient has any of the following risk factors: enhanced corticosteroid use for rejection; vascular, urinary, or drainage catheters; total parenteral nutrition; suspicion of gastrointestinal inflammation or perforation; or diabetes mellitus.

Pneumonia

Diagnostic specimens for posttransplantation pneumonia include blood, sputum, tracheal suction in ventilated patients, broncho-alveolar lavage (BAL) fluid, transthoracic fine-needle aspirate, and, occasionally, lung biopsy. Blood cultures may assist in the etiologic diagnosis of pneumonia because 10% to 15% of patients with pneumonia have bacteremia. Fiberoptic bronchoscopy with BAL and transbronchial biopsy are valuable in the diagnosis of infectious pneumonia and accessible pulmonary lesions. Atypical nosocomial pathogens, such as *Legionella* species, can be cultured from respiratory specimens on charcoal media, and specific *Legionella* nucleic acid probes or direct fluorescent antibodies of antigens in respiratory specimens are useful for detection. Serologic analysis and urinary antigen detection of *Legionella pneumophila* group 1 are adjunctive tests for legionellosis. Fungal cultures of respiratory specimens, pleural fluid, or fine-needle aspirates and pulmonary or extrapulmonary biopsy specimens should be obtained and immediately stained for fungal or hyphal elements by sensitive methods, such as calcofluor staining. For *Pneumocystis carinii,* a fluorescein-labeled monoclonal antibody increases the sensitivity of BAL or sputum specimens. *Nocardia* species can be presumptively diagnosed if modified acid-fast staining reveals delicately branching, gram-positive, beaded filaments. Acid-fast staining of respiratory specimens, biopsy specimens, nodules, and lymph nodes may reveal mycobacterial forms. Culturing methods, however, are necessary for final speciation, and specific mycobacterial DNA probes are useful for species confirmation.

Chest computed tomography (CT) scanning has proved valuable in the diagnosis of infectious pneumonia and to guide percutaneous or thoracoscopic biopsy of suspected lesions. Because of the concurrent immunosuppression and attenuated inflammatory response in transplant recipients, however, the usual radiographic presentation of common infectious pneumonia may appear atypical. These studies must also be interpreted in the context of noninfectious causes of pulmonary infiltrates. The differential diagnosis should include atelectasis, aspiration, contusion, hemorrhage, infarction or emboli, capillary leak, or pulmonary edema.

Although more commonly observed in the later posttransplantation period, CMV infection should be considered (see later); diagnostic studies include shell-vial culture and early-antigen detection (i.e., PCR, DNA-hybridization) from blood, respiratory specimens, or other suspected fluids.

Urinary Tract Infection

For UTIs, a clean-catch midstream urine specimen should be submitted for quantitative culture. In renal transplant recipients, lower levels of bacteriuria may be a significant risk factor for systemic infection. The tips of genitourinary stents should be cultured for bacterial and fungal pathogens. If ureteral stents are required in the posttransplantation setting, infections may be more difficult to eradicate without their removal because microbicidal concentrations may not be achievable in this environment and immune function may be impaired.

Wound and Other Infections

Diagnosis of wound infections, skin nodules, or necrotic tissues should include aspiration of any drainable material, a swab specimen from the site, and a biopsy specimen when appropriate; Gram stain, aerobic and anaerobic bacterial culture, and fungal and acid-fast staining with culture should be ordered. Percutaneous or open drainage may be necessary in case of infected perigraft collections, hematomas, or urinomas. Furthermore, culture of fluid collections (e.g., intraabdominal, pleural, mediastinal, genitourinary, pericardial, and vascular or catheter site) is useful in patients who exhibit unexplained fever or other signs and symptoms in the early postoperative period. Localization and aspiration can be facilitated under ultrasound or CT guidance. In most circumstances, percutaneous or open drainage of infected fluid collections or hematomas is necessary for symptom resolution. Intravascular catheter tips should be cultured after access catheters have been removed. Stool specimens for *Clostridium difficile* detection should be obtained from patients with diarrhea, colitis, or abdominal symptoms who have received antibiotic therapy.

Approach to the Kidney Transplant Recipient With Fever

Fever in the kidney transplant recipient assumes a similar, although expanded, differential diagnosis compared with the non-immunocompromised patient. This includes infection (i.e., bacterial, viral, fungal, parasitic), graft rejection, medication adverse effect, or a systemic inflammatory response. Fever may accompany episodes of acute rejection; however, with current immuno-suppressive drugs, patients are often afebrile. Temperature elevations may occur during treatment of rejection with both OKT3 and the polyclonal antibodies as a result of cytokine release (see Chapter 4). Other reported adverse effects of antibody treatment that can be confused with infectious symptoms include cephalalgia, photophobia, aseptic meningitis, and pulmonary infiltrates (edema).

MICROBIAL ETIOLOGY, TREATMENT PRINCIPLES, AND SPECIFIC THERAPY

Bacterial Infections

The predominant bacterial pathogens in the early posttransplantation period tend to be similar both in transplant recipients and transplantation centers (Tables 10.4 and 10.5). This observation undoubtedly reflects the fact that similar organisms and nosocomial pathogens infect nontransplantation surgical patients in the early postoperative period. The antibiotic sensitivity patterns and incidence of a particular pathogen reflect specific hospital antibiotic usage and epidemiologic patterns. In the early posttransplantation period, Enterobacteriaceae, *Staphylococcus,* and *Pseudomonas* species are the most commonly isolated pathogens. In bacteremic kidney transplant recipients, aerobic gram-negative bacilli constitute nearly half of all pathogens found by blood culture, with a 2-week mortality rate after bacteremia of 11%. Bacterial pathogens causing secondary bacteremia were similar to the predominant bacterial isolates responsible for the primary infected site (i.e., lung, abdomen, surgical wound, and
(*text continues on page 238*)

Table 10.5.   Pathogens, sites of infection, and antimicrobial treatment

Organisms	Common Site	Preferred Antibiotic	Alternative Regimen
Aerobic gram-negative rods			
Escherichia coli, *Proteus mirablis*	Blood, intra-abdominal, wound, urinary tract infection	TGC(4), ampicillin (if sensitive), ampicillin, TMP/SMX (7), Cephs (4), APPN (2)	AG (1), TMP/SMX (7), FQ (5), FGC (4), SGC (4) FQ (5), aztreonam
Klebsiella pneumoniae, *Klebsiella oxytoca*	Blood, intra-abdominal, lung, Urinary tract infection	TGC (4), TMP/SMX (7), Cephs (4)	TMP/SMX (7), FQ (5), AG (1), APPN (2), BLI (6) AG (1), BLI (6), FQ (5)
Enterobacter aerogenes, *Enterobacter cloacae*	Urinary tract, lung, blood, GI tract, abdomen	Imipenem, meropenem, AG (1), TMP/SMX (7)	FQ (5), FTHGC (4), APPN (2)
Serratia marcesens	Urinary tract, blood, lung	TGC (4)	TMP/SMX (7), APPN (2)+/– AG (1), FQ (5), imipenem
Citrobacter freundii	Blood, wound, lung	AG (1), TMP/SMX (7), FQ(5)	Imipenem, meropenem APPN (2), TGC (4)
Pseudomonas aeruginosa	Intra-abdominal, lung, blood	AG (1) + ceftazidime or APPN (2)	Imipenem +/– AG (1), FQ (5), aztreonam +/– AG (1)
Acinetobacter anitratus	Blood, lung	Imipenem, AG (1) + ceftazidime or APPN (2)	FQ (5), TGC (4), ampicillin/ sulbactam (?)
Haemophilus influenzae	Paranasal, sinuses, blood, lung	Ampicillin, amoxicillin +/– clav, TMP/SMX (7) SGC, TGC (4), TMP/SMX	Erythromycin, FQ (7), BLI (6)
Legionella species	Lung, blood	Erythromycin (+/– rifampin)	Clarithromycin, azithromycin, TMP/SMX (7), FQ (5)

ESBL-producing gram-negative bacilli	Blood, intra-abdominal, wound, lungs	Imipenem, meropenem, BLI (6), FTHGC (4)	FQ (5), AG (1), TMP/SMX (7)
Anaerobic gram-negative rods			
Bacteroides fragilis, Fusobacterium species	Abdominal, liver abscess, blood	Metronidazole, clindamycin, cefoxitin	APPN (2), BLI, clindamycin, imipenem
Anaerobic gram-positive rods			
Clostridium perfringens	Skin, wound, abdomen, blood	Penicillin	Clindamycin, metronidazole, APPN (2), imipenem
Clostridium difficile	GI tract	Vancomycin (oral), metronidazole (oral)	Bacitracin (oral), cholestyramine, lactobacilli (post treatment)
Anaerobic gram-positive cocci			
Peptococcus, Peptostreptococcus sp.	Abdomen, skin, wound, blood	Penicillin, ampicillin, amoxicillin, BLI (6)	Clindamycin, metronidazole Cephs (4), erythromycin, vancomycin, imipenem
Aerobic gram-positive cocci			
Staphylococcus, aureus (MS)	Blood, lung, wound, line site	PRP (3), FGC, SGC (4)	BLI(6), vancomycin, imipenem, clinda/erythro(?)
S. aureus (MR)		Vancomycin +/– rifampin or gentamicin	Doxycycline, Quinapristin/dalfopristin, Teicoplanin, TMP/SMX (7)
S. epidermidis	Blood, line site	Vancomycin	Doxycycline, TMP/SMX + rifampin, PRP (3), imipenem

continued

Table 10.5. *(continued)*

Organisms	Common Site	Preferred Antibiotic	Alternative Regimen
Enterococcus faecalis (group D streptococcus)	Wound, intra-abdominal sepsis	Ampicillin	Vancomycin, penicillin + AG (1), imipenem
	Urinary tract	Ampicillin, amoxicillin	Vancomycin, penicillin + AG (1)
	Endocarditis	Penicillin/ampicillin + gentamicin or streptomycin	Vancomycin + gentamicin or streptomycin
VRE	Blood, wound, intra-abdominal, urinary tract	Quinapristin/dalfopristin[a]; ampicillin or penicillin + AG (1) *if susceptible* because many VRE isolates are resistant to one or both of these agents; teicoplanin + AG (if VanB phenotype); linezolid	Chloramphenicol, doxycycline, rifampin, novobiocin, bacitracin, FQ (7), nitrofurantoin (or combinations of above); Evernimomycins
Streptococcus pneumoniae (pneumococcus)	Blood, CNS, lungs, endocarditis	Penicillin	Cephs (4), vancomycin, clindamycin, erythromycin
Alpha-hemolytic *Streptococcus viridans*		Penicillin + gentamicin or streptomycin	Vancomycin
PRSP	Blood, CNS, lungs	Ceftriaxone, cefotaxime (if not resistant), high-dose intravenous penicillin (e.g., 20 MU/day), vancomycin, 2nd generation FQ	Imipenem, meropenem (not meningitis), rifampin, clindamycin (in otitis media if susceptible strain)

Listeria monocytogenes	Blood, CNS	Ampicillin or penicillin +/− gentamicin	TMP/SMX (7)
Corynebacterium sp.	Blood, wound	Penicillin	Erythromycin
Nocardia sp.	Lung, abscess—skin, CNS	TMP/SMX (7)	Imipenem +/− amikacin, amikacin +/− sulfa

ESBL, extended spectrum beta-lactamase; VRE, vancomycin-resistant enterococcus; PRSP, penicillin-resistant *Streptococcus pneumoniae.*

[a] Only for *E. faecium; E. faecalis* intrinsically resistant to Quinapristin/dalfopristin

1. Aminoglycoside (AG) = gentamicin, tobramycin, amikacin; therapy of choice for serious enterococcal infections, but many VREs are resistant to one or both agents.
2. Antipseudomonal penicillin = piperacillin, mezlocillin, ticarcillin
3. Penicillinase-resistant penicillins: methicillin, nafcillin, oxacillin, dicloxacillin
4. Cephalosporins
    1st generation (FGC): cefazolin, cephalexin
    2nd generation (SGC): cefuroxime, cefoxitin
    3rd generation (TGC): cefotaxime, ceftizoxime, ceftriaxone, ceftazidime
    4th generation (FTHGC): cefepime
5. Fluoroquinolones (FQ):
    1st generation FQ: ciprofloxacin, norfloxacin, ofloxacin
    2nd generation FQ: levofloxacin, gatifloxacin, moxifloxacin
6. Beta-lactamase inhibitor: piperacillin/tazobactam, ampicillin/sulbactam, amoxicillin/clavulanate
7. Trimethoprim sulfamethoxazole

urinary tract). Bacteremia and disseminated infection due to pathogens with increased antimicrobial resistance can be seen (Fig. 10.2). Infections due to vancomycin-resistant *Enterococcus faecium* (VRE) have also been reported in kidney transplant recipients. These patients had received more preoperative antibiotics and were more likely to have received vancomycin preoperatively and to have been hospitalized in the intensive care unit. Aerobic gram-negative bacilli (Enterobacteriaceae, *Escherichia coli, Pseudomonas aeruginosa*) account for most cases of pneumonia. Additional pathogens include *S. aureus,* enterococci, streptococci (*S. pneumoniae*), and *Legionella* species (*L. pneumophila, L. bozemanii, L. micadadei*). Gram-negative bacilli with transferable resistance to extended-spectrum cephalosporins have been reported with increased frequency among hospitalized patients and nosocomial infections. Most of these strains, predominantly *Klebsiella pneumoniae* and *E. coli,* are generally resistant to all beta-lactam antimicrobials except carbapenems.

Enteric gram-negative bacilli are responsible for most UTIs in kidney transplant recipients, but other pathogens include enterococci, staphylococci, and *P. aeruginosa.* Bacterial organisms causing wound infection after solid organ transplantation vary depending on the surgical complications at the operative site. Predominant pathogens include gram-positive bacteria, such as *Staphylococcus* and *Streptococcus* species; aerobic gram-negative bacteria, especially *E. coli, Enterobacter* species, and *Pseudomonas* species; and last in frequency, enterococci, polymicrobial species, and anaerobes such as *Bacteroides fragilis.*

Among all kidney transplant recipients who develop infective endocarditis in the early posttransplantation period, *S. aureus,* coagulase-negative staphylococci, *E. coli, Acinetobacter* species, *Enterococcus faecalis,* and *Pseudomonas* species have been reported. Fungal infections predominate as causes of infective endocarditis in the early posttransplantation period. Most of these episodes are associated with previous hospital-acquired infection, notably, venous access and wound infections.

Other infrequently encountered bacterial pathogens reported in the early posttransplantation period include *Nocardia, Mycobacterium,* and *Salmonella* species; *Mycoplasma hominis, Ureaplasma urealyticulum,* and *Rhodococcus equi.*

Listeriosis

In renal transplant recipients, infection with *L. monocytogenes* most commonly manifests as meningoencephalitis or septicemia but may also cause febrile gastroenteritis. Infection typically occurs more than months after transplantation. Intravenous ampicillin (200 mg/kg in divided doses every 4 hours for 2 weeks) should be used for the treatment of bacteremia. High-dose ampicillin and gentamicin for 3 weeks should be used for meningitis, and repeat lumbar puncture should be performed. A substantial proportion of sporadic cases of listeriosis are associated with ingestion of processed meats; patients should be instructed to eat only properly cooked meats and pasteurized dairy products.

Nocardiosis

Although the prophylactic use of TMP/SMX has decreased the incidence of disease, *Nocardia* species remains a source of infection

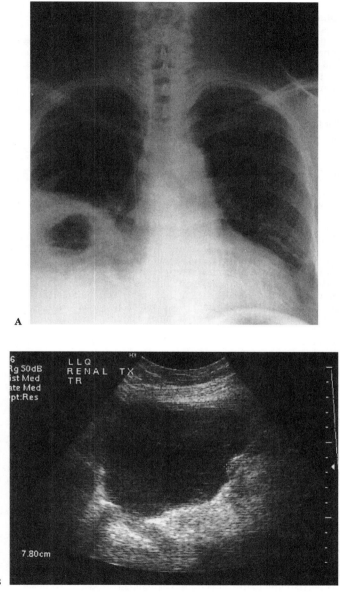

Fig. 10.2.   Disseminated infection with methicillin-resistant *Staphylo-coccus aureus* (MRSA). A: Cavitary pneumonia on chest radiograph after bacteremic disease. B: Perigraft collection with MRSA in same patient.

after renal transplantation. Risk factors include early rejection, enhanced immunosuppression, neutropenia, and uremia. Infection most commonly presents as acute or subacute pneumonia, but hematogenous spread to the brain, skin and subcutaneous tissues, bone, and eye has also been observed. TMP/SMX at high doses (2.5 to 10 mg/kg twice daily, depending on the severity of illness) is the treatment of choice for most *Nocardia* species infections. Imipenem, amikacin, cephalosporins (ceftriaxone, cefotaxime, cefuroxime), minocycline, and quinolones may be used in combination when treating serious nocardial infection. Because of the risk for relapse, treatment should be for a minimum of 12 months.

Clostridium difficile Infection

The true incidence of *C. difficile* infection in the kidney transplant population is unknown, although the similar risk factors for *C. difficile* acquisition and disease in nontransplantation patients presumably apply to transplant recipients. *C. difficile*–associated syndromes include asymptomatic carriage, diarrhea, intestinal obstruction, *C. difficile* culture–positive pelvic abscess, and pseudomembranous colitis; colectomy can be required for severe toxic megacolon. Most *C. difficile* infections are acquired nosocomially (i.e., through environmental transmission and prolonged hospital stay), and antimicrobial therapy is the greatest risk factor. In addition, the use of immunosuppressive agents has been suggested as one of the predisposing factors for fulminant *C. difficile* infection. *C. difficile* diarrhea is the most common bacterial infection in the first 2 weeks after transplantation among kidney transplant recipients younger than 2 years of age with intraabdominal kidneys. Colonic dysregulation subjects the patient to additional fluid and electrolyte disorders and, potentially, to malabsorption of immunosuppressive medications. Oral vancomycin is the preferred treatment for severe *C. difficile* infection; orally administered metronidazole can be used in less severe or vancomycin-intolerant cases.

Legionella species Infection

Legionella species infections have been described in kidney transplant recipients. Risk factors include multiple corticosteroid boluses, the number of days on a ventilator, and contamination of hospital water supplies despite superheating and hyperchlorination. Pneumonia is usually a manifestation of *L. micadadei* and *L. pneumophila*, but extrapulmonary sites of involvement have been reported (renal, hepatic, central nervous system). Systemic manifestations of *L. pneumophila* include a nonproductive cough, temperature–pulse dissociation, abnormalities in hepatic enzymes, diarrhea, hyponatremia, myalgias, and confusion; radiologic findings include alveolar or interstitial infiltrates, frank cavities, pleural effusions, or lobar consolidation. Intravenous erythromycin should be started with the addition of rifampin for severe disease. TMP/SMX, ciprofloxacin, doxycycline, and the macrolides (clarithromycin and azithromycin) have demonstrated some efficacy in *Legionella* species infections. The macrolides may increase the blood levels of the calcineurin inhibitors, necessitating dose modification (see Chapter 4).

Mycobacterial Infection

Mycobacterial and nontuberculous mycobacterial (NTM) infections can represent a serious problem in renal allograft recipients and can present as early as the first posttransplantation month. The incidence of active tuberculosis in this population has been estimated to be 1% to 4% and will probably increase as a reflection of the overall escalation of tuberculosis reported in the general population. Pulmonary presentations of *M. tuberculosis* and NTM *(M. kansasii, M. xenopi, M. avium–intracellulare, M. fortuitum)* can appear as multilobar disease, focal infiltrates and nodularity, empyema, pleuritis, or a combination of findings.

Unusual presentations of *M. tuberculosis* and NTM disease in the transplant population may delay diagnosis and contribute to overall morbidity. Transplant recipients with a prior history of mycobacterial infection, with old granulomatous disease, or from countries with increased mycobacterial exposure should be investigated for reactivation disease. Disseminated disease in kidney transplant recipients is observed in about 40% of patients at the time of diagnosis, with involvement of the skin, skeletal (bone and joint), and central nervous system. The presence of granuloma in peripheral tissues is suggestive of disseminated disease. Historically, tuberculosis has been effectively treated in kidney transplant recipients; however, with the increase in multidrug-resistant (MDR) strains, appropriate therapy should include a minimum of four antituberculous agents until sensitivities are known.

Initial drug regimens should include 2 months of oral isoniazid (INH), rifampin (RIF), pyrazinamide (PZA), and ethambutol (EMB) or intramuscular streptomycin (SM). Of these, at least two agents should be continued for an additional 4 to 10 months according to susceptibility results (e.g., continue only INH and RIF if susceptible). Although there are no controlled clinical trials in kidney transplant recipients to determine the adequacy of treatment, therapy should last for a total of 12 months. Adverse effects associated with antituberculous agents include hepatitis (INH > PZA > RIF), neuritis and optic neuropathy (INH, EMB), hearing loss, azotemia (SM), and abdominal discomfort (INH, RIF, EMB, PZA). Both INH and RIF affect the cytochrome P450 enzyme system. INH may lead to accumulation of cyclosporine, whereas RIF is a P450 inducer and lowers calcineurin inhibitor concentrations, thus increasing the risk for rejection due to subtherapeutic levels. These interactions are usually predictable and may occur within 1 to 3 days of initiating antituberculous therapy; appropriate dosage adjustments and monitoring are required.

Atypical nontuberculous pathogens have been reported in renal transplant recipients, including *M. kansasii, M. chelonei, M. xenopi, M. marinum,* and *M. haemophilum.* These pathogens can be cultured from infected lungs, skin, bone, and disseminated sites (Fig. 10.3). Treatment of atypical mycobacterial disease can include combinations of standard antituberculous agents and specific antibiotics determined by sensitivity testing. However, atypical mycobacteria may be resistant to classic antituberculous agents.

Mixed Infections

Bacterial, fungal, and viral pathogens may be encountered concurrently in infectious syndromes, each participating in the patho-

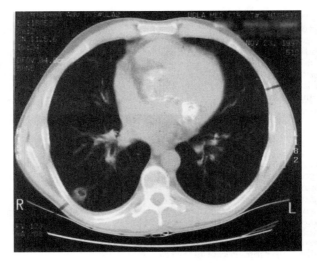

Fig. 10.3.   Chest CT scan from patient treated for several episodes of rejection; both nodular and cavitary infiltrates are observed. Broncho-alveolar lavage from this patient revealed *Aspergillus fumigatus*, cytomegalovirus, and *Mycobacterium fortuitum*. Combination therapies with amphotericin B lipid complex (ABLC), ganciclovir, and antimycobacterial agents were required for resolution.

physiology of the infection. This scenario can reflect (1) a significant net state of immunosuppression due to multiple courses of rejection treatment with corticosteroids and anti–T-cell preparations; (2) nosocomial acquisition of multiple pathogens; or (3) immuno-modulation by CMV or other viruses facilitating opportunistic infections by multiple pathogens. Figure 10.3 illustrates a case of pneumonia caused by multiple pathogens in a kidney transplant recipient.

Treatment

The implementation antibacterial therapy can be considered under the following categories:

Surgical prophylaxis: antimicrobial agents used to prevent a commonly encountered infection in the immediate postoperative period

Empiric therapy: antimicrobials initiated without identification of the infecting pathogen

Specific therapy: antimicrobials administered to treat a diagnosed pathogen

SURGICAL PROPHYLAXIS.   Perioperative prophylaxis reduces the frequency of wound infection in the immediate postoperative setting. Generally, prophylactic antibiotics should be directed against skin pathogens (e.g., staphylococci, streptococci) and urinary tract pathogens (*E. coli, Klebsiella* and *Proteus* species). Cefazolin is useful perioperatively and is discontinued after 24 hours to minimize the risk for superinfection with resistant bacterial organisms or development of antibiotic-associated *C. difficile* colitis, although this is more commonly observed with more prolonged antibiotic therapy. Cephalosporins, quinolones, or beta-lactam plus beta-lactamase inhibitor combinations have activity against common urinary tract gram-negative pathogens (e.g., *E. coli, Klebsiella* and *Enterobacter* species), but choosing the precise antimicrobial should be based on institution-specific susceptibility patterns. The duration of broad-spectrum prophylaxis should be minimized to reduce the risk for suprainfection and cost.

EMPIRICAL THERAPY.   For patients with suspected bacterial sepsis, a number of antimicrobials can be selected for empirical treatment. Empirical therapy should be guided by the available clinical information, including the suspected anatomic site of infection, the probable bacterial flora and institution-specific susceptibility patterns, any previously administered antimicrobial therapy, the time since transplantation, the severity of renal and hepatic dysfunction, and the net state of immunosuppression. Initial empirical therapy should be broad spectrum. The duration of empirical therapy is based on the resolution of clinical signs and symptoms of bacterial infection, sterilization of infected sites, and tolerance of the agent. After a specific pathogen is isolated and sensitivities are available, a narrow-spectrum agent with appropriate antibacterial activity is substituted to avoid the risk for suprainfection. Commonly used agents for empirical therapy include broad-spectrum penicillins (piperacillin), third-generation cephalosporins (ceftizoxime), and beta-lactam plus beta-lactamase inhibitor combinations (ampicillin/sulbactam, ticarcillin/clavulanate, or piperacillin/tazobactam).

SPECIFIC THERAPY.   With the isolation of a specific organism, therapy is focused on the specific pathogen to minimize the risk for suprainfection. Examples of specific microbial agents, syndromes, and antimicrobial agents used to treat bacterial pathogens are listed in Table 10.5, with dosage adjustments in Table 10.6. Specific treatment options for infectious pneumonia are listed in Table 10.7. Antimicrobial and immunosuppressant drug interactions are discussed in Chapter 4. Nosocomial gram-negative bacteria are associated with an increase in mortality in allograft recipients, and these pathogens warrant additional attention. Organisms such as *Enterobacter cloacae* may be resistant to third-generation cephalosporins; effective therapies for this pathogen include carbapenems, fluoroquinolones, TMP/SMX, piperacillin, and piperacillin/tazobactam. Aminoglycosides, although generally active against *E. cloacae,* and most other gram-negative bacteria, should be used judiciously in renal allograft recipients because of the risk for increased nephrotoxicity. When *P. aeruginosa* is suspected or cultured, combination therapy using an antipseudomonal penicillin (piperacillin), carbapenem, or ceftazidime plus an aminoglycoside or fluoroquinolone is recommended for synergistic bactericidal activity and the prevention of resistance.

Fungal Infections

Although the incidence of fungal infections in renal transplant recipients is less than that reported for other solid organ trans-

(*text continued on page 249*)

Table 10.6.   Dosages of selected antimicrobial agents in renal insufficiency

Antimicrobial	Usual Adult Dose	CLCR 20–50 mL/min	CLCR 10–19 mL/min	CLCR <10 mL/min
Antibacterials				
Amikacin	7.5 mg/kg IV q 12 h	q 12–q 24 h	q 24–q 48 h	q 48–q 72 h
Ampicillin	2 g IV q 6 h	q 6–8 h	q 12 h	0.5–1 g q 12 h
Ampicillin/ sulbactam	3 g IV q 6 h	q 8 h	q 12 h	1.5 g q 12 h
Azithromycin	0.5 g IV q 24 h (500 mg PO q 24 h, then 250 mg PO q 4 days)			
Aztreonam	1 g IV q 8 h	Same	q 12 h	0.5–1 g q 24 h
Cefazolin	1 g IV q 8 h	q 12 h	0.5–1 g q 12 h	0.5–1 g q 24 h
Cefoxitin	1 g IV q 6 h	q 8 h	0.75 mg q 12–24 h	0.5–1 g q 12–24 h
Ceftazidime	1 g IV q 8 h	q 12 h	q 24 h	0.5–1 g q 24 h
Ceftizoxime	1 g IV q 8 h	q 12 h	0.5–1 g q 12 h	0.5–1 g q 24 h
Ceftriaxone	1–2 g IV/IM q 24 h			
Cefuroxime	0.75 g IV q 8 h	q 12 h	0.75 g q 24 h	0.75 mg q 24 h
Cefepime	2.0 g IV q 12 h	Same	2.0 g q 16–24 h	2.0 g q 24–48 h
Ciprofloxacin	0.25–0.75 g PO q 12 h 0.2–0.4 g IV q 12 h	Same	Same	q 24 h
Clarithromycin	0.5–1.0 g PO q 12 h	Same	0.5 g PO q 12 h	0.5 g PO q 24 h
Clindamycin	0.6 g IV q 8 h/ PO 150–450 q 8 h	Same	Same	Same
Erythromycin	0.5–1.0 g IV q 6 h	0.5–1 g q 6 h	0.5–1 g q 6 h	0.5 g q 6 h
Gentamicin	1–2 mg/kg IV q 8–12 h	1.2–1.5 mg/kg q 12–24 h	1.5 mg/kg q 24–48 h	1–1.5 mg/kg q 48–72 h

Drug				
Gatifloxacin	400 mg IV/PO q 24 h	400 mg q 24 h	200 mg q 24 h	200 mg q 24 h
Imipenem	0.5 g IV q 6–8 h	q 8–12 h	q 12 h	0.25 g q 12 h
Levofloxacin	0.5 g IV q 24 h	Same	0.25 g q 24 h	0.125 g q 24 h
Linezolid	0.2–0.6 mg q 12 h	Same	Same	Same
Meropenem	1.0 g IV q 8 h	1.0 g q 12 h	1 g q 24 h	0.5 g q 24 h
Metronidazole	0.5 g IV q 8–12 h; 0.5 g PO q 8–12 h	Same	q 12 h	q 12 h
Mezlocillin	1.5–4 g IV q 4–6 h	Same	1.5–4.0 g q 6–8 h	1.5–4 g q 8 h
Moxifloxacin	400 mg PO q 24 h	Same	Same	Same
Ofloxacin	0.4 g IV q 12 h	Same	0.4 g q 24 h	0.2 g q 24 h
Oxacillin	1–2 g IV q 6 h	No dosage adjustment		
Penicillin G	1–2 million U IV q 4 h	q 6 h	q 8 h	q 12 h
Piperacillin	3–4 g IV q 4–6 h	3–4 g IV q 4–6 h	3g IV q 6–8 h	3 g IV q 8 h
Piperacillin/tazobactam	3.375 g IV q 6 h	3.375 g IV q 6 h	2.25 g IV q 6 h	2.25 g IV q 8 h
Quinupristin, dalfopristin	7.5 mg/kg IV q 8–12 h	No dosage adjustment		
Tobramycin	1–2 mg/kg IV q 8–12 h	See gentamicin		
TMP	10 mg/kg/day (TMP) IV q 6–12 h; PCP dosage = 15–20 mg/kg/day (TMP) divided q 6 h	5–7.5 mg TMP/kg/day q 12 h	2.5–5.0 mg TMP/kg/day q 24 h	1.25–2.5 mg TMP/kg/day q 25 h
Vancomycin	1 g IV q 12 h; 0.125–0.5 mg PO q 6–8 h (PO for *Clostridium difficile* colitis)	10–15 mg/kg q 24–48 h	10–15 mg/kg q 48–72 h	10–15 mg/kg q 4–7 days

continued

Table 10.6. *(continued)*

Antimicrobial	Usual Adult Dose	CLCR 20–50 mL/min	CLCR 10–19 mL/min	CLCR <10 mL/min
Antivirals				
Acyclovir	5–10 mg/kg IV q 8 h[a]	5–10 mg/kg IV q 12 h	5–10 mg/kg IV q 24 h	2.5 mg/kg IV q 24 h
Amantadine	0.1 g PO BID	0.1 g PO 24–48 h	0.1 g PO 48–72 h	0.1 g PO 48–72 h
Cidofovir	5 mg/kg IV Q wk × 2 wk	1–1.5 mg/kg IV q wk × 2 wk	0.5 mg/kg IV q wk × 2 wk	0.5 mg/kg IV q wk × 2 wk
Famciclovir	0.5 g PO q 8 h	0.5 g PO q 12 h	0.25–0.5 g PO q 24 h	0.25 g PO q 48 h
Foscarnet (induction)	60 mg/kg IV q 8 h × 2–3 wk	40–50 mg/kg IV q 8–12 h	50–60 mg/kg IV q 24 h	Avoid
Ganciclovir	5 mg/kg IV q 12 h	2.5 mg/kg IV q 12 h	2.5 mg/kg IV q 24 h	1.25 mg/kg IV q 24 h
Lamivudine	1 g PO t.i.d.	0.5–1.0 g PO b.i.d.	0.5 g PO q.d.	0.5 g PO 3 times/wk
Oseltamivir	0.15 g PO b.i.d.	0.15 g PO q.d.	0.1 g PO q.d.	0.025–0.05 g PO q.d.
Rimantadine	75 mg PO b.i.d. × 5 days	0.1 g PO q.d.–b.i.d.	0.1 g PO q.d.–b.i.d.	0.1 g PO q.d.
Valaciclovir	0.1 g PO b.i.d.	1 g PO q 12 h	1 g PO q 24 h	0.5 g PO q 24 h
Zanamivir	1 g PO t.i.d.			
	10 mg b.i.d. × 5 days by inhaler			

Antifungals				
Amphotericin B	Nonlipid: 0.3–1.5 mg/kg IV qD ABLC: 3.5–5 mg/kg IV qD (>5–12 mg/kg: higher doses under study) L-AB: 3–5 mg/kg IV qD (lower dose "empirical" for neutropenic fever)	Same	Same	q 24–48 h
Fluconazole	0.2–0.4 g PO/IV q 24 h	0.05–0.2 g PO/IV q 24 h	0.05–0.1 g PO/IV q 24 h	0.05–0.1 g PO/IV q 24–48 h
Flucytosine	12.5–37.5 mg/kg IV q 6 h	12.5–37.5 mg/kg IV q 12 h	12.5–37.5 mg/kg IV q 24 h	12.5–25 mg/kg IV q 24 h
Itraconazole	0.1–0.2 g PO q 12 h	Same	Same	0.1–0.2 g PO q 24 h

CLCR, creatine clearance; PCP, *Pneumocystis carinii*; TMP, Trimethoprim sulfamethoxazole; ABLC, Amphotericin B Lipid Complex; L-AB, Liposomal Amphotericin B.

[a] Dosage for herpes simplex virus is 200 mg PO five times daily or 400 mg t.i.d; dosage for varicella zoster virus is 12.5–15 mg/kg q 8 h; oral: 800 mg five times daily for 7 days.

Table 10.7.   Pneumonitis in the kidney transplant recipient

Pathogens	Suggested Therapy
Bacteria	
Staphylococcus aureus	Oxacillin, nafcillin, first-generation cephalosporin, vancomycin
Methicillin-resistant *S. aureus*	Vancomycin
Enteric gram-negative bacilli	Third-generation cephalosporin, antipseudomonal penicillin +/– aminoglycoside, ciprofloxacin, carbapenem, TMP/SMX
Streptococcus pneumoniae	Penicillin G, second- or third-generation cephalosporin; evofloxacin, vancomycin, or imipenem may be required for intermediate to penicillin resistant pneumococci
Legionella pneumophilia	Erythromycin (+/– rifampin), clarithromycin, azithromycin (mild disease), fluoroquinolone
Mycobacteria tuberculosis	Isoniazid, rifampin, and pyrazinamide or ethambutol; alternative agent directed by sensitivities and/or intolerance (fluoroquinolone, streptomycin)
Nocardia asteroides	TMP/SMX, sulfisoxazole, minocycline, or amikacin and imipenem or third-generation cephalosporin (ceftriaxone)
Fungi	
Cryptococcus neoformans	Amphotericin B +/– flucytocine, fluconazole, itraconzale, lipid-based formulation
Aspergillus species	Amphotericin B, lipid-based formulation, itraconazole, voriconazole
Coccidioides immitis	Amphotericin B, fluconazole, lipid-based formulation
Histoplasma capsulatum	Amphotericin B, itraconazole, lipid-based formulation
Candida albicans	Amphotericin B, fluconazole, lipid-based formulation
Non-albicans *Candida* sp.	Amphotericin B, lipid-based formulation, fluconazole (susceptible *Candida* sp. only and higher doses may be necessary), itraconazole
Pneumocystis carinii	TMP/SMX, pentamidine, dapsone + trimethoprim, atovaquone

Table 10.7.   (*continued*)

Pathogens	Suggested Therapy
Viruses	
Cytomegalovirus	Ganciclovir, foscarnet, cidofovir or fomivirsen (retinitis)
Herpes group (non-CMV)	Acyclovir, ganciclovir, famciclovir, valacyclovir, penciclovir (topical for orolabial herpes simplex virus)
Varicella zoster	Acyclovir, famciclovir, valacyclovir
Respiratory syncytial virus	Ribavirin (aerosolized)
Influenza (A/B activity)	Oseltamivir (A/B), zanamivir (A/B), amantadine (A), ramantidine (A)

CMV, cytomegalovirus; TMP/SMX, trimethoprim-sulfisoxazole.

plant recipients, the mortality from fungal infections remains high. Predisposing factors include the following:

- Use of corticosteroids, particularly the large doses used to treat rejection episodes
- Administration of broad-spectrum antibiotics
- Overall state of immunosuppression
- Use of indwelling catheters
- Duration and the number of surgical procedures
- Disruption of intestinal or bladder mucosa, vascular complications, and hyperglycemia

Most fungal infections involve nosocomially or environmentally acquired pathogens, such as *Candida, Aspergillus, Zycomycosis (Mucor, Rhizopus)*, and *Cryptococcus* species and the geographically restricted mycoses (coccidioidomycosis, histoplasmosis, blastomycosis, and paracoccidioidomycosis), presenting as either reactivation disease or newly acquired disease (Table 10.4).

In the immediate postoperative period, candidiasis of the oropharyngeal, vaginal, or intertriginous areas may be seen. Opportunistic fungal infections are most common between 1 and 6 months after transplantation. The following fungal syndromes are observed:

- Candidiasis: mucocutaneous, disseminated, UTI, obstructing fungal elements ("fungal ball") of the genitourinary system, pneumonia, hepatosplenic infection, peritonitis, endocarditis, and central nervous system). All species of *Candida* have been implicated in clinical disease, including *C. albicans, C. tropicalis, C. parapsilosis, C. kruseii, C. lusitaniae,* and *C. (Torulopsis) glabrata.* Speciation is important because of varying sensitivity to azoles and amphotericin B.
- Cryptococcosis: central nervous system, pulmonary, dermatologic, skeletal, organ-specific disease

- Aspergillosis: pneumonia and other tissue-invasive forms, including genitourinary, central nervous system, rhinocerebral, sinus, gastrointestinal, skin, and musculoskeletal as well as other, more rare disseminated forms
- Zycomocoses: *Rhizopus* and *Mucor* species
- Coccidioidomycosis: pneumonia, meningitis, musculoskeletal, and skin involvement
- Histoplasmosis: pneumonia, disseminated disease
- Pneumocystosis: pneumonia
- *Penicillium marneffei* infection: pneumonia
- Scedosporiosis: pneumonia, disseminated disease

Other fungal pathogens observed in renal transplant recipients include the dermatophytes (*Trichophyton, Microsporum, and Epidermophyton* species), hyalohyphomycosis (*Fusarium* species), and phaeohyphomycosis (*Phialophora parasitica*), which may present locally as cutaneous lesions or, rarely, with disseminated disease. *Trichophyton mentagrophytes* is the most common dermatophyte described. The prevalence of dermatomycoses may vary according to immunosuppressive and rejection history, diabetes mellitus, and environmental exposures.

The diagnosis of fungal infection remains problematic and frequently leads to delays in clinical recognition. Biopsy of suspected lesions is often required for confirmation. Table 10.8 summarizes the techniques for the diagnosis of *Candida* and *Aspergillus* species infections. The isolation of yeasts (e.g., *Candida* species) from surveillance cultures of stool, respiratory, and urine samples may be common in kidney transplant recipients taking corticosteroids and broad-spectrum antibiotics and does not necessarily correlate with

Table 10.8.   Laboratory methods for the detection of invasive fungal infection associated with *Aspergillus* and *Candida* species

Species	Method	Description	Comments
Aspergillus	Culture	Respiratory or sterile site specimen	Specificity of culture from nonsterile site limited
	Nucleic acid detection	PCR detection of *Aspergillus* DNA from BAL, serum, or CSF	Research method Methods not standardized
	Antigen detection	Detection of galactomannan in serum, urine, or CSF by latex agglutination, ELISA, EIA, or other method	Research method Wide variability in sensitivity but specific for invasive disease

Table 10.8. (*continued*)

Species	Method	Description	Comments
			May be useful for monitoring response to therapy and detecting relapse
	Antibody detection	Serum or CSF IgG, IgM, or total antibody	Antibody often absent in immunocompromised patients
	Histopathology	Direct visualization	Permits assessment of tissue invasiveness
Candida	Culture	Blood or other sterile site specimen preferred	Limited specificity of isolation from nonsterile site
			Identify to species level to direct therapy
	Nucleic acid detection	PCR detection of *Candida* DNA from BAL, serum, or CSF	PCR contamination problematic because of the ubiquity of *Candida*
		Direct detection by DNA probe	Species-specific DNA probes in development
	Antigen detection	Detection of mannan or other protein in serum by latex agglutination, EIA, RIA, or other method	Interlaboratory differences in sensitivity and specificity
			Sensitivity improved by serial measurements
	Antibody detection	Serum or CSF IgG, IgM, or total antibody	Limited usefulness
			Most people have antibody
	Histopathology	Direct visualization	Useful for detection of deep tissue infection

PCR, polymerase chain reaction; BAL, bronchoalveolar lavage; CSF, cerebrospinal fluid; ELISA, enzyme-linked immunosorbent assay; EIA, enzyme-immunoassay; Ig, immunoglobulin; RIA, radioimmunoassay.

disease. Repeatedly positive fungal cultures from single sites or from multiple sites, however, may be a harbinger of invasive or systemic disease in the appropriate clinical setting. Patients with genitourinary tract stents and recurrent urinary fungal isolates may require removal of foreign body to eradicate fungal infection. In a kidney transplant recipient with repeatedly positive *Aspergillus* respiratory cultures (particularly *A. fumigatus* and *A. terreus*), a search for invasive disease should be initiated. High-resolution chest CT with biopsy of suspected pulmonary lesion may be useful. Radiologic appearances of pulmonary aspergillosis in kidney transplant recipients include nodules, diffuse or wedge-shaped opacities, empyema, cavitary forms, tracheobronchitis, or a combination of parenchymal lesions.

Prophylaxis

Prophylaxis of mucocutaneous candidal infection during induction immunosuppression or enhanced corticosteroid use can include oral or topical preparations (e.g., troches, solutions, powders), such as clotrimazole or nystatin. Routine antifungal prophylaxis with systemic antifungal agents after uncomplicated renal transplantation is not routinely recommended. However, renal transplant recipients receiving broad-spectrum antibiotics for bacterial infections may warrant antifungal prophylaxis, assuming the absence of concomitant fungal infection. Antifungal agents, including azoles, conventional lower-dose amphotericin B, and lipid-based amphotericin preparations, are administered for a duration proportional to the risk for fungal infection. Prophylaxis may also be associated with the emergence of less susceptible or resistant fungal pathogens, such as non-*albicans Candida* or *Aspergillus* species.

Renal transplant recipients with evidence of prior-treated endemic mycoses and old "healed" granulomatous lesions (e.g., coccidioidomycosis) may benefit from long-term azole prophylaxis with fluconazole or itraconazole. The cyclosporine and tacrolimus dosages should be adjusted.

Treatment

Fungal infections require aggressive therapy with conventional amphotericin B deoxycholate, a lipid-based amphotericin B preparation, or an appropriate azole antifungal agent. Amphotericin B has traditionally been the drug of choice for systemic fungal infections, including candidiasis, cryptococcosis, coccidioidomycosis, histoplasmosis, and aspergillosis. It can be given with flucytosine for cryptococcal disease. For fungal infections due to aspergillosis, amphotericin B should be initiated at high doses (e.g., 1 to 1.5 mg/kg/day).

The toxicity of amphotericin B is of particular concern in kidney allograft recipients. Nephrotoxicity, hypokalemia, hypomagnesemia, and acidosis occur frequently. In addition, infusion-related toxicity commonly occurs as a result of release of tumor necrosis factor and interleukin-1. This often necessitates dose reduction or the addition of premedications such as corticosteroids, diphenhydramine, acetaminophen, meperidine, or combinations of these agents. Additive toxicity occurs with concurrent use of other nephrotoxic agents, or with alterations in allograft perfusion.

Several lipid-based amphotericin B formulations associated with lower risk for nephrotoxicity have become available for the treatment of fungal infections in solid organ transplantation, and experience with their use is increasing. These agents include amphotericin B lipid complex (Abelcet), liposomal amphotericin B (AmBisome), and amphotericin B colloidal dispersion (Amphotec). These agents were originally approved for the treatment of fungal infections refractory to or intolerant of conventional amphotericin B. They produce less nephrotoxicity and metabolic derangements and milder infusion-related adverse effects. Higher therapeutic concentrations can be administered, and broad-spectrum anti-fungal activity is generally maintained. Figure 10.4 demonstrates the utility of a lipid-based amphotericin B formulation (ABLC) in the treatment of pulmonary aspergillosis in a kidney transplant recipient. Although the cost of these agents may be higher, the consequences of delayed therapeutic response, conventional amphotericin-induced organ toxicity, or development of renal failure or fungal sepsis-induced organ failure also carries significant medical costs.

Itraconazole has demonstrated good *in vitro* activity against *Aspergillus* species, although its activity may vary with select fungal pathogens. An acid gastric environment is necessary for optimal absorption. After satisfactory treatment of an invasive *Aspergillus* species infection with an amphotericin preparation, some transplantation centers use itraconazole as posttreatment "maintenance" therapy for an indefinite period. Ketoconazole, fluconazole, and itraconazole are useful for treating mucocutaneous fungal infection and infection of the genitourinary tract, gastrointestinal system, lungs, and, under specific conditions, central nervous system. The use of fluconazole at standard doses may be

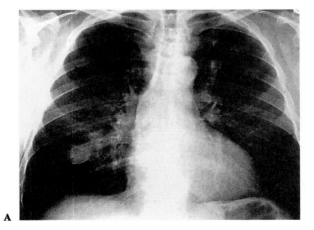

A

Fig. 10.4.   Pulmonary aspergillosis after kidney transplantation.
A: Multiple pulmonary nodules with hilar adenopathy are seen
on chest radiograph. B: Thoracic CT showing nodules some with
central cavitation. C: Chest radiograph showing resolution of
pulmonary nodules after amphotericin B lipid complex (ABLC) and
subsequent itraconazole therapy.

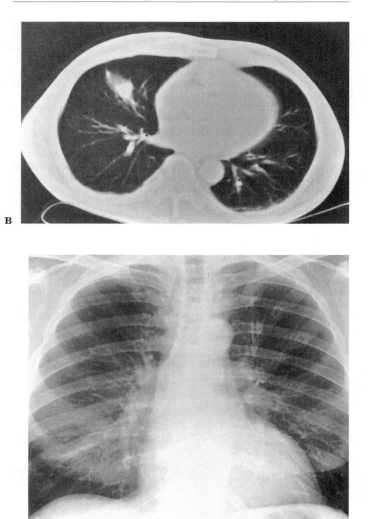

Fig. 10.4.   *Continued*

associated with the development of fungal resistance or tolerance and also with the risk for fungal superinfection with *C. glabrata, C. kruseii,* or *C. tropicalis.* Fluconazole may be a primary therapeutic agent or posttreatment preventative agent for coccidioidomycosis in renal transplant recipients. Itraconazole can be used in the treatment of histoplasmosis, blastomycosis, sporotrichosis, paracoccidioidomycosis, and aspergillosis. For serious and tissue-invasive aspergillosis, however, initial therapy usually should include amphotericin B or a lipid-based preparation.

All of the triazole antifungals impair calcineurin inhibitor metabolism and increase blood levels (see Chapter 4). This effect is most consistent with ketoconazole, and its use may permit a reduction in cyclosporine or tacrolimus dose of up to 80%.

The development of any serious fungal infection in a transplant recipient demands a critical evaluation of the immunosuppressive regimen. The corticosteroid dose should be minimized, the blood levels of cyclosporine and tacrolimus should be kept in the low therapeutic range, and adjunctive agents can often be temporarily discontinued. Failure of clinical response to an antifungal regimen may require discontinuation of immunosuppression even at the cost of abandoning the graft.

Pneumocystosis

Pneumocystis carinii pneumonia occurs 1 to 6 months after transplantation. It typically presents with fever, nonproductive cough, arterial–alveolar mismatching, and diffuse interstitial infiltration or focal air-space consolidation. BAL with transbronchial biopsy is a highly sensitive method of identifying pulmonary disease. First-line treatment is with TMP/SMX for 14 to 21 days. Second-line agents include intravenous pentamidine (3 to 4 mg/kg/day) and dapsone/trimethoprim (100 mg dapsone daily with trimethoprim 15 mg/kg/day). Adverse effects of trimethoprim include nephrotoxicity, pancreatitis, and marrow suppression; dapsone is associated with hemolytic anemia in glucose-6-phosphate dehydrogenase deficiency. Mild to moderate *P. carinii* pneumonia can be treated with atovaquone (750 mg orally thrice daily for 21 days) in patients intolerant to TMP/SMX. Prophylactic agents, in order of efficacy, include TMP/SMX, bimonthly intravenous or aerosolized pentamidine, dapsone, or possibly atovaquone.

Viral Infections

Viral infections are a major problem in allograft recipients, particularly 1 to 6 months after transplantation. Clinical disease may occur later, especially after intensification of immunosuppression or physiologic insults that increase the net state of immunosuppression. EBV-related PTLD is discussed in Chapter 9.

Cytomegalovirus

CMV infection occurs primarily after the first month of transplantation with an estimated incidence of 30% to 78%, depending on the serological status of the donor and recipient (Table 10.3). The seronegative recipient of a seropositive donor graft is at the greatest risk, particularly after the use of antilymphocytic preparations, which can reactivate latent infection.

Primary CMV infection represents infection in the previously uninfected seronegative host and may be asymptomatic. *CMV dis-*

ease refers to symptomatic or tissue-invasive acute CMV infection responsible for virus-associated morbidity or mortality. Symptomatic CMV infection may be further differentiated into the *CMV syndrome* (fever, leukopenia, and an increased CMV antigen titer) and *invasive CMV disease* (e.g., pneumonitis, hepatitis, and gastrointestinal involvement). *Secondary CMV infection* represents infection in previously infected seropositive hosts caused by either reactivation of latent endogenous virus or reinfection or supra-infection with new virus. *Active CMV infection* is a primary or secondary infection that may be asymptomatic or symptomatic and is characterized by viral replication and shedding with a specific immune response to CMV. *Latent CMV infection* represents lifelong persistence of virus without replication in healthy seropositive host. Factors predisposing to CMV infection in kidney transplant recipients include donor CMV seropositive status; recipient CMV seropositive status; the use of blood products from CMV seropositive donors; episodes of acute rejection; the net state of immunosuppression; retransplantation; and antilymphocyte preparations, which have the capacity to convert latent to active infection.

CMV is associated with immunomodulatory derangements (e.g., reduced helper/suppressor cell ratio) that can lead indirectly to opportunistic superinfections, allograft injury or rejection, and development of PTLD. CMV may incite proinflammatory cytokines (e.g., tumor necrosis factor), which can bind to a latently infected cell, generating nuclear transcription factors that initiate CMV replication. CMV infection induces antiendothelial cell antibodies, which may be risk factors for both acute and chronic rejection.

CMV can produce a variety of clinical syndromes. The most common presents with fever and malaise, leukopenia, and transaminitis. CMV pneumonitis is the most serious sequela, manifested by dyspnea, hypoxemia, interstitial infiltrates, and the detection of CMV antigens, nucleic acids, or inclusion bodies on BAL. CMV upper and lower gastrointestinal disease manifests as esophagitis, cholecystitis, duodenitis, hepatitis, and colitis. Diagnostic endoscopy can reveal solitary or multiple ulcerations and hemorrhage; biopsy material should be examined by immunohistochemical methods or cytology for CMV antigens or inclusion bodies, respectively. CMV hepatitis is accompanied by cytologic or immunohistochemical analysis and transaminitis. CMV retinitis can be diagnosed by fundoscopy. Central nervous system CMV disease (e.g., meningitis, encephalitis, myelitis) may be more difficult to diagnose. Neurologic disease caused by other neurotropic opportunistic pathogens should be simultaneously investigated. Multiorgan involvement can be observed in disseminated CMV disease; criteria for specific visceral involvement were listed previously. *Recurrent CMV disease* is defined as clinical manifestations meeting the previously listed criteria shortly after cessation of anti-CMV therapy. *Refractory CMV disease* may reflect viral resistance resulting from mutations in CMV strains or a depressed net state of immunosuppression.

DIAGNOSIS.   Table 10.9 summarizes methods for the diagnosis of CMV infection and disease. Specific CMV antigens or nucleic acid in tissue or white blood cells can be identified. CMV can be isolated from an initial culture of various clinical specimens, and a monoclonal antibody against early viral antigens can be used to confirm

Table 10.9.   Current diagnosis of cytomegalovirus infection

Method	Description	Comments
Nucleic acid detection, antigen detection, culture	PCR DNA hybridization Antigenemia Buffy coat isolation, shell vial centrifugation; tube cell culture techniques	Detection of CMV from throat swabs, urine, or saliva may not support the presence of CMV disease. Specialized equipment & labor required for PCR, hybridization, antigenemia
Serology	Acute, convalescent CMV IgG or single CMV IgM titer	Serologic response may be slow or absent in primary infection; false-positive reactions or interference may occur; potential variability in kit standardization
Immunopathology, histopathology	Microscopic examination of tissue for inclusion bodies Immunohistochemical staining with anti-CMV specific–labeled antibody Electron microscopic examination of biopsy specimens for CMV	Insensitive; inclusion bodies may be present only in advanced infection Specialized equipment required

PCR, polymerase chain reaction; CMV, cytomegalovirus; Ig, immunoglobulin

the presence of CMV in conventional cell culture or shell vial. Serologic detection of a persisting CMV IgM or IgG in a previously seronegative patient can be performed by EIA or other serologic assay. Clinical correlation is necessary in the interpretation of serologic assays because of differences in the sensitivity and specificity of laboratory assays, variability in commercially available kits, and interfering substances. CMV DNA assays involve a signal-amplified hybridization assay for detection and quantitation of CMV DNA in peripheral white blood cells, using a specific probe to eliminate cross-reactivity with other herpesvirus sequences. The CMV antigenemia assay detects the presence of CMV antigens in white blood cells. Delays in processing blood used for these assays may result in a significant decrease in the sensitivity of selected tests. CMV DNA detection by PCR has been used clinically with enhanced sensitivity. Even after effective treatment of sympto-matic CMV disease, however, this method may continue to detect CMV DNA despite the disappearance of antigenemia.

TREATMENT. The availability of effective agents for CMV pro-phylaxis and treatment has considerably diminished the morbid-ity and mortality associated with CMV infection. Treatment of active CMV disease includes reduction in the immunosuppressive regimen, as tolerable, and the administration of intravenous gan-ciclovir. An additional period of treatment may be necessary in selected patients. Frequent monitoring for signs and symptoms of CMV disease may be warranted after a treatment course of gan-ciclovir in selected high-risk renal transplant recipients because ongoing risk factors for CMV may be present. Maintenance gan-ciclovir therapy has been suggested in certain patients; monitor-ing may be preferred in lower-risk patients. Adverse effects of ganciclovir include reversible dose-related granulocytopenia and thrombocytopenia, fever, rash, seizures, nausea, myalgias, abnor-malities in liver enzyme determinations, and, rarely, pancreati-tis. Drug interactions include an increased seizure risk when used in combination with acyclovir and imipenem, and additive marrow suppression with azathioprine and TMP/SMX.

Experience in treating refractory CMV disease suggests that the addition of CMV hyperimmune globulin or intravenous pooled gamma-globulin may improve the response to ganciclovir. Some transplantation centers have advocated the use of CMV hyper-immune globulin in conjunction with high-dose acyclovir for the prophylaxis and treatment of CMV disease. Foscarnet has been used to treat ganciclovir-resistant CMV isolates; however, its use is associated with considerable nephrotoxicity.

PROPHYLAXIS. A rational way to minimize severe CMV infec-tion would be to avoid transplanting CMV-positive kidneys into CMV-negative recipients. Such a policy has been implemented in some transplantation centers but has been made largely imprac-tical by the competing need for HLA matching and the shortage of cadaveric kidneys. Several prophylactic strategies have been employed to reduce CMV infection and disease in kidney allograft recipients (Table 10.10). By recognizing the CMV serologies of the donor and recipient before transplantation, and by assessing the net state of immunosuppression, CMV prophylactic strategies can be optimized to limit the incidence of CMV and, subsequently, improve overall patient and allograft survival.

CMV prophylaxis regimens described in the literature include monotherapy with antiviral agents such as acyclovir or ganci-clovir, monotherapy with CMV immune globulin or hyperimmune serum, or a combination of antiviral agents and CMV immune globulin. Although there is no consensus regarding which agents are superior, several kidney transplantation centers continue to use these regimens in routine prophylaxis or as part of a pre-emptive treatment approach. High-dose oral acyclovir has been reported to reduce the risk for CMV disease in lower-risk patients but may be ineffective in high-risk patients. Oral ganciclovir has been demonstrated to provide effective CMV prophylaxis in recip-ients of seropositive kidneys.

CMV-positive patients who are treated with OKT3 or the poly-clonal antibodies have a high incidence of symptomatic CMV disease. So-called preemptive daily ganciclovir therapy (2.5 to

Table 10.10. Regimens for cytomegalovirus (CMV) prophylaxis

Prophylactic Regimens	CMV Serologies		
	Donor+, Recipient–	Recipient+	Donor–, Recipient–
Acyclovir PO		X	X
Acyclovir IV/ PO + CMVIG	X	X	
CMVIG	X	X	
Ganciclovir PO	X	X	X
Ganciclovir IV followed by acyclovir PO		X	X
Ganciclovir IV followed by DHPG PO	X	X	X
Ganciclovir IV/ PO + CMVIG	X	X	

Other agents
Cidofovir[a], foscarnet[a], valacyclovir[b], valganciclovir (investigational)

CMVIG, cytomegalovirus immune globulin.
[a] Used for treatment of documented ganciclovir-resistant CMV isolates.
[b] Increased risk for hemolytic-uremic syndrome is solid organ transplant recipients.

5 mg/kg/day) administered during antibody treatment courses can reduce this incidence. Preemptive ganciclovir treatment presumably inactivates latent virus that has the potential for reactivation when immunosuppression is intensified. Kidney transplant recipients who require multiple treatment for rejection may require additional periods of CMV prophylaxis to diminish the occurrence of CMV disease. Strategies include preemptive intravenous ganciclovir, as described previously, followed by an additional period of reduced-frequency intravenous ganciclovir (e.g., five times per week) or oral ganciclovir (1 to 3 g/day, dose adjusted for the level of renal function and white blood cell count). Patients should be assessed clinically for their risk for reactivation of CMV as a function of their cumulative net state of immunosuppression.

Additional antiviral agents, such as cidofovir or foscarnet, have been used to treat ganciclovir-resistant CMV isolates; however, the risk for additive nephrotoxicity with calcineurin blockers precludes their use as part of routine prophylaxis. Clinical trials should also provide information regarding the efficacy, safety, and drug interactions of newer antiviral agents such as valaciclovir or valganciclovir, which have greater bioavailability than oral acyclovir or ganciclovir.

Herpes Simplex Virus and Varicella Zoster Virus
HSV infection predominates in mucosal surfaces and typically manifests within the first 6 weeks after transplantation; infection

can occasionally disseminate to visceral organs. Atypically, lesions are common in kidney transplant recipients. Both acyclovir and ganciclovir are active against herpesviruses *in vitro,* and both are useful in the treatment or prophylaxis of HSV. Alternative agents include valaciclovir and famciclovir. Acyclovir can be given intravenously or orally for mucocutaneous infections. For treatment of HSV encephalitis, a higher dosage (Table 10.6) is given by slow infusion to prevent crystallization within the renal tubules.

Herpes zoster develops in about 10% of organ transplant recipients and may involve two or three adjoining dermatomes. Acyclovir, famciclovir, and valaciclovir can be all be used for herpes zoster and varicella. Disseminated VZV, usually as a result of primary VZV infection, is fortunately rare but may cause pneumonia, encephalitis, disseminated intravascular coagulation, and graft dysfunction. Antiviral treatment for varicella or zoster in immunocompetent patients includes intravenous acyclovir (10-15 mg/kg every 8 hours in a slow infusion) for severe or disseminated cases. Ganciclovir and foscarnet are also active against VZV.

Other Human Herpesviruses

Human herpesvirus (HHV) types 6, 7, and 8 are ubiquitous and may be isolated from immunocompromised patients and renal transplant recipients. HHV-6 and HHV-7 can cause persistent infection in their hosts. HHV-6 may reactivate during episodes of acute rejection or calcineurin inhibitor toxicity and has been associated with CMV infection, encephalitis, and bone marrow suppression in immunocompromised patients. Transmission of HHV-8 from kidney donors to recipients has been documented, and infection with this virus has been associated with the development of symptomatic Kaposi's sarcoma after kidney transplantation. Diagnosis is supported by morphologic study and by the presence of HHV-8 DNA sequences in involved tissue.

Adenovirus

Adenovirus may cause a self-limiting hemorrhagic cystitis after transplantation, or it may disseminate, causing pneumonia and hepatitis. Treatment options are limited, and reduction in immunosuppression may be of some benefit. Treatment with intravenous ribavirin has been used in clinical trials.

Papovaviruses

The so-called BK and JC viruses (BKV and JCV) belong to the human papovavirus family. Reactivation of virus can occur and has been implicated as a cause of ureteral stricture, progressive multifocal leukoencephalopathy, and interstitial nephritis (see Chapters 8 and 13). The differentiation among the viral inclusions of BKV, JCV, CMV, HSV, and adenovirus can be difficult. Specific *in situ* hybridization and polymerase chain reaction techniques can demonstrate papovavirus. No specific therapy for human papovavirus infection is available, and reduction of immunosuppression offers the best therapeutic option.

Influenza Types A and B, Parainfluenza
Virus, and Respiratory Syncytial Virus

Community respiratory viruses may cause significant morbidity and mortality in renal transplant recipients. These seasonal viruses can be transmitted by virus-laden respiratory droplets and aerosols through the environment and person-to-person contact. Noso-comial transmission can occur, with infected hospitalized or intensive care unit patients spreading viruses to adjacent patients through respiratory secretions, fomites, or inadequate infection control measures among staff personnel. Renal transplant recipients may act as the "sentinel" cases for a community influenza outbreak. Community respiratory virus disease usually presents with upper respiratory tract symptoms, progressing to systemic symptoms such as high fever, myalgias, arthralgias, anorexia, and mucosal inflammation. The spectrum of illness includes mild upper respiratory illness, bronchiolitis, and pneumonia with respiratory failure.

The diagnosis of respiratory virus illness is facilitated by the rapid detection of virus-laden upper respiratory cells (e.g., nasopharyngeal washing, bronchoalveolar fluid) by virus-specific fluorescent-labeled antibody probes. Progressive viral infection can lead to fatal pneumonia or death from suprainfection with bacterial pathogens such as *S. aureus, Streptococcus* species, nosocomial gram-negative bacilli, or fungal pathogens; simultaneous CMV reactivation may occur as a result of immunomodulation.

Immunization with influenza vaccine is the optimal method of prevention in healthy patients but may be ineffective in immunosuppressed patients because of their reduced antibody response. A novel vaccine antigen-delivery system (virosome) may be immunogenic when administered by the intranasal route. Treatment of influenza A includes early administration of amantadine or rimantadine. Prophylaxis with amantadine or rimantadine can be used in institutional outbreaks. Neither agent is effective against influenza B. Newer agents, such as oseltamivir and zanamivir, are neuraminidase inhibitors that, if started within 30 to 36 hours after onset of symptoms, can shorten the duration of illness and decrease some upper respiratory complications. Both agents can be used as prophylaxis in preventing influenza illness.

Respiratory syncytial virus (RSV) pneumonitis may respond to aerosolized ribavirin delivered in a controlled contained administration system given over 24 hours. RSV immunoglobulin or RSV monoclonal antibody may have benefit for RSV infection in conjunction with aerosolized ribavirin before respiratory failure, although their use has not been studied in renal transplant recipients.

Parvovirus

Human parvovirus B19 can cause a variety of clinical manifestations, including fifth disease in healthy children. In transplant recipients, parvovirus infection is an occasional cause of refractory severe anemia, pancytopenia, and thrombotic microangiopathy. Infection is recognized by the finding of typical giant proerythroblasts in the bone marrow, followed by confirmation by a PCR assay. Treatment with intravenous immunoglobulin may be dramatically effective. Most infected patients have been taking tacrolimus, and alternative agents can be used if the therapeutic response is inadequate.

Acute Viral Exposures

Renal transplant recipients who are susceptible to VZV are candidates for VZV immune globulin (VZIG) if exposure is considered to be significant (e.g., continuous household or social contact, hospital contact in adjacent beds, or prolonged contact with an infectious patient). The complication rate in immunocompromised patients who contract varicella is substantially greater than that in healthy individuals. Fortunately, however, more than 90% of adults are seropositive for VZV and are not at risk for primary infection. VZIG is of maximal benefit if administered quickly after the presumed exposure but may be effective given as late as 96 hours after exposure. VZV vaccine should not be administered to patients receiving immunosuppressive therapy. During outbreaks of documented influenza A, vaccination with influenza vaccine and administration with antiviral prophylaxis are useful.

SELECTED READINGS

Delmonico FL, Snydman DR. Organ donor screening for infectious diseases. *Transplantation* 1998;65:603.

Fishman JA, Rubin RH. Infections in organ-transplant recipients. *N Engl J Med* 1998;338:1741.

Ho M. Human herpesvirus 8: let the transplant physician beware. *N Engl J Med* 1998;339:1391.

Jassal SV, Roscoe JM, Zalzman JS, et al. Clinical practice guidelines: prevention of cytomegalovirus disease after renal transplantation. *J Am Soc Nephrol* 1998;9:1696.

Jha V, Sakhuja V, Gupta D, et al. Successful management of pulmonary tuberculosis in renal allograft recipients in a single center. *Kidney Int* 1999;56:1944.

Lowance D, Neumayer HH, Legendre CM, et al. Valacyclovir for the prevention of cytomegalovirus disease after renal transplantation. *N Engl J Med* 1999;340:1462.

Meier-Kriesche HU, Friedman G, Jacobs M, et al. Infectious complications in geriatric renal transplant patients. *Transplantation* 1999;68:1496.

Murer L, Zacchello G, Bianchi D. Thrombotic microangiopathy associated with parvovirus B19 infection after renal transplantation. *J Am Soc Nephrol* 2000;11:1132.

Nickiliet V, Hirsch HH, Binet IF, et al. Polyomavirus infection in renal allograft recipients: from latent infection to manifest disease. *J Am Soc Nephrol* 1999;10:1080.

Patterson JE. Epidemiology of fungal infection in solid organ transplant recipients. *Transplant Infect Dis* 1999;1:229.

Pizzo PA. Fever in immunocompromised patients. *N Engl J Med* 1999; 341:893.

Rubin RH. Infectious diseases in transplantation: pre- and posttransplantation. In: Douglas NJ, Suki WN, eds. *Primer on transplantation*. Thorofare, NJ: American Society of Transplant Physicians, 1998:141;152.

Rubin RH. Infection in the organ transplant patient. In: Rubin RH, Young LS, eds. *Clinical approach to infection in the compromised host*. New York: Plenum, 1994:629–669.

Walsh TJ, Finberg RW, Arndt C, et al. Liposomal amphotericin B for empirical therapy in patients with persistent fever and neutropenia. *N Engl J Med* 1999;340:764.

Hepatitis in Kidney Transplantation

Fabrizio Fabrizi and Paul Martin

Of the five major hepatotropic viruses, only two have major clinical impact on the management of patients with end-stage renal disease (ESRD): hepatitis B and hepatitis C.

The potential for worsening of liver disease as a result of viral hepatitis after renal transplantation was first recognized in patients with chronic hepatitis B virus (HBV) infection. This led to a reluctance in some centers to offer renal transplantation to HBV-infected patients. Chronic hepatitis C virus (HCV) is typically an indolent disease, and early reports implied that its presence did not affect survival of infected recipients. More recently, however, it has been observed that there is also significant morbidity and mortality related to liver disease in these patients. Thus, appropriate evaluation of the renal transplantation candidate with chronic viral hepatitis now includes assessment of viral replication, liver histology, and consideration of antiviral therapy.

RENAL TRANSPLANT RECIPIENTS WITH VIRAL HEPATITIS

Hepatitis B

Interpretation of Diagnostic Tests

In acute HBV infection, hepatitis B surface antigen (HBsAg) is the first viral marker detectable in serum (Table 11.1). By the time clinical hepatitis is present after an incubation period of up to 140 days, other serum markers of HBV infection have appeared in serum, including antibody to the hepatitis B core antigen (anti-HBc). Hepatitis B core antigen, a marker of viral replication found in infected hepatocytes, does not circulate in serum, but the corresponding antibody (anti-HBc) does. Persistence of HBsAg in serum for more than 6 months is indicative of chronic HBV, with a low likelihood of spontaneous resolution. Chronic HBV is confirmed by the absence of immunoglobulin M (IgM) anti-HBc in serum. Initially anti-HBc is predominantly an IgM antibody that serves as a marker of acute or recent acute hepatitis B and persists for about 6 months; IgG anti-HBc, however, persists indefinitely. With successful resolution of acute hepatitis B, protective antibody directed against HBsAg (anti-HBs) appears, signifying immunity against HBV. Additional HBV markers detectable by routine testing include HBV DNA and hepatitis e antigen (HBeAg), both of which are evidence of active viral replication. Any patient who is HBsAg positive is potentially infectious, but a patient who is also HBeAg positive is more so because of higher viral levels.

Natural History

Somewhat less than 5% of infected immunocompetent adults fail to clear acute HBV infection and develop chronic HBV infection.

Table 11.1.   **Hepatitis B virus (HBV) tests**

Test	Interpretation
Hepatitis B surface Antigen (HBsAg)	HBV infection
Hepatitis B core Antibody (anti-HBc)	
IgM anti-HBc	Acute or recent HBV infection
IgG anti-HBc	Chronic or remote HBV infection
Hepatitis B surface antibody	Immunity to HBV (vaccine induced or due to prior infection)
Hepatitis B e antigen, HBV DNA	Markers of active replication

Chronicity is more likely in uremic patients, elderly people, and others with a less vigorous immune response, such as very young children. There are two phases of chronic HBV infection. In the initial months and years of chronic HBV infection, active viral replication persists with high levels of HBV DNA and HBeAg in serum. This *replicative phase* of chronic HBV infection is often accompanied by necroinflammatory changes in the liver and elevated serum aminotransferase levels. The second phase of chronic HBV infection is the *nonreplicative phase,* which follows either spontaneous or therapy-induced HBeAg loss; this phase is often heralded by a transient rise in aminotransferase levels. With loss of HBeAg, antibody to HBeAg may or may not appear in serum, but HBV DNA levels decrease significantly, and liver disease activity subsides both biochemically and histologically. Infectivity is much reduced after HBeAg is lost, although minute concentrations of HBV DNA may remain detectable in serum by polymerase chain reaction (PCR). The persistence of the replicative phase of chronic HBV infection is linked to a higher risk for progression to cirrhosis. HBsAg persistence with normal aminotransferase activity was previously referred to as the *healthy carrier state.* These patients, however, may have had many years of active replication, with the potential for significant liver injury and complications, including hepatocellular carcinoma (HCC), and are best described as having *low-level replication.*

The association between chronic HBV infection and HCC is strong; the risk for HCC is 10 to 390 times higher in patients with chronic HBV than in uninfected controls. Hepatocellular carcinoma due to HBV infection is usually associated with cirrhosis. HCC represents the most common cause of death due to malignancy in populations with high HBV prevalence. Various mutant forms of HBV have been identified in which amino acid substitution at crucial sites in the viral genome exist, including the precore mutant characteristic by its failure to secrete HBeAg despite active viral replication and abundant HBV DNA present in serum. Its presence has been associated with more severe liver disease. More recently recognized HBV mutants have occurred as a result of lamivudine therapy. Administration of long-term hepatitis B immunoglobulin therapy to prevent HBV recurrence after liver transplantation has also been associated with mutant formation.

The control of spread of HBV infection in dialysis units has been one of major triumphs in the management of ESRD. Patients with chronic HBV, however, continue to enter the population pool of dialysis patients and transplant candidates.

Disease Progression After Renal Transplantation

Although HBV-related liver disease often appears clinically mild, with only modest elevations of aspartate (AST) and alanine aminotransferase (ALT) levels before transplantation, progressive deterioration has been observed after transplantation. The outcome of HBV-infected transplant recipients is less favorable than that of noninfected transplant recipients. Patients with chronic HBV who continue dialysis treatment generally do not suffer clinically obvious worsening of their liver disease; thus, the decision to proceed with transplantation must be made with great care.

Immunosuppressive agents are clearly permissive for HBV replication. Increased viral replication with reappearance or increase in serum HBV DNA and HBeAg occurs, and reappearance of serum HBsAg after apparent clearance of previous HBV has been reported. Cyclosporine and other immunosuppressives may directly enhance HBV replication. Withdrawal of azathioprine may favorably alter the clinical course of chronic HBV. Impairment of host response may also contribute to enhanced HBV replication. In addition, the HBV genome contains a glucocorticoid-responsive element, which increases HBV replication when steroids are used.

The adverse effect of immunosuppressive therapy on HBV infection has been recognized in several other settings. Reactivation of HBV infection has been well described in HBsAg-positive patients receiving cytotoxic cancer therapy, and death from liver failure has been observed. Liver transplantation in HBV-infected patients is associated with frequent liver graft reinfection followed by progressive liver disease if some form of immunoprophylaxis is not given.

The effects of HBV infection on graft survival after renal transplantation remain unclear, although the detrimental effect of HBsAg-positive status on patient survival is well established.

Role of Pretransplantation Liver Biopsy
and Current Recommendations

Liver biopsy should be incorporated in the evaluation of the renal transplant candidate with HBsAg (Fig. 11.1). A decision regarding transplant candidacy in HBV-infected patients should be based on both liver histology and assessment of evidence of HBV replication in serum (i.e., HBV DNA and HBeAg). Nevertheless, the absence in serum of HBV DNA or HBeAg before transplantation does not preclude reactivation of HBV infection after transplantation. Patients with severe chronic hepatitis with bridging fibrosis (stage III), a precursor of cirrhosis, or established cirrhosis (stage IV) on liver biopsy are at particular risk for frank hepatic decompensation after transplantation, and renal transplantation is not recommended. In patients with less histologically severe liver disease, transplantation is not precluded. All patients

HBV Infected Candidate

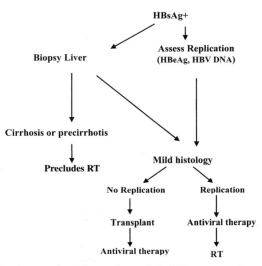

Fig. 11.1.   Approach to the work-up of the kidney transplant candidate with viral hepatitis B. RT, renal transplant.

infected with HBV, however, must be cautioned that even histologically mild disease has the potential to deteriorate under the influence of immunosuppression. The advent of effective antiviral therapies offers the opportunity to prevent posttransplantation progression of HBV. If active replication is present (i.e., positive HBeAg or HBV DNA), antiviral therapy should be started before transplantation to slow progression of liver disease. All patients with HBV should be placed on antiviral therapy after transplantation.

Antiviral Strategies
Although there is only limited information on monotherapy with interferon-alpha (IFN-alpha) in renal transplant recipients with chronic HBV, it appears that the response rate to IFN-alpha therapy is similar to that of immunocompetent hosts, with normalization of serum aminotransferase activity and clearance of HBV DNA from serum in responders. The most significant concern regarding posttransplantation use of IFN-alpha is precipitation of graft rejection, which is frequently irreversible and steroid resistant. IFN-alpha therapy may also compromise graft function by other mechanisms, such as direct nephrotoxicity, acute interstitial nephritis, and induction of cytokines. Thus, the role of IFN-alpha in treating HBV in transplant recipients is limited. The use of IFN-alpha before transplantation in patients with ESRD may be limited by relative host immunocompromise. The efficacy of

IFN-alpha in clearing HBV is strongly related to its ability to enhance intrinsic immune reactivity to HBV.

The most promising agent for use in renal transplant recipients with HBV is lamivudine, another nucleoside analogue. It is highly efficacious and has potent antiviral activity against HBV, even in immunocompromised patients. It causes premature termination of the viral DNA chain during reverse transcription. In renal transplant recipients, lamivudine has been effective in suppressing HBV replication, with clearance of HBV DNA from serum and improvement in liver chemistries; HBsAg positivity, however, persists. Lamivudine is well tolerated. In contrast to IFN-alpha, it has no proven immunomodulatory effect and is administrated orally. The major limitation to its use is the emergence of "escape" mutants. These mutants are less lamivudine responsive than the so-called wild-type HBV and may be associated with clinical worsening of liver disease. As additional nucleoside analogues become available, patients with chronic HBV will probably be treated with a combination of agents to lessen the risk for viral resistance. Both ganciclovir and famciclovir have been used in the treatment of HBV in kidney transplant recipients.

Hepatitis C

Interpretation of Diagnostic Tests

Although the accuracy of diagnostic testing has evolved rapidly since the recent identification of HCV, concern remains about lack of sensitivity of anti-HCV ELISA serologic testing in patients with ESRD (Table 11.2). The recombinant immunoblot assay (RIBA), which is a supplemental test to improve specificity in anti-HCV–positive people, is mainly of use in low-risk populations, such as blood donors. Direct detection of HCV RNA by the PCR may be necessary to completely exclude HCV infection in patients with ESRD. A variety of PCR-based tests are available, which vary in their sensitivity and ability to quantify viral load. Improper collection, handling, and storage of samples may also result in considerable variability in results. The occurrence of HCV viremia in a small but significant minority of ESRD patients, negative by serologic testing, suggests that a PCR test should be considered if there is clinical suspicion of HCV infection despite negative serologies. Quantitative PCR tests measure viral load, whereas the more sensitive qualitative tests can detect even low-level viremia. A variety of

Table 11.2. Hepatitis C virus (HCV) tests

Test	Interpretation
Anti-HCV	An ELISA test, indicates infection not immunity
RIBA test	Improves specificity of anti-HCV testing
HCV RNA	By PCR, indicates viremia, can be quantitative (for viral load) or qualitative (for detecting low viral levels)
Genotype	Predictor of interferon responsiveness

ELISA, enzyme-linked immunosorbent assay; RIBA, recombinant immunoblot assay. PCR, polymerase chain reaction.

PCR tests are available but lack standardization, which leads to difficulty comparing results from one system to another. It is important to know whether the test is quantitative or qualitative to interpret the results obtained.

The evaluation of HCV infection in transplant candidates is complicated by the finding that even the mild aminotransferase elevations typical of chronic HCV are frequently absent in patients with ESRD. Thus, the absence of an elevated ALT in a patient with ESRD does not preclude active viral infection as a result of HCV. Chronic HCV infection has a typically indolent progression, but cirrhosis and other complications such as HCC do occur in a subset of patients. An important predictor of disease progression is alcohol abuse.

Because the natural history of HCV extends over decades rather than years, the adverse consequences of chronic HCV infection in patients followed for a shorter period of time may not be apparent, particularly in a population of patients with ESRD who have a high mortality rate from nonhepatic causes.

Disease Progression After Renal Transplantation

The frequency of HCV infection among renal transplant candidates reflects its prevalence in chronic hemodialysis patients. This prevalence is related to a variety of factors, including duration and type of dialysis, blood transfusion requirements, and prior transplants. Most transplant recipients with anti-HCV antibody have detectable serum HCV RNA, which is persistent in almost all cases. Posttransplantation HCV infection may or may not be associated with elevated aminotransferase activity, although HCV RNA levels increase significantly.

The effect of renal transplantation on the progression of HCV-related liver disease has been the source of much debate. Initial reports had suggested that no excess of liver morbidity or mortality occurred in HCV-infected recipients. However, a number of reports have identified an increased attrition rate as a result of hepatic decompensation within 5 to 10 years of transplantation. Because liver disease caused by HCV may be clinically silent even in the presence of cirrhosis, the absence of a pretransplantation liver biopsy may lead to a failure to recognize significant liver disease.

HCV infection acts more aggressively in renal transplant recipients who first acquire HCV infection at the time of transplantation, probably because acute hepatitis develops while the patient is receiving maximal immunosuppression. It may occasionally lead to rapidly progressive liver failure. It is unclear whether the choice of immunosuppressive agents affects HCV progression, although azathioprine and the antilymphocytic agents have been implicated in clinically more severe liver disease.

HCV infection in renal transplant recipients has been associated with the development of membranoproliferative glomerulonephritis and mixed cryoglobulinemia. The lesion is similar to that seen with chronic HCV infection in the nontransplant situation.

Role of Liver Biopsy Before Renal Transplantation

The severity of preexisting liver disease on pretransplantation liver biopsy provides useful prognostic information (Fig. 11.2).

HCV Infected Candidate

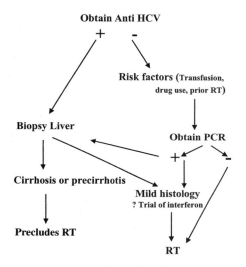

Fig. 11.2. Approach to the work-up of the kidney transplant candidate with viral hepatitis C. RT, renal transplant.

Liver biopsy is essential to assess the severity of liver damage in patients with chronic HCV; severity cannot be inferred from routine liver chemistries or virologic testing.

Current Status of Antiviral Therapy
As in any patient with chronic viral hepatitis, excessive immunosuppression should be avoided. IFN-alpha therapy for chronic HCV in transplant recipients is not advised because of concern about precipitating graft dysfunction and low efficacy. There are, however, encouraging reports of successful antiviral therapy for HCV in ESRD patients with responses persisting even after transplantation.
    Ribavirin is a synthetic guanosine analogue that enhances IFN-alpha response rates in HCV therapy. It has activity against a spectrum of DNA and RNA viruses. Ribavirin monotherapy is not recommended because it has no convincing efficacy against HCV and may accumulate in the presence of renal insufficiency, leading to increased toxicity. Its major side effect is hemolytic anemia, which is clearly a concern in patients with ESRD who are anemic at baseline; this side effect effectively precludes its use in this population.

Current Recommendations
PCR testing should be obtained in seronegative candidates with risk factors for HCV or elevated aminotransferases to exclude false-negative serologies. All HCV-infected patients should undergo liver biopsy. Patients with minimal changes to mild chronic hepati-

tis (stage I, II) can be offered renal transplantation, and a trial of antiviral therapy should be considered. Patients with cirrhosis should not undergo transplantation because of the risk for post-transplantation hepatocellular failure. Combined transplantation (orthotopic liver and kidney transplantation) in these patients may be a consideration if they subsequently develop decompensated cirrhosis (see Chapter 6). In patients whose histology precludes renal transplantation yet whose hepatic function is too well compensated to require liver transplantation, it is safer to remain on dialysis.

KIDNEY DONOR WITH POSITIVE HEPATITIS SEROLOGIES

Effects on Recipient

Transmission of HCV during solid organ transplantation from infected donor to HCV naive recipient has been unequivocally demonstrated, and occasional cases of severe, acute HCV infection with a fatal outcome have been reported. The risk for HCV transmission may be related to several factors, including donor viral load and the method used for organ preservation. The rate of transmission of HCV by organ transplantation has been much higher when the kidneys have been preserved in slush rather than pulsatile perfusion (see Chapter 5). The use of renal grafts from HCV-infected donors in recipients with documented HCV infection does *not* appear to result in a greater burden of liver disease and is a reasonable consideration.

HBsAg positivity precludes kidney donation. HBV infection may potentially be transmitted from a donor with negative HBsAg but a positive anti-HBc antibody. This serologic profile indicates prior resolved HBV infection. In hepatic allograft recipients, *de novo* HBV infection has occasionally occurred, presumably because of amplification of minute residual viruses in the graft itself despite the absence of HBsAg. For renal transplant recipients, isolated donor anti-HBc positivity does not appear to represent a risk for HBV transmission, although IgM anti-HBc indicates recent acute HBV infection and viremia and suggests a higher rise of HBV transmission.

SELECTED READINGS

David-Neto E, Americo da Fonseca J, Jota da Paula F, et al. The impact of azathioprine on chronic viral hepatitis in renal transplantation: a long-term single-center, prospective study on azathioprine withdrawal. *Transplantation* 1999;68:976.

Degos F, Lugassy C, Degott C, et al. Hepatitis B virus and hepatitis B related viral infection in renal transplant recipients: a prospective study of 90 patients. *Gastroenterology* 1988;94:151.

Fornairon S, Pol S, Legendre C, et al. The long-term virologic and pathologic impact of renal transplantation on chronic hepatitis B virus infection. *Transplantation* 1996;62:297.

Glicklich D, Thung SN, Kapoian T, et al. Comparison of clinical features and liver histology in hepatitis C positive dialysis patients and renal transplant recipients. *Am J Gastroenterol* 1999;94:159.

Knoll GA, Tankersley MR, Lee JY, et al. The impact of renal transplantation on survival in hepatitis C-positive end-stage renal disease patients. *Am J Kidney Dis* 1997;29:608.

Legendre C, Garrigue V, Le Bihan C, et al. Harmful long-term impact of hepatitis C virus infection in kidney transplant recipients. *Transplantation* 1999;65:667.

Martin P, Friedman LS. Chronic viral hepatitis and the management of chronic renal failure. *Kidney Int* 1995;47:1231.

Martin P, Carter D, Fabrizi F, et al. Histopathological features of hepatitis C in renal transplant candidates. *Transplantation* 2000; 69:1–6.

Mathurin P, Mouquet C, Poynard T, et al. Impact of hepatitis B and C virus on kidney transplantation outcome. *Hepatology* 1999;29:257.

Parfrey PS, Forbes RDC, Huchinson TA, et al. The impact of renal transplantation on the course of hepatitis B liver disease. *Transplantation* 1985;39:610.

Pereira BJG, Natov SN, Bouthot BA, et al. Effect of hepatitis C infection and renal transplantation on survival in end-stage kidney disease. *Kidney Int* 1998;53:1374.

Diagnostic Imaging in Kidney Transplantation

Peter Zimmerman, Nagesh Ragavendra,
Carl K. Hoh, and Zoran L. Barbaric

The clinician evaluating a patient with renal transplant dysfunction has the choice of a variety of imaging procedures, including ultrasound (US), nuclear medicine studies, computed tomography (CT), magnetic resonance imaging (MRI), and excretory urography. Imaging evaluation is usually initiated either with duplex US, which provides cross-sectional imaging and physiologic information quickly, noninvasively, and portably; or with nuclear medicine studies, which provide physiologic information and some anatomic information. CT provides superb anatomic information but involves the use of iodinated contrast medium and lacks portability. MRI provides superb anatomic information, can noninvasively image large vessels, and can evaluate function using relatively nonnephrotoxic contrast medium (gadolinium). MRI, however, is not portable, is expensive, and requires special equipment for guided interventions. This chapter emphasizes the use of US and nuclear medicine studies in renal transplantation, although CT, MRI, and urography may, on occasion, be the optimal imaging modalities for certain clinical problems encountered in renal transplant recipients.

RADIOLOGIC EVALUATION OF THE LIVING DONOR

The process of evaluation of a potential living donor is discussed in Chapter 5. The radiologic studies used in potential living donors are done to ensure that after nephrectomy, the donor is left with an anatomically and functionally normal kidney. They also permit the surgeon to make appropriate technical decisions regarding the choice of kidney (right or left) and type of vascular anastomosis (see Chapter 7). The traditional donor radiologic work-up typically consisted of an intravenous urogram followed by angiography.

Computed Tomographic Angiography and Urography

The helical, or spiral, CT scan, followed in the same session by several postcontrast radiographs, produces a modified intravenous urogram, usually called a *computed tomographic urogram* (CTU). This technique is replacing the traditional work-up in many centers. *Computed tomographic angiography* (CTA) differs from usual CT in that intravenous contrast is injected rapidly (4 to 5 mL/sec), imaging begins at peak contrast concentration in the aorta (20 seconds after injection), the beam is collimated to 3 mm, and reconstruction is at 2-mm intervals. The images are usually viewed using *maximal intensity projection* (MIP). MIP is a computer rendition of all data made to look like a projectional angiogram that can be rotated along various planes (Fig. 12.1). The technique of

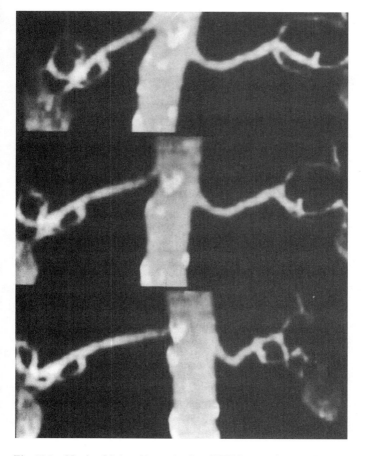

Fig. 12.1. Maximal intensity projection (MIP) is one of several ways to present a multitude of these axial computed tomography images. An MIP image can be rotated along any axis.

surface shading renders the surface of the kidney, aorta, and renal arteries totally opaque, such that is it impossible to see intrarenal details. Artificial shading is applied to give the structures a three-dimensional appearance. *Pseudo-cine,* or rapid scrolling through a stack of axial images, is probably the least expensive and most accurate method to search for supernumerary renal arteries. The rapid, cinelike mode allows the radiologist to integrate successive images in his or her brain, and the multiple renal arteries are almost always identified. This method has replaced renal angiography for the purpose of identifying renal arteries and renal veins in the renal donor evaluation in most institutions (Fig. 12.2).

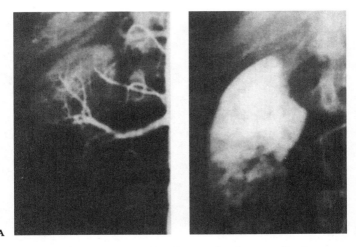

A   B

**Fig. 12.2.   A: The donor renal angiogram showing a small polar
artery. B: Selective renal arteriogram of the main renal artery
(nephrogram phase) demonstrates just how much renal parenchyma
could be lost if the upper polar artery were ligated during harvest.**

The urographic images of the CTU permit an evaluation of
the anatomy of the collecting system, ureters, and bladder. The
entire urinary tract is seen at a glance, so that supernumerary
ureters, ureteropelvic junction obstruction, papillary necrosis,
calyceal diverticula, extrarenal pelves, ureteroceles, urolithiasis,
and other abnormalities may be discovered.

Magnetic Resonance Angiography and Urography

Along similar lines, it is possible to use magnetic resonance imaging to achieve almost identical results to CTA and CTU. The draw-
back is the relative insensitivity of MRI in detecting small kidney
stones. This technique is still under investigation.

Radiologic Techniques in the Early Posttransplantation Period

The indications for radiologic investigations in the early posttransplantation period are discussed in Chapter 8.

Allograft Size

Renal transplant size increases in most acute processes and is thus
a nonspecific indicator of renal dysfunction. Some studies have
shown that an increase in graft cross-sectional area of more than
10% (measured by US) is suggestive of acute rejection, but the finding is too nonspecific to be clinically reliable. Practical use of allograft size is also limited by the fact that a normally functioning
graft may be increased in size by up to 30% at 2 months after transplantation. The volume of a normal renal transplant usually stabilizes by 6 months.

Collecting System Dilation

Collecting system dilation may be obstructive or nonobstructive. The degree of dilation is often expressed using a grading system (grades I to IV) for US or excretory urography or as mild, moderate, or severe; however, both of these systems are subjective. Obstruction of the transplant collecting system may occur secondary to extrinsic processes (e.g., peritransplantation fluid collection); ureteral stricture (due to vascular insufficiency or rejection); or intraluminal lesions, such as kidney stone, blood clot, or sloughed papilla (Fig. 12.3). A mild, self-limited obstruction may result from early postoperative edema at the ureteroneocystotomy site, and minimal dilation may persist despite resolution of obstruction. Other causes of nonobstructive collecting system dilation include a full bladder, rejection, infection, and resolved, prior obstruction. This latter cause of nonobstructive dilation is particularly relevant in the transplanted kidney because the collecting system is denervated and has no tone.

Use of the resistive index (RI; see Acute Rejection) to distinguish obstructive from nonobstructive pyelocaliectasis has been proposed, but data regarding its reliability have been inconclusive. The absence of collecting system dilation does not entirely exclude the possibility of obstruction. The most reliable noninvasive method to diagnose obstruction is progressive collecting system dilation on serial sonograms. Antegrade pyelography, a mini-nephrostomy, or a Whitaker pressure-flow study may be necessary to determine whether collecting system dilation has an obstructive or nonobstructive cause. Ureteral obstruction on a nuclear medicine technetium-99m (^{99m}Tc) diethylenetriaminepentaacetate (DTPA), mer-

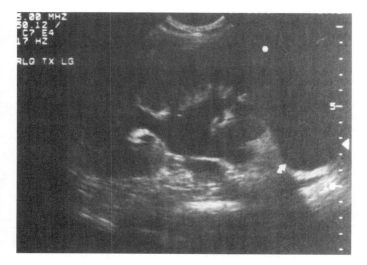

Fig. 12.3. Sonogram demonstrating hydronephrosis secondary to peritransplantation fluid collection *(arrow).*

captoacetyltriglycine (^{99m}Tc MAG3), or iodine-131 (^{131}I) orthoiodohippurate (OIH) image (Table 12.1) typically shows normal perfusion and parenchymal uptake but prolonged pelvic retention of activity.

PERITRANSPLANTATION FLUID COLLECTIONS

Peritransplantation fluid collections may be produced by lymphoceles, urinomas, hematomas, and abscesses; all of these may compress the ureter and iliac veins, resulting in hydronephrosis and lower extremity edema. They all manifest as fluid collections on cross-sectional imaging studies (US, MRI, CT) or as photopenic regions on scintigrams. Although there are imaging features suggestive of the nature of the fluid collection, their appearance is usually not sufficiently specific; imaging-guided aspiration is often necessary.

Hematomas

Hematomas are common in the immediate postoperative period, may be extrarenal or subcapsular in location, and usually resolve spontaneously. They may also occur after a biopsy or result from rupture of a graft pseudoaneurysm. On occasion, the hematoma may be large enough to obstruct the ureter. The US appearance of a hematoma varies with time, being echogenic in the acute phase and decreasing in echogenicity as clot lysis occurs. An acute hematoma is of high attenuation on CT and also decreases with time. The signal intensity of a hematoma on MRI is variable.

Urinomas

Urinomas resulting from extravasation of urine from the renal pelvis, ureter, or ureteroneocystostomy usually occur in the first 1 to 3 weeks after transplantation and may be due to disruption of the ureterovesical anastomosis, incomplete bladder closure, ischemia of the collecting system, postbiopsy injury, or severe obstruction.

US reveals a nonspecific, usually nonseptated, fluid collection, often adjacent to the lower pole of the transplant. The CT appearance of a urinoma is a peritransplantation fluid collection that may contain contrast-opacified fluid that is isodense to collecting system fluid if the leak is active at the time of the scan. MRI reveals a fluid collection that has identical signal characteristics to urine in the bladder. The leak may be extraperitoneal, intraperitoneal, or both, and in the latter circumstance, ascites may also be present. Characterization of the fluid can be achieved by obtaining a sample using US-guided aspiration and then determining the creatinine concentration (see Chapter 8).

Cystography is the examination of choice to confirm or exclude the bladder as the source of leak. If the bladder is not the source, the extravasation must be from above the ureterovesical anastomosis. If kidney function is adequate, a nuclear medicine study or a urogram may visualize the urinoma, although the precise location of the leak may be difficult to identify. The nuclear medicine images typically show abnormal accumulations of activity outside the collection system (Fig. 12.4). Occasionally, this finding may be confused with ureteral stasis, in which case the abnormal accumulation will resolve when the patient voids or is given intra-

Table 12.1. Radiopharmaceuticals used in the evaluation of renal transplants

Isotope Carriers	Physiologic Property
^{99m}Tc or ^{111}In DTPA (diethylenetriaminepentaacetate)	>95% excreted by glomerular filtration, <5% excreted by tubular secretion, no resorption; therefore, useful for assessing the GFR.
^{51}Cr EDTA (ethyldiaminetetraacetic acid)	>95% excreted by glomerular filtration, however, unable to image due to ^{51}Cr energy; therefore, useful in nonimaging scintillation methods (not available in the United States).
^{131}I or ^{123}I OIH (orthoiodohippurate)	20% excreted by glomerular filtration, 80% excreted by tubular secretion on a first pass; therefore, useful for assessing ERFF, Disadvantage: Increased radiation dose to patient with obstruction or renal failure.
^{99m}Tc MAG 3 (mercaptoacetyltriglycine)	Similar to OIH but labeled with ^{99m}Tc, which is a better isotope for imaging than with ^{131}I.
^{99m}Tc DMSA (dimercaptosuccinate)	Only 7–14% excreted into urine, binds to sulfhydryl groups in perfused renal cortical tubule cells; therefore, useful in imaging regions of functioning versus infarcted renal cortex tissue.
^{99m}Tc GHA (glucoheptonate)	>50% excreted by glomerular filtration, <50% excreted by tubular secretion, 10% bound to tubular cells like DMSA: therefore, useful for assessing a combination of GFR, ERPF, and the amount and shape of functioning renal cortical tissue. Disadvantage: More difficult to accurately estimate GFR or ERPF.
^{111}In white blood cell ^{111}In lymphocytes ^{111}In platelets ^{125}I or ^{131}I fibrinogen ^{67}Ga	Localizes in inflammatory tissue; therefore, maybe useful in detecting transplant rejection.

Cr, chromium; Ga, gallium; I, iodine; In, indium; OIH, orthoiodohippurate; Tc, technetium; DMSA, dimercaptosuccinate; GFR, glomerular filtration rate; ERPF, effective renal plasma flow.

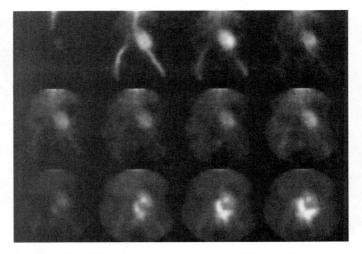

Fig. 12.4. ⁹⁹ᵐTc DTPA images of a transplanted kidney with urinary
extravasation seen as an enlarging irregular activity between
the kidney and urinary bladder.

venous furosemide. Antegrade pyelography is the most accurate
and definitive method for determining the extravasation site.

Lymphoceles

Lymphoceles are the most common type of peritransplantation
fluid collection and are the product of extraperitoneal or renal lym-
phatic disruption at surgery or during graft harvesting (see Chapter 7). They usually occur several weeks to months after surgery.
Small lymphoceles are common and are usually asymptomatic,
but larger ones can cause obstruction.

The typical US appearance of a lymphocele is a fluid collection
inferior and medial to the transplant that often contains septations
and low-level echoes (Fig. 12.5). The MRI signal characteristics of
a lymphocele tend to be of low signal intensity on T1-weighted
images and of high signal intensity on T2-weighted images.

Abscesses

A peritransplantation abscess is usually secondary to infection of
a preexisting fluid collection and generally occurs 4 to 5 weeks
after transplantation. The US appearance is a fluid collection that
contains debris, low-level echoes, and occasionally gas; the latter
manifests as mobile, nondependent, echogenic foci with "dirty"
shadowing or "ring-down" artifact.

The CT appearance is a heterogeneous fluid attenuation lesion
(Fig. 12.6) that may contain gas. In the acute setting, cross-
sectional imaging techniques (US, CT) allow rapid diagnosis and
potential treatment of a suspected abscess by providing guidance
for aspiration and drainage. The absence of any imaging features
suggestive of an abscess does not exclude the presence of infection.

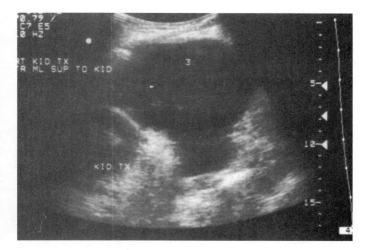

Fig. 12.5. Sonogram demonstrating lymphocele (3) with septations (arrowhead).

Radiopharmaceutical agents, such as indium-111 (^{111}In) white blood cells, ^{111}In lymphocytes, ^{111}In platelets, ^{131}I fibrinogen, or gallium-67 (^{67}Ga) localize in inflammatory tissue and may be helpful in detecting a renal or perirenal abscess; a rejecting transplant, however, may also "light up." With these nuclear medicine techniques, the radiopharmaceutical is injected and allowed to accumulate. Images are acquired 1 to 2 days after injection for ^{111}In-labeled blood products and up to 3 days after injection for [67]Ga.

ACUTE REJECTION

A variety of morphologic alterations may occur with acute rejection. All of these abnormalities may be seen with other medical complications of transplantation. Many are subjective; therefore, these findings are not sufficiently sensitive or specific to diagnose rejection definitively and obviate the need for biopsy. These US abnormalities include graft enlargement, obscured corticomedullary definition, decreased echogenicity of the renal sinus, thickened urothelium, prominent hypoechoic medullary pyramids, increased or decreased cortical echogenicity, and scattered heterogeneous areas of increased echogenicity, the latter probably representing foci of hemorrhage (Fig. 12.7).

With the advent of duplex US (combining gray-scale imaging with Doppler capability), it was hoped that the physiologic parameters that could be measured with this technique would be diagnostic of rejection. The major parameter studied was vascular resistance (impedance), which is quantified by the RI (RI = peak systolic velocity [PSV] minus end-diastolic velocity divided by PSV) or the pulsatility index (PI = PSV minus end-diastolic velocity divided by the mean velocity). These indices are often elevated in rejection (Fig. 12.8), but because any cause of renal dysfunction

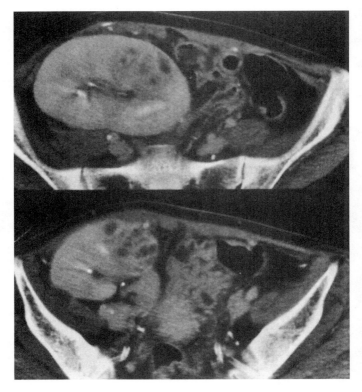

Fig. 12.6.   Abscess in a renal allograft. There is a heterogeneous mass on contrast-enhanced computed tomography. Many small compartments preclude percutaneous drainage. Renal function was surprisingly well preserved. Abscess resolved after intensive antibiotic therapy.

may increase vascular resistance in the kidney, the finding of an elevated RI is nonspecific. Elevation of the RI (greater than 0.9) has been reported in rejection, severe acute tubular necrosis (ATN), renal vein obstruction, pyelonephritis, extrarenal compression, obstruction, and cyclosporine toxicity.

Duplex Ultrasonography

Duplex US (or, more accurately, "triplex," if color, pulsed, and gray-scale are employed simultaneously) combines a two-dimensional image with flow information, the latter being in the form of color, pulsed, and most recently, power Doppler. These techniques employ the same sound waves as real-time imaging but measure the frequency and energy of the Doppler shift from the echoes interacting with flowing blood, allowing determination of flow presence, velocity, and direction (power Doppler does not assess the latter

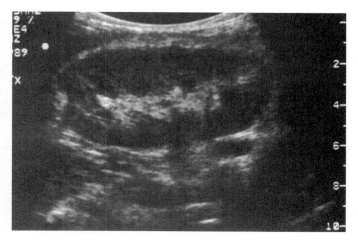

A

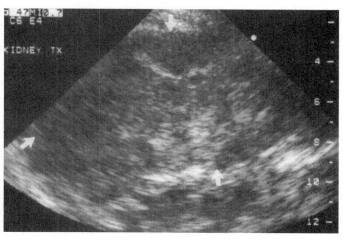

B

Fig. 12.7.   A: Sonogram of normal transplant kidney. B: Sonogram of transplant undergoing rejection reveals graft enlargement, decreased echogenicity of renal sinus (compare to echogenic sinus in A, and obscured corticomedullary delineations. Margins of graft marked by arrows.

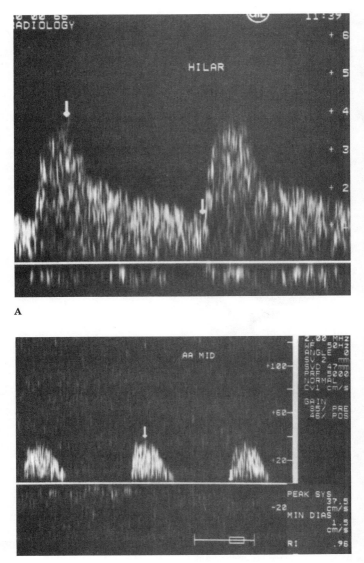

Fig. 12.8. A: Normal pulsed-gate Doppler spectrum from kidney transplant with considerable flow throughout diastole and normal resistive index (RI = 0.65). B: Doppler spectrum of graft undergoing acute rejection with no diastolic flow (RI = 1). This is a nonspecific indicator of graft dysfunction.

two). Color Doppler US provides an estimate of the mean velocity and direction of flow within a vessel by color-coding the information and displaying it superimposed on the gray-scale image. Power Doppler (also known as *amplitude* or *energy map*) measures the power of the Doppler signal and displays a greater range of signal strengths, thus allowing improved sensitivity to flow and visualization of smaller vessels. Power Doppler is displayed as a single color map of flow superimposed on a gray-scale image but does not provide directional or velocity information as does color Doppler. Pulsed Doppler allows a sampling volume to be positioned in a vessel visualized on the gray-scale image and provides a spectrum, or graph, of velocities of blood within the gate plotted as a function of time. A read-out of absolute velocities and calculation of the RI and PI are obtained using a spectrum from pulsed Doppler. Because the Doppler equation uses the angle between the beam axis and the vessel to calculate the velocity (performed by the machine software) and this angle is estimated by the ultrasonographer, incorrect angle correction may yield spurious velocities.

Nuclear Medicine Evaluation of Graft Dysfunction

Transplant dysfunction can be evaluated with filtered or tubular-secreted radiopharmaceuticals using a three-phase approach. The first phase assesses the perfusion and is also known as the *angiographic phase* or the *first-pass study*. The second phase is the *parenchymal phase,* during which the accumulation of tracer in the renal parenchyma reflects the physiologic mode of clearance of that radiopharmaceutical (i.e., filtered or secreted). The third phase is the excretory phase, which reflects the glomerular filtration rate (GFR) and permits an assessment of the integrity of the ureteral system.

Typically, acute rejection appears on nuclear medicine ^{99m}Tc DTPA, ^{99m}Tc MAG3, or ^{131}I OIH scans as delayed transplant visualization (decreased perfusion) on the first-pass renal scintiangiography phase, with poor parenchymal uptake and high background activity (poor renal function and clearance) in the second and third phases (Fig. 12.9). Transplant rejection may also be detected by several static imaging techniques. Increased uptake can be seen with ^{67}Ga, ^{131}I-labeled or ^{125}I-labeled fibrinogen, ^{99m}Tc sulfur colloid, or ^{111}In-labeled blood components. Unfortunately, the low specificity of uptake of these agents prevents them from being of much value in the differential diagnosis of graft dysfunction.

Acute Tubular Necrosis

On nuclear medicine imaging studies, ATN typically shows good renal perfusion on the first-pass phase with ^{99m}Tc DTPA, ^{99m}Tc MAG3, or ^{131}I OIH. On the second and third phases, ^{99m}Tc DTPA shows poor parenchymal accumulation and wash-out of the radiotracer as a result of decreased glomerular filtration (Fig. 12.10). In addition, high surrounding tissue background activity is seen as a result of poor overall plasma clearance of the radiotracer. With ^{99m}Tc MAG3 and ^{131}I OIH radiopharmaceuticals, preserved parenchymal accumulation is seen in the second phase because of relatively preserved renal blood flow and tubular secretion. In the third phase, however, there is a similar poor wash-out of the accumulated renal parenchymal activity as a result of diminished glomerular filtration. These findings are consistent with the patho-

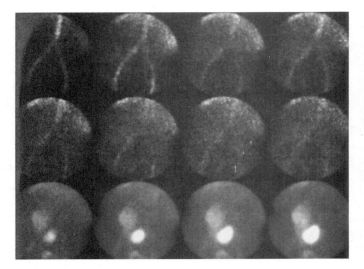

Fig. 12.9. ^{99m}Tc MAG3 images of a transplanted kidney with severe acute rejection. Note the poor perfusion to the transplant (delayed renal visualization) in the initial images. Overall reduction in glomerular filtration is represented by high surrounding background tissue activity, poor parenchymal wash-out of accumulated tracer in the tubules, and reduced collecting system or urinary bladder activity.

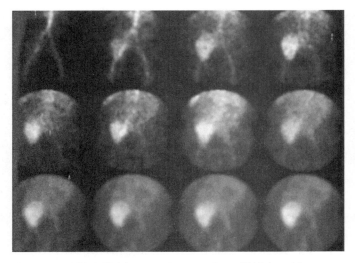

Fig. 12.10. ^{99m}Tc DTPA images of a transplanted kidney with acute tubular necrosis. Note the well-preserved perfusion in the transplant (prompt renal visualization) in the initial stages. Overall reduction in glomerular filtration is represented by high surrounding background tissue activity, poor parenchymal wash-out of accumulated tracer in the tubules, and no collecting system or urinary bladder activity. A similar pattern is seen with ^{99m}Tc MAG3 in acute tubular necrosis.

physiology of ATN, in which renal blood flow is preserved relative to glomerular filtration.

POSTTRANSPLANTATION VASCULAR COMPLICATIONS

Arterial Thrombosis

Renal arterial thrombosis is an uncommon complication of transplantation and usually occurs in the early postoperative period. The most common causes are faulty surgical anastomoses, severe acute rejection, and progression of a stenosis to thrombosis. The findings in color and pulsed Doppler imaging consist of absent arterial and venous blood flow within the graft. There is some controversy regarding the necessity of further imaging to confirm this diagnosis because there are several reported cases in which no flow was demonstrated by Doppler but digital subtraction angiography revealed patent vessels. Power Doppler should, in theory, reduce false-positive results, but this remains to be proved.

The ^{99m}Tc DTPA flow scan shows lack of perfusion, absent visualization of the transplanted kidney, poor background clearance of activity, and sometimes a photopenic space in the transplant bed (Fig. 12.11). Renal vein thrombosis, acute cortical necrosis, and hyperacute rejection may all have similar scintigraphic findings.

Infarction

Acute segmental infarction may be diagnosed with Doppler US by demonstration of lack of flow to the infarcted parenchymal region. This diagnosis is facilitated by use of color and power Doppler,

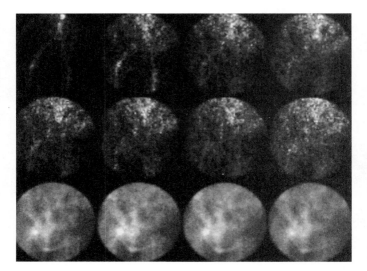

Fig. 12.11. ^{99m}Tc DTPA images of a transplanted kidney with renal artery thrombosis. Note the absence of renal blood flow (nonvisualization of the transplant in the images) and absence of filtration (no collecting system activity and high background tissue activity).

which both provide a global evaluation of flow to the organ, and help to identify segmental arteries, which can then be interrogated individually with pulsed Doppler.

Segmental renal infarction on ^{99m}Tc dimercaptosuccinate (DMSA), ^{99m}Tc MAG3, or ^{99m}Tc glucoheptanoic acid (GHA) scan (see Table 12-1) appears as a wedge-shaped, "cold" defect. DMSA radiopharmaceutical binds to sulfhydryl groups in perfused renal cortical tubule cells, allowing the visualization of the mass of functioning renal tissue.

Renal Vein Thrombosis

Renal vein thrombosis is an uncommon complication of transplantation that usually occurs in the first postoperative week. The US diagnosis is mainly dependent on the Doppler portion of the examination because the gray-scale diagnosis is limited by the difficulty of direct visualization of the anechoic or hypoechoic acute thrombus and the nonspecificity of the frequently associated graft swelling and hypoechogenicity. The combination of Doppler findings of high-impedance renal arterial waveforms with reversed, prolonged diastolic flow, a spikelike systolic component, and no detectable venous flow in the graft is highly suggestive of renal vein thrombosis (Fig. 12.12). Reversal of diastolic flow is a nonspecific finding that is reflective of increased arterial impedance in the graft. It may also be seen in ATN, acute rejection, and severe obstruction.

Chronic Rejection

In chronic rejection, there is gradual deterioration of kidney function, and the allograft is usually decreased in size. Angiographic findings include decreased blood flow and reduction of the number

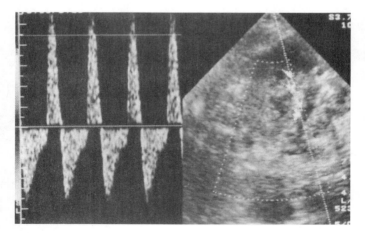

Fig. 12.12.   Duplex sonogram of transplant renal vein thrombosis demonstrates reversed flow in diastole and a spikelike systolic peak. No venous flow was detectable in the kidney, renal hilum, or location of the renal vein.

of arteries, which may be narrow and irregular. The nephrogram is patchy. US findings include decreased size of kidney, cortical thinning, and altered cortical echogenicity, often with increased echogenicity. Doppler US may show a nonspecific elevation in resistive index.

Renal Artery Stenosis

Renal scintangiography may be useful in the diagnosis of renal artery stenosis (RAS) in a native kidney because the contralateral kidney acts as a control for comparison. In the transplanted kidney with RAS, there may be a delayed blush on scanning, but in the absence of a paired kidney, this finding is too nonspecific to be diagnostically reliable.

The diagnosis of RAS by Doppler US is made by demonstration of a focal, segmental region of flow abnormality, characterized by elevated PSV and turbulent flow (Fig. 12.13). Various threshold values for PSV have been proposed for optimal detection of RAS, ranging from 100 to 300 cm/sec; reported sensitivities and specificities range from fair to excellent. Because the normal range of PSV in the transplant renal artery may be variable, a ratio of PSV in the renal artery compared with the external iliac artery may be more useful. The accurate calculation of velocity by the machine's software, however, is highly dependent on the accuracy of the operator's estimate of the angle of insonation, and errors in this regard can yield spuriously elevated velocities. The accuracy of this estimate (*angle correction*) is dependent on the adequacy of delineation of the course of the renal artery, which is often small

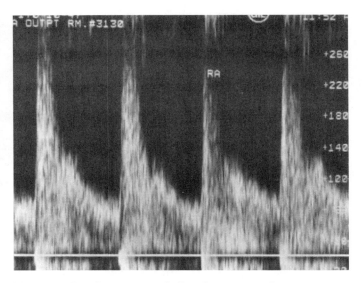

Fig. 12.13.   Renal artery stenosis. Doppler spectrum demonstrates focal elevated peak systolic velocity (faster than 260 cm/sec) with mild spectral broadening at the anastomosis.

and tortuous. Color and power Doppler, by providing a map of the vascular anatomy, are helpful in tracing a vessel and therefore in determining the appropriate angle. A confident diagnosis of RAS using Doppler US can be made if the characteristic findings occur in a well-delineated vessel, allowing accurate angle correction. Conversely, high velocities without associated turbulence in a region where the accuracy of angle correction is equivocal must be viewed with skepticism.

Angiography remains the gold standard for diagnosis of RAS, and the threshold for performance of this study remains a matter of clinical judgment (see Chapters 7 and 9). CO_2 angiography provides a useful alternative to nephrotoxic iodinated contrast agents, but it may be less reliable than standard angiography.

Arteriovenous Fistulas

Postbiopsy arteriovenous fistulas most often resolve spontaneously but can produce persistent hematuria or hypertension. Gray-scale US cannot identify these small vascular communications, but they are readily demonstrated on color Doppler as an area of artifactual color assignment in the renal parenchyma (Plate 2). This finding is believed to be due to high-velocity flow in the fistula, which results in localized turbulence and vessel wall vibrations that are transmitted to the perivascular tissues. The vibrating interfaces in the perivascular tissue produce phase shifts in the reflected sound wave and result in random color assignment in this region. This phenomenon is essentially the Doppler equivalent of a bruit.

After an area of suspicion is identified, the fistulized vessels may be visualized on color Doppler by virtue of their high-velocity flow. Confirmation of the presence of an arteriovenous fistula is achieved by performing waveform analysis with pulsed Doppler and by demonstrating high-velocity, low-resistance flow in the supplying artery, and arterialization (highly pulsatile flow) of the waveform in the draining vein. A focal, intrarenal arterial stenosis can produce high-velocity flow and tissue vibration, thereby mimicking a fistula, but no changes in the venous waveform should occur.

Doppler US is readily able to demonstrate many fistulas and should be the initial, primary imaging modality. If no fistula can be demonstrated by US in a patient with persistent gross hematuria and hypertension, angiography may be necessary. Angiography is the examination of choice for defining the extent of the fistula and for treatment planning. Superselective occlusion of the segmental or interlobar branches is possible using a variety of occlusive devices, including steel coils and detachable balloons.

Pseudoaneurysms

Pseudoaneurysms in a renal transplant may be intrarenal, usually secondary to a biopsy, or less commonly, extrarenal, usually due to faulty surgical anastomosis or perianastomotic infection. Extrarenal pseudoaneurysms have a much higher risk for spontaneous rupture and are therefore treated as a relative surgical emergency. Arteriovenous fistulas may be associated with pseudoaneurysms. The US findings are the same for intrarenal and extrarenal pseudoaneurysms and consist of a spherical fluid collection that may or may not contain thrombus. Color Doppler reveals swirling internal flow (Plate 3) and occasionally adjacent tissue vibrations.

Measurement of Glomerular Filtration Rate

Clinicians generally rely on the serum creatinine level as a marker of graft function, and although this simple test is indisputably invaluable in transplant management, its accuracy as a marker of GFR is inconsistent. In chronic renal failure with proteinuria, tubular secretion of creatinine may form a significant percentage of total creatinine excretion and overestimation of GFR results. Radiolabeled DTPA, ethylene diamine tetraacetic acid (EDTA), and iothalamate are all accurate filtration markers that, like inulin, reach the urine by filtration but without any element of tubular secretion or reabsorption. The clearances of these compounds are equivalent to the classic chemical inulin clearance. They are more convenient to use than inulin because their plasma and urine levels can be measured with a scintillation counter.

The best isotopic techniques for measuring GFR are true clearance techniques during which, after intravenous injection and bladder emptying, serial blood and urine samples are taken over several hours and GFR is calculated from the standard clearance formula. GFR can also be extrapolated from the disappearance curve of the plasma isotope concentration, the so-called plasma clearance.

SELECTED READINGS

Bude RO, Rubin JM. Detection of renal artery stenosis with Doppler sonography: it is more complicated than originally thought. *Radiology* 1995;196:612.

Budihna NV, Milcinski M, Kajtna-Koselj M, et al. Relevance of ^{99m}Tc DMSA scintigraphy in renal transplant parenchymal imaging. *Clin Nucl Med* 1994;19:782.

Cochran ST, Krasny RM, Danovitch GM, et al. Helical CT angiography for examination of liver renal donors. *Am J Roentgenol* 1997; 168:1569–1573.

Grant EG, Perrella RR. Wishing won't make it so: Duplex Doppler sonography in the evaluation of renal transplant dysfunction. *Am J Roentgenol* 1990;153:538.

Harrison KL, Nghiem HV, Coldwell DM, et al. Renal dysfunction due to arteriovenous fistula in a transplant recipient. *J Am Soc Nephrol* 1994;5:1300.

Kuo PC, Peterson J, Semba C, et al. CO_2 angiography: a technique for vascular imaging in renal allograft dysfunction. *Transplantation* 1996;61:652.

Loubeyre P, Abidi H, Cahen R, et al. Transplanted renal artery: detection of stenosis with color doppler US. *Radiology* 1997;203:661–665.

Middleton WD, Kellman GM, Melson GL, et al. Post biopsy renal transplant arteriovenous fistulas: color Doppler US characteristics. *Radiology* 1989;171:253.

O'Neill WC. Sonographic evaluation of renal failure. *Amer J Kid Dis* 2000;35:1021.

Phillips AO, Deane C, O'Donnell P, et al. Evaluation of Doppler ultrasound in primary non-function of renal transplants. *Clin Transplant* 1994;8:83.

Slakey DP, Florman S, Lovretich J, et al. Utility of CT angiography for evaluation of living kidney donors. *Clin Transplant* 1999;13:104.

Swierzewski SJ III, Konnak JW, Ellis JH. Treatment of renal transplant ureteral complications by percutaneous techniques. *J Urol* 1993;150:1115.

Pathology of Kidney Transplantation

Cynthia C. Nast and Arthur H. Cohen

Structural abnormalities in the transplanted kidney may be assessed by either of two methods: (1) standard tissue histopathology of a biopsy or transplant nephrectomy or (2) cytologic evaluation of cells aspirated from the graft using a thin needle (Table 13.1). The core biopsy is typically regarded as the gold standard, whereas aspiration cytology, although clinically valuable and quite accurate in experienced hands, is somewhat limited as a procedure by the lack of trained clinicians to interpret the material. In this chapter, these techniques are considered separately, although the information obtained from them is often complementary, and certain important concepts and actual lesions described for one method bear directly on an understanding of the other.

KIDNEY TRANSPLANT HISTOPATHOLOGY

Core Needle Biopsy

Indications and Technique

Kidney transplant biopsies are most frequently performed at times of graft dysfunction when the etiology cannot be accurately elucidated by clinical or noninvasive means. Protocol biopsies are performed at predetermined intervals after transplantation at some centers in an attempt to recognize so-called subclinical rejection (see Chapter 8); they may also be required as part of clinical trials for the evaluation of new immunosuppressive drugs (see Chapter 4). More precise clinical indications for biopsy are reviewed in Chapters 8 and 9. Transplantation programs vary in their reliance on biopsies and the clinical setting in which biopsies are performed.

Preparations for transplant biopsy are similar to those for biopsy of the native kidney. Informed consent is required from patients, who should be specifically warned of the risk for bleeding and occasional damage to the graft (see Complications). Before biopsy, coagulation studies are usually performed, although in the absence of liver disease, use of anticoagulants, thrombocytopenia, or a clinical history of bleeding, these may not be necessary. The blood pressure should be controlled at a level of less than 160/100 mm Hg.

The locations of the graft and biopsy site can be determined by palpation or by ultrasound guidance. A small pillow or towel roll in the small of the patient's back may facilitate palpation. Ultrasound offers the advantage of more precise localization of the graft, and its depth, and may reduce the frequency of inadequate specimens. Ultrasound may detect perinephric fluid collections or hydronephrosis. It is unwise to perform biopsy through a fluid collection because of the inability to tamponade the biopsy site adequately. Significant hydronephrosis should be relieved before the

Table 13.1. Diagnostic capabilities of histologic and cytologic techniques for evaluation of kidney transplants

Lesion	Fine-needle Aspiration	Core Biopsy
Acute cellular rejection	Yes	Yes
Acute vascular rejection	No	Yes
Acute cyclosporine toxicity	Yes	Yes
Acute tubular necrosis	Yes	Yes
Viral infection	Yes	No
Allograft rupture	No	No
Bacterial infection	Yes	Yes
Infarction	Yes	Yes
Chronic transplant rejection	No	Yes
Chronic cyclosporine toxicity	No	Yes
Glomerular lesions	No	Yes
Recurrent nonglomerular disorders	No	Yes

biopsy is performed because it may be the cause of the graft dysfunction; a small blood clot after the biopsy may exaggerate the degree of obstruction. Generally, the upper or lower poles of the transplant are sought, depending on which is more easily palpated or near the surface. If the location of the biopsy site is difficult to ascertain or if the kidney is deep, it is wise to use real-time ultrasound with visual guidance or a fixed biopsy guide device (see Chapter 12).

Disposable automatic spring-loaded needles (18-gauge is usually adequate) have largely replaced the traditional modified 14-gauge Vim-Silverman needle and may be less traumatic to the kidney. The site chosen for the biopsy is locally anesthetized with 1% lidocaine, and a small stab wound in the skin is made to facilitate the passage of the needle. Precise instructions for use of the newer needles are provided in the package inserts. The needles are advanced up to the depth assigned by ultrasound or until an increase in resistance is felt as the needle makes contact with the kidney. When the automatic needles are used, it may be advisable to withdraw the needle slightly before taking the sample to avoid excessive depth.

Two biopsy cores should be adequate. It is advisable to inspect the specimen immediately with a stereomicroscope to ensure adequacy. As soon as the needle is withdrawn, hemostasis should be augmented by manual compression or with a sandbag. Postbiopsy orders should include observation of the patient's vital signs every 15 minutes for at least 2 hours and then hourly for several hours. Patients should initially be immobile; in the absence of macroscopic hematuria, ambulation can begin after 6 to 8 hours. Many transplantation centers permit outpatients to go home the same day as the biopsy.

Complications
Core needle biopsy is an invasive technique and is not risk free; these risks must be weighed against the benefit gained from the

information obtained from the procedure. Careful assessment of potential risks and benefits must precede every decision to subject a patient to a biopsy.

All major complications after needle biopsy manifest as perinephric or urinary bleeding. Transient macroscopic hematuria is common and is of little clinical significance. Macroscopic hematuria follows about 3% of biopsies and may prolong hospitalization or lead to blood transfusion or placement of a bladder catheter for clot drainage. Ureteral obstruction occasionally occurs, requiring placement of a percutaneous nephrostomy; massive hemorrhage necessitating surgical exploration, graft nephrectomy, or angiographic embolization is rare. Postbiopsy arteriovenous fistulas may sometimes be detected by Doppler ultrasound and can usually be treated expectantly. Angiographic embolization may occasionally be required, and graft loss has been reported.

Specimen Handling

Detailed methods for handling tissue specimens are beyond the scope of this chapter. For all specimens, portions are obtained for each of the three traditional methods of evaluating renal parenchyma: light microscopy, electron microscopy, and immunofluorescence. For the initial biopsy, all methods should be used; for subsequent biopsies, electron and immunofluorescent microscopy are performed only if indicated. This approach allows the pathologist to obtain maximal diagnostic and prognostic information. In selected instances, rapid processing or frozen sections can be performed on the tissue placed in fixative for light microscopy when an immediate assessment of the changes in the graft is necessary for initiating or modifying therapy.

Transplant Rejection

Traditionally, three major forms of rejection are recognized: hyperacute, acute, and chronic. Each has reasonably distinctive changes, although acute and chronic rejection may be present simultaneously, resulting in a mixture of histopathologic features. Pathologic findings in the major lesions responsible for functional impairment of the graft are shown in Table 13.2.

Hyperacute Rejection

Hyperacute rejection is produced by preformed cytotoxic antibodies and is an infrequent event so long as the pretransplantation crossmatch is negative (see Chapters 3 and 5). It may manifest shortly after vascular anastomoses are established or may be delayed up to 2 to 3 days. It is characterized by rapid and widespread vascular thrombosis, predominantly affecting arteries, arterioles, and glomeruli, often with polymorphonuclear leukocytes incorporated in the thrombi. The kidney is usually cyanotic, slightly edematous, and flaccid, and urine production suddenly ceases or does not begin at all. If the kidney is not removed immediately, extensive cellular necrosis ensues, followed after 24 hours by numerous cortical and medullary infarcts. Immunofluorescence may disclose capillary and arterial wall immunoglobulin G (IgG) or IgM, C3, and fibrin, with fibrin also in the thrombi. Electron microscopy in the early lesions indicates degeneration and early necrosis of vascular endothelium.

Table 13.2. Histopathologic findings in the major causes of allograft dysfunction

Type	Interstitium	Tubules	Glomeruli	Arteries
Acute cellular rejection	Edema, lymphocytes	Lymphocytes, cell degeneration	Capillary lymphocytes	Swollen endothelium, lymphocytes, foam cells
Acute humoral rejection	Hemorrhage, zonal necrosis (infarction)	Necrosis	Neutrophils, thrombosis	Necrosis, neutrophils, thrombosis
Acute tubular necrosis	Edema	Cell degeneration, necrosis, mitotic figures	Normal	Normal
Acute cyclosporine toxicity	Edema	Isometric vacuoles	Normal	Normal
Chronic rejection	Fibrosis, lymphocytes	Atrophy, drop-out	Chronic transplant glomerulopathy	Fibrosis, lymphocytes, narrowed lumina
Chronic cyclosporine toxicity	"Striped" fibrosis	Atrophy	Ischemic collapse	Arteriolopathy, hyalinization

Hyperacute rejection needs to be differentiated from other circumstances in which extensive vascular thrombi occur. The differential diagnosis includes physical perfusion-related injury to vascular endothelium and injury caused by cold-reacting IgM antibodies against blood cells. Both of these conditions rarely may manifest in the immediate posttransplantation period and may produce entrapment of leukocytes in thrombi. It is only in hyperacute rejection, however, that polymorphonuclear leukocytes are typically and regularly incorporated in the thrombi. Recurrent hemolytic-uremic syndrome and a thrombotic microangiopathy associated with administration of the calcineurin inhibitors (discussed later) are characterized by thrombi, usually without leukocytes, and are generally later-occurring lesions.

Acute Rejection

Two immunopathologic mechanisms are responsible for acute rejection: cell-mediated immunity and humoral (antibody) immunity.

CELL-MEDIATED ACUTE REJECTION.   Cell-mediated acute rejection is the most common form of early rejection. Light microscopy represents the major diagnostic procedure, although at times, immunofluorescence and electron microscopic evaluation may be helpful for the differential diagnosis. The major lesion is in the interstitium, which is diffusely edematous and infiltrated by numerous leukocytes, most of which are mature and transformed lymphocytes (T4, T8) with fewer monocytes and plasma cells (Fig. 13.1). Eosinophils are either absent or found focally in small numbers; polymorphonuclear leukocytes are not a regular feature. Peritubular capillaries are dilated and filled with lymphocytes that may be seen migrat-

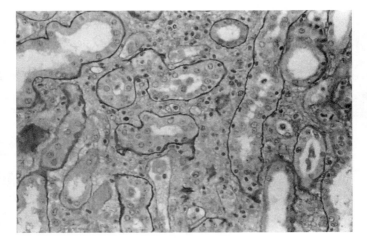

Fig. 13.1.   Acute cell-mediated interstitial rejection. There is interstitial edema with lymphocytes in both the interstitium and tubular walls in association with tubular cell degeneration. (Periodic acid–methenamine silver stain, ×200.)

ing into the interstitium. A characteristic lesion, called *tubulitis,* occurs, whereby lymphocytes and monocytes extend into the walls and lumina of tubules, with associated degenerative changes of epithelial cells. The cells and basement membranes of tubular walls may be damaged and discontinuous. When this lesion affects cast-containing distal tubules, cast matrix (Tamm-Horsfall protein) may be found in the interstitium and occasionally in peritubular capillaries and small veins. For tubulitis to have diagnostic significance, the inflammation should be documented in normal (nonatrophic) tubules. The significance of tubulitis in atrophied tubules only is not known.

Acute transplant glomerulopathy is a form of glomerular cell-mediated rejection in which lymphocytes and monocytes accumulate in glomerular capillary lumina and mesangial regions (Fig. 13.2). Endothelial and mesangial cells are swollen, and capillary walls display subendothelial lucencies, with occasional segmental peripheral mesangial migration and interposition on ultrastructural examination. In cell-mediated vascular rejection, lymphocytes, monocytes, and foam cells may undermine arterial endothelium but rarely extend into the muscularis (Fig. 13.3). The endothelial cells are swollen and often vacuolated, but arterial wall necrosis is not a feature of this type of acute rejection. When acute cellular rejection is treated successfully, the interstitial inflammatory infiltrate diminishes, whereas edema, tubular inflammation, and tubular cell damage may persist for some time. Immunofluorescence typically discloses fibrin in the interstitium; segmental linear or granular IgM, C3, and fibrin may be found in glomerular capillary walls in acute transplant glomerulopathy. Ultrastructural examination usually confirms the light

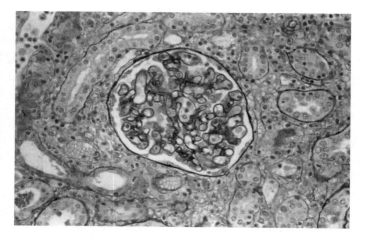

Fig. 13.2.   Acute transplant glomerulopathy. Glomerular capillary lumina contain monocytes and lymphocytes. There are also lymphocytes in tubular walls and interstitial rejection with interstitial edema and inflammation. (Periodic acid–methenamine silver stain, ×200.)

Interstitial
inflammation
and edema

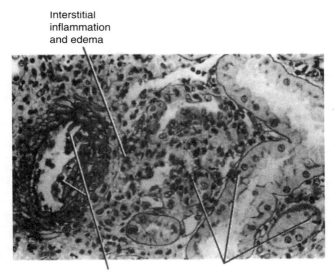

Vascular   Tubular
inflammation   inflammation

Fig. 13.3.   Acute cell-mediated vascular rejection. A small artery contains lymphocytes in the lumen and in the intima beneath swollen endothelial cells. Note the interstitial edema and infiltration by lymphocytes, which are also in the walls of tubules. (Periodic acid–Schiff stain, ×220.)

microscopic findings and provides additional diagnostic information only for the glomerular lesion.

ANTIBODY-MEDIATED ACUTE REJECTION.   Antibody-mediated acute rejection is an uncommon form of rejection and is characterized primarily by necrotizing arteritis, with mural fibrinoid necrosis and variable inflammation, including a proliferation of lymphocytes, monocytes, and neutrophils (Fig. 13.4). Endothelial cells are severely damaged or absent, and luminal thrombosis is common. This lesion typically results in cortical infarction with focal interstitial hemorrhage. Immunofluorescence discloses IgG and sometimes IgM accompanied by C3 in the walls of arteries. In these structures, fibrin may be intramural and intraluminal and may also be in the interstitium when hemorrhage is present. Diffuse peritubular capillary staining for the complement component C4d has been described as a marker for humoral rejection.

Some investigators consider intimal arterial lymphocytic infiltration, described previously for cell-mediated rejection, to be a part of the vascular pathology of antibody-mediated rejection. It is believed that the two forms of arterial inflammation are distinct and unrelated to one another. *Vascular rejection* is therefore an imprecise term that signifies merely inflammation of arteries, which can result from either cell-mediated or humorally mediated immu-

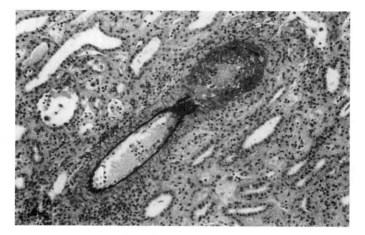

Fig. 13.4.   Acute humoral rejection. The arterial wall is infiltrated by neutrophils and lymphocytes and has segmental fibrinoid necrosis. There are edema and inflammation in the adjacent interstitium. (Elastic–van Gieson stain, ×200.)

nity. When arterial inflammation is present, it should be further categorized to indicate the etiologic mechanism. The humoral form is characterized by arterial mural necrosis, neutrophilic infiltrate, and luminal thrombosis and represents a more severe lesion that is poorly responsive to therapy.

DIFFERENTIAL DIAGNOSIS OF ACUTE CELL-MEDIATED REJECTION. Other forms of acute interstitial nephritis may have many of the same structural lesions as acute rejection, including infectious interstitial nephritis (viral, bacterial) and drug-induced acute hypersensitivity interstitial nephritis. Certain viral and bacterial interstitial nephritides may be characterized by a mononuclear, rather than polymorphonuclear, infiltrate, thereby simulating rejection. Glomerular inflammation and arterial inflammation, when present, indicate rejection. Because of the negligible role of polymorphonuclear leukocytes in acute cellular rejection, their presence should be taken to signify acute infection, especially when antibody- mediated rejection with fresh infarction is excluded. Acute hypersensitivity lesions induced by drugs may have a prominent component of eosinophils and sometimes granulomas. Some biopsy specimens with calcineurin inhibitor toxicity may have small focal interstitial lymphocytic infiltrates that do not extend into tubules. These infiltrates are not usually associated with diffuse edema.

Subclinical rejection describes a morphologic pattern of acute cell-mediated rejection that may occur in up to 30% of patients without clinical signs or symptoms of rejection or after apparently successful treatment of rejection. The significance of this asymptomatic inflammatory process relative to short-term or long-term renal function is discussed in Chapter 8.

DIFFERENTIAL DIAGNOSIS OF ANTIBODY-MEDIATED REJECTION. The
arterial inflammation may be indistinguishable from a systemic
necrotizing arteritis, but recurrence of vasculitic lesions in the
transplant is rare. The effects of vascular occlusion, infarction,
and parenchymal hemorrhage may be manifestations not only of
arteritis but also of arterial occlusion from other causes, including
surgical ligation of a large artery and emboli of any nature.

Chronic Allograft Nephropathy

Chronic allograft nephropathy is the preferred term to the more
loosely used "chronic rejection" (see Chapter 9). It is characterized
by chronic changes in arteries, tubules, interstitium, and glomeruli. The pathogenesis is mixed; it may be the result of repeated
episodes of overt or covert acute rejection (allogeneic factors) exaggerated by nonimmunologic factors related to the kidney donor and
recipient (nonallogeneic factors). From both the clinical and pathologic standpoints, the umbrella term chronic allograft nephropathy
is a better term than chronic rejection because many of the chronic changes may be evident in several different forms of immunologically and nonimmunologically mediated chronic injury to the
transplant, including chronic rejection, chronic calcineurin inhibitor toxicity, nephrosclerosis, partial obstruction, reflux, and chronic infection.

The pathologic changes are primarily cortical. There is patchy
interstitial fibrosis with infiltrates of lymphocytes, plasma cells,
and mast cells associated with *tubular atrophy,* or drop-out. There
may be neoexpression of the alpha$_3$ chain of type IV collagen and
laminin B2 in the proximal tubular basement membranes. The
walls of arteries are thickened with intimal fibrosis and sometimes
with medial fibrosis, variable mononuclear leukocyte inflammation
(including foam cells), and disruption and duplication of the internal elastic lamina, all resulting in luminal narrowing (Fig. 13.5).
Immunofluorescence may document IgG, IgM, C3, and fibrin in the
walls of arteries. In addition, juxtaglomerular apparatus hyperplasia may be present and is indicative of large artery involvement.

The glomeruli are often abnormal and exhibit a variety of
changes, many of which constitute the lesion of *chronic transplant glomerulopathy,* which may occur as early as 4 months after
transplantation (Fig. 13.5). This abnormality probably represents
chronic glomerular rejection and most likely evolves from acute
transplant glomerulopathy. Capillary walls are thickened with a
double-contoured appearance; mesangial matrix, mesangial cells,
or both are increased. The glomeruli may have a lobular appearance, and segmental sclerosis can occur. *Mesangiolysis,* or dissolution of mesangial matrix, is occasionally seen, with resulting
capillary microaneurysms. Immunofluorescence usually discloses
mesangial and capillary wall granular deposits of IgM, C1q, and
C3, with linear fibrin along capillary walls. When segmental sclerosis is also present, these same immune reactants are in a segmental distribution in a coarsely granular-to-amorphous pattern.
Electron microscopy reveals a variety of abnormalities, including
peripheral migration of mesangium, subendothelial new basement membrane formation, subendothelial flocculent material,
and, infrequently, subendothelial and mesangial electron-dense
deposits. The basement membranes of peritubular capillaries are

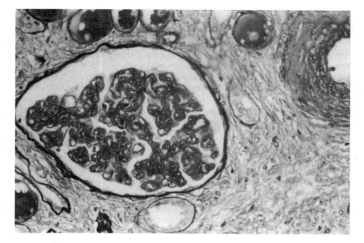

**Fig. 13.5.   Chronic rejection with chronic transplant glomerulopathy.
The arterial wall is thickened and the lumen narrowed due to intimal
fibrosis. Glomerular capillary walls often display "double contours,"
and monocytes are within widened mesangial regions and few capillary lumina. (Periodic acid–methenamine silver stain, ×200.)**

often thickened and *multilayered*; this change has been correlated
with the presence of chronic transplant glomerulopathy.

As with other forms of chronic renal parenchymal diseases,
acquired cystic disease has been documented in the chronically
rejected transplant. In an attempt to provide prognostic information and standardization of the pathologic changes of chronic
allograft failure, a *Chronic Allograft Disease Index* has been developed. Its use may permit prognostication and evaluation of therapeutic interventions for chronic allograft failure, although its
reliability has not yet been fully validated.

DIFFERENTIAL DIAGNOSIS.   As noted previously, the parenchymal
changes of chronic rejection need to be differentiated from those of
hypertension and chronic calcineurin inhibitor toxicity. The presence of transplant glomerulopathy and arterial fibrosis with or
without inflammation suggests chronic allograft nephropathy. In
the absence of these findings, these lesions may be difficult to differentiate from one another.

Calcineurin Inhibitor Nephrotoxicity

Cyclosporine and tacrolimus produce similar renal structural and
functional effects, and the pathologist cannot differentiate between
the nephrotoxic affects of these two drugs. The mechanism of calcineurin inhibitor nephrotoxicity is discussed in Chapter 4.

Acute Toxicity

Few structural abnormalities are evident in acute calcineurin
inhibitor toxicity; the dysfunction likely relates to calcineurin

inhibitor–induced alterations in renal blood flow. There may be tubular dilation, tubular cell flattening, and occasional individual tubular cell necrosis, all with little or no interstitial edema or inflammation. Giant mitochondria and focal tubular calcification also may be present. Unlike the lesions of acute rejection, lymphocytes, when present, are usually restricted to peritubular capillaries and small foci in the interstitium. They are rarely observed in tubules and are not in any other vascular location. Uniform, clear, small isometric vacuoles may be seen in a variable number of proximal tubular cells, often involving many cells of only few tubular profiles (Fig. 13.6).

Vascular Effects

A number of structural lesions of the vasculature are ascribed to the calcineurin inhibitors. *Arteriolopathy* consists of a variety of abnormalities that occur separately or together. There is necrosis of individual myocytes, often with massive accumulation of plasma protein precipitates; these insudates (hyalinization) are characteristically on the adventitial aspect of arteriolar walls (Fig. 13.7). In contrast, in hypertension and diabetes mellitus, the insudative lesions more typically are subendothelial or within the muscularis. Cessation of or reduction in cyclosporine administration has resulted in amelioration or clearing of the arteriolopathy in some patients.

Thrombotic microangiopathy (TMA), or hemolytic-uremic syndrome, is an uncommon but well-recognized complication of calcineurin inhibitor administration; its clinical diagnosis and man-

Isometrically vacuolated
tubular cells

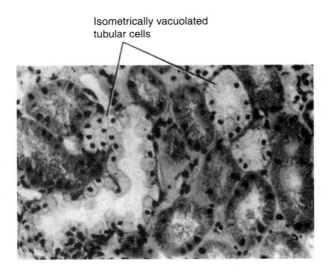

Fig. 13.6. Cyclosporine toxicity with tubular cell isometric vacuoles. The cells of the lighter-staining tubules contain numerous closely packed uniform vacuoles. Note the lack of interstitial edema or inflammation. (Hematoxylin & eosin stain, ×200.)

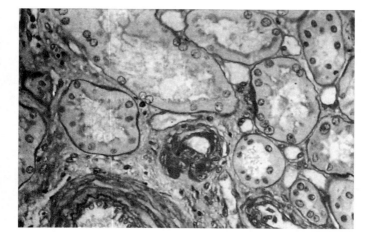

Fig. 13.7. Cyclosporine-associated arteriolopathy. The arteriole has plasma protein insudates ("hyalinization") along the outer aspect of the hypertrophied muscularis. There is no significant edema or inflammation in the interstitium. (Periodic acid–Schiff stain, ×285.)

ifestations are discussed in Chapters 4 and 8. In its mildest form, bland thrombi are present within lumina of arterioles and glomerular capillaries. These lesions are rarely widespread or associated with extensive tissue necrosis. If severe and prolonged, however, TMA may result in more severe arterial and arteriolar alterations with extensive cortical necrosis similar to that observed in the hemolytic-uremic syndrome. In patients whose original disease is hemolytic-uremic syndrome, it may be impossible to differentiate between these two lesions. The pronounced intimal changes ("onion-skin" lesions) of interlobular arteries seen in the hemolytic-uremic syndrome are not regular features of the calcineurin inhibitor-associated process. Hepatitis C virus infection has been linked to anticardiolipin antibodies, which may induce TMA in allograft recipients.

Chronic Toxicity

The changes of chronic calcineurin inhibitor toxicity are similar to chronic renal ischemia. In their purest form, they consist of focal fibrosis, or "striped" *interstitial fibrosis,* and tubular atrophy without inflammation. The interstitium may show a generalized increase of collagen types I and III. Glomerular ischemic collapse or complete sclerosis is also present. These features appear not to be a consequence of intrarenal arterial narrowing because the arteries are largely unremarkable; therefore, the combination of normal arteries with a vascular pattern of parenchymal fibrosis is highly suggestive of chronic calcineurin inhibitor nephrotoxicity. Juxtaglomerular apparatus hyperplasia may be pronounced.

DIFFERENTIAL DIAGNOSIS. The differentiation among chronic allograft nephropathy, nephrosclerosis, and chronic calcineurin inhibitor nephrotoxicity may be difficult. Perhaps the most salient feature permitting this distinction in ideal circumstances is the status of the arteries (interlobular, arcuate), which are often fortuitously included in the biopsy. Normal arteries usually indicate chronic calcineurin inhibitor nephrotoxicity. Intimal and medial fibrosis of arteries, often with lymphocytic infiltrates, are diagnostic for chronic allograft nephropathy. If the arteries disclose the usual features of hypertension, nephrosclerosis is likely. These three lesions may coexist and cloud the picture. In addition, characteristic findings may be present in large (large arcuate and interlobar) arteries only and may not be included in a core biopsy specimen, further causing diagnostic difficulty.

Other Pathologic Transplant Lesions
Acute Tubular Necrosis

Acute tubular necrosis in transplants is similar histologically to the lesion found in native kidneys, although there may be more overt necrosis of epithelial cells and sloughing of nonpyknotic epithelium into tubular lumina (Fig. 13.8). It is most often encountered in a biopsy performed within the first month or so after transplantation because of delayed graft function (see Chapter 8). In addition to the usual changes of tubular necrosis, focal interstitial lymphocytic infiltrates may be present.

Flattened
tubular cells

Necrotic
tubular cells

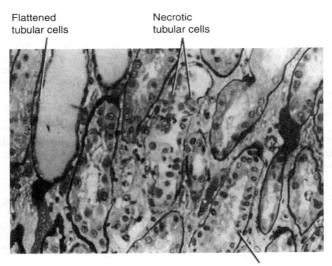

Mitotic
figure

Fig. 13.8. Acute tubular necrosis. The tubule in the center is incompletely lined by epithelial cells; sloughed cells and cellular debris are in the lumen. There is mild interstitial edema with few accompanying lymphocytes. (Periodic acid–methenamine silver stain, ×175.)

Infections

Although the transplanted kidney may be the site of various infections, it may be difficult to diagnose them on the basis of tissue examination. This is not the case for usual forms of acute bacterial interstitial nephritis (acute pyelonephritis), in which the predominant interstitial and tubular infiltrating cells are polymorphonuclear leukocytes. Some uncommon nonsuppurative bacterial infections, however, are characterized by mononuclear leukocytic tubular and interstitial infiltrates. Viral infections typically produce a mononuclear tubulointerstitial nephritis, which may be morphologically similar to cell-mediated acute rejection. Specific agents, such as cytomegalovirus (CMV), may be difficult to diagnose because intranuclear or cytoplasmic inclusions are rare.

Human polyomavirus BK has become a more frequently recognized infectious agent in immunosuppressed patients. It presents clinically as a severe acute rejection that appears unresponsive to intensification of immunosuppression. It may also be associated with ureteric stenosis (see Chapter 7). In biopsy specimens with severe tubulointerstitial nephritis, its presence is suggested by the finding of large basophilic intranuclear inclusions, occasionally with central clearing in enlarged tubular epithelial cells. Special staining with polyomavirus monoclonal antibody confirms the diagnosis, which may have critical therapeutic repercussions.

De Novo Glomerulopathies

De novo membranous glomerulonephritis is found in up to 10% of kidneys in place for more than 1 year, and the capillary wall deposits are not infrequently combined with lesions of chronic transplant glomerulopathy. Membranous glomerulonephritis is often clinically silent or mild and is usually detected as an incidental finding. Focal and segmental glomerulosclerosis, including the usual and collapsing types, may occur as an independent lesion, although it often accompanies transplant glomerulopathy and may be associated with heavy proteinuria. Other forms of *de novo* glomerulonephritis are uncommon. The most reliable manner in which to diagnose this lesion is with immunofluorescence and electron microscopy because the deposits and basement membrane changes are often not readily visible by light microscopy or are overshadowed by transplant glomerulopathy.

Recurrent Lesions

GLOMERULAR LESIONS.   Although many glomerulonephritides may recur in the posttransplantation course, the recurrences may be of immunopathologic rather than clinical significance and do not necessarily affect graft survival or function (see Chapter 9). These lesions include IgA nephropathy, membranoproliferative glomerulonephritis type II (dense deposit disease), and, occasionally, membranous glomerulonephritis. Focal and segmental glomerulosclerosis may recur early after engraftment and is the recurrent lesion that is most likely to be responsible for graft loss. Anti–glomerular basement membrane disease rarely recurs but can arise in a normal kidney transplanted into a patient with Alport's syndrome (see Chapter 6). The vasculitides may recur after transplantation.

OTHER LESIONS.   Amyloidosis, multiple myeloma, light-chain deposit disease, fibrillary nephropathy, and oxalosis can recur, often with significant graft dysfunction. The structural changes of diabetic nephropathy have been noted to recur in the transplanted kidney but are infrequently responsible for graft loss (see Chapter 14). Nodular glomerulosclerosis and arteriolar hyalinization are the usual morphologic manifestations of the recurrent lesion.

Classification Schema

In an attempt to develop an organized and consistent approach to the classification and grading of the various structural lesions in the transplanted kidney, a series of conferences was held in Banff, Canada. The resulting schema, known as the *Banff classification,* was then combined with a separately developed classification resulting from a National Institutes of Health–sponsored study (Cooperative Clinical Trials in Transplantation). Although there remain some differences in the schemata, the combined approach, termed *Banff 97,* defines the abnormalities of rejection and assigns them a numeric score.

There are two parts to the schema: (1) the diagnostic classifications and (2) the grading of each pathologic component in the tissue sample. The grading is somewhat cumbersome and involves assigning a degree of severity to changes affecting the tubules, interstitium, vessels, and glomeruli. The diagnostic categories include antibody-mediated hyperacute and accelerated acute rejection; a borderline lesion; grade I (Fig. 13.1), grade II (Fig. 13.3), and grade III (Fig. 13.4) acute rejection; acute tubular necrosis; acute cyclosporine or FK506 toxicity; grade I (mild), grade II (moderate), and grade III (severe) chronic rejection (chronic nephropathy); and other lesions (e.g., infection, glomerulonephritides, posttransplantation lymphoproliferative disorder). A summary of the important aspects of the Banff 97 classification is provided in Table 13.3.

Table 13.3.   Selected features of the Banff 97 classification

Grade	Criteria
Acute rejection	
I	Interstitial inflammation (>25% of parenchyma)
	Tubulitis (>4 lymphocytes per tubular cross-section)
II	Intimal arteritis (mild to severe)
III	Transmural arteritis and/or arterial fibrinoid necrosis
Chronic rejection (includes chronic vascular and glomerular changes)	
I	Mild interstitial fibrosis and tubular atrophy
II	Moderate interstitial fibrosis and tubular atrophy
III	Severe interstitial fibrosis and tubular atrophy or drop-out

According to the Banff 97 classification, mild interstitial edema, patchy (10% to 25%) interstitial lymphocytic infiltration, and mild tubulitis (one to four lymphocytes per tubular cross-section) in the absence of arterial intimal inflammation are considered *borderline lesions,* suspicious for acute rejection. There remains some controversy regarding the significance of borderline lesions; some studies have shown these lesions to be associated with treatment-responsive clinical acute rejection. The grade III rejection criteria do, however, appear to correlate with more severe clinical rejections, which may be unresponsive to treatment with high-dose steroids alone (see Chapter 4). Further work is required to clarify the clinical usefulness of the Banff 97 classification, and classification schemata with specific quantifiable criteria require further validation in clinical studies.

KIDNEY DONOR HISTOPATHOLOGY

The ever-widening gap between the supply and demand for cadaveric kidneys has led to the increasing use of organs from "marginal" donors (see Chapters 3 and 5). Histopathology of these kidneys is often requested as a guide to the wisdom of transplanting them. The most common clinical situations in which donor pathology is requested are for older donors, donors with a history of hypertension or vascular disease, or donors with preharvesting evidence of renal dysfunction. Baseline histology may be required in the clinical trials evaluating new immunosuppressive drugs.

The time constraints imposed by the need for rapid decision making prevent routine histopathologic processing of biopsy material. Use of frozen tissue may impair diagnostic precision and rapid-processing techniques are preferred. A superficial wedge biopsy specimen is often provided; however, the subcapsular parenchyma often has chronic changes and may not be representative of the whole organ. Additionally, arteries may be absent from superficial biopsy specimens, precluding adequate evaluation for nephrosclerosis. The number and percentage of sclerosed glomeruli should be determined and an assessment made of the degree of tubulointerstitial and vascular disease. Transplantation teams tend to give more prognostic credence to numeric values that may reflect the degree of nephrosclerosis, and kidneys with more than 20% sclerosed glomeruli are often discarded. Interstitial and vascular changes, however, which are more difficult to quantitate, may have more prognostic importance.

FINE-NEEDLE ASPIRATION CYTOLOGY

Aspiration cytology is a relatively new technique for assessing intrarenal events in allografts, performing a qualitative and quantitative comparison of the cells within the graft and peripheral blood. Transplant aspiration was first used clinically by Hayry and von Willebrand as a minimally invasive procedure for monitoring immunologic processes in renal allografts. There is little morbidity associated with aspiration, and it may be performed daily on an outpatient basis. It allows for close monitoring of the immunologic status of the graft and its response to therapeutic interventions. Aspiration cytology is a valuable tool for the investigation of transplant biology, providing intragraft cells for culture or characterization by immunohistochemistry and *in situ* hybridization.

Indications

Aspiration is usually performed within the first several months after transplantation for episodes of acute graft dysfunction. The procedure is best used in a serial fashion to follow changes in the graft cell population, and a baseline sampling performed within the first posttransplantation week is useful for comparison with subsequent aspirates. It may be done successfully up to 6 to 12 months after transplantation. After this time, fibrosis in the interstitium tends to prevent adequate numbers of cells from being aspirated, and inadequate samples are frequently obtained.

Diagnostic Uses

Aspiration cytology may be used in the assessment of graft dysfunction due to acute cellular (interstitial) rejection, acute tubular necrosis, acute cyclosporine nephrotoxicity, bacterial infection (pyelonephritis), viral infection, or renal infarction. Aspirate material can also be obtained in a serial manner for following response to therapy by evaluation of the numbers and types of intragraft cells.

Diagnostic Limitations

Several renal allograft abnormalities cannot be diagnosed with aspiration. Vascular inflammation cannot be assessed because the anatomic location of the aspirated inflammatory cells is not ascertainable. Chronic rejection and chronic calcineurin inhibitor nephrotoxicity are fibrotic processes and usually result in inadequate specimens because cells within scar tissue cannot be aspirated. Graft rupture, intraparenchymal hemorrhage, and obstruction result in inadequate aspirates that mimic blood contamination of the sample. Glomeruli are infrequently obtained and, when present, are not interpretable in the usual cytologic preparations. Their presence merely serves to prove the cortical location of the aspirate.

Aspirate Handling and Interpretation

TECHNIQUE.   The patient is supine and rotated contralaterally to the allograft, with the contralateral knee bent and the ipsilateral knee straight. This position tends to make the graft more prominent. After sterile preparation, a 25-gauge spinal needle is inserted into the graft, the trocar removed, and the needle attached to a 10-mL syringe containing 4 mL of tissue culture medium, which is fitted into an aspiration gun. Suction is then applied, the needle is rotated and removed quickly, and the sample and medium are expressed through the needle into a culture tube. The procedure is repeated two to four times, and each aspirate is placed into a separate tube. A finger-stick blood sample is obtained simultaneously and placed separately in 2 mL of medium. All samples must be immediately refrigerated and processed within 24 hours to prevent cellular degeneration. Routine preaspiration coagulation studies are not required, and the patient may ambulate immediately after the procedure.

PROCESSING.   The aspirate and blood specimens are handled similarly. Samples are centrifuged, resuspended in medium, and cytocentrifuged onto glass slides. Aspirates containing similar quantities of blood contamination are pooled before cytocentrifugation to allow preparation of the maximal number of slides. The cytospin preparations are air-dried and stained with May-Grünwald-Giemsa stain or stored in a desiccator for additional staining procedures.

INTERPRETATION. Qualitative and quantitative assessments of aspirate leukocytes, parenchymal cells, and blood leukocytes are performed for routine evaluation of the specimens.

Leukocytes. The entire aspirate cytospin preparation is screened to assess the total number of T- and B-cell immunoblasts and plasma cells. A 100-cell differential count is then performed separately on the aspirate and peripheral blood samples. The peripheral blood count is subtracted from the aspirate count, resulting in increments for each type of leukocyte observed; negative increments are not included. Immunoblasts and plasma cells observed in the peripheral blood differential count are added to those in the aspirate, rather than subtracted, to give a higher blast increment. The increments are multiplied by correction factors, which give added weight to those cell types more strongly associated with acute rejection (Table 13.4). The corrected increments are then added to give the total corrected increment (TCI). The TCI and total immunoblast and plasma cell count are used to evaluate the status of immune activation in the graft.

Parenchymal Cells. Tubular and endothelial cells are assessed to determine parenchymal injury in the graft and to determine aspirate adequacy, which is defined as a minimum of seven parenchymal cells per 100 leukocytes. Endothelial cells may be either normal or swollen. Tubular cells may appear normal, swollen, irregularly vacuolated, isometrically vacuolated, phagocytic, degenerated, or necrotic, in increasing order of injury. Phagocytosis is an *in vitro* event occurring in the test tube after aspiration wherein injured tubular cells ingest erythrocytes or leukocytes. Parenchymal cells are often artifactually smashed; only intact cells are evaluated qualitatively, although all parenchymal cells are used for adequacy determination.

Table 13.4. Correction factors for leukocytes within aspirate preparations[a]

Leukocyte	Correction Factor
Immunoblast	1.0
Plasma cell	1.0
Macrophage	1.0
Activated lymphocyte	0.5
Large granular lymphocyte	0.2
Monocyte	0.2
Lymphocyte	0.1
Neutrophil	0.1
Basophil	0.1
Eosinophil	0.1

[a] Used for calculation of the total corrected increment (see text).

Acute Cellular Rejection

May-Grünwald-Giemsa Stain

Immune activation is defined as more than four immunoblasts, plasma cells, or both in the aspirate; a TCI of more than 3; or both. The degree of activation often correlates with the amount of inflammation observed in corresponding core biopsy specimens. Tubular cells may be swollen, irregularly vacuolated, phagocytic, and degenerated. Severe rejection is associated with high TCI and blast counts and the presence of intragraft macrophages and peripheral blood immunoblasts (Fig. 13.9). Resolution of rejection is reflected by fewer immunoblasts, a decreasing TCI, and less tubular cell injury and can be evaluated by serial aspiration during and after antirejection therapy.

Immunochemical Stains

In acute rejection, there is up-regulation of tubular cell major histocompatibility complex (MHC) class II antigens that are not constitutively expressed. This can be used to improve diagnostic sensitivity of aspiration by immunostaining aspirate samples for class II antigens; they are found in 30% or more of tubular cells after the onset of acute rejection. This staining decreases incrementally after successful treatment of rejection but may not disappear for up to 2 weeks after therapy.

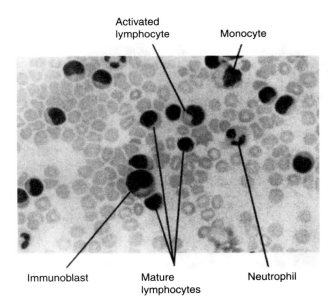

Fig. 13.9.   **Fine-needle aspirate from a patient with severe acute interstitial (cellular) rejection. There are many mononuclear leukocytes, including immunoblasts, activated lymphocytes, and mature lymphocytes, with relatively few neutrophils. (May-Grünwald-Giemsa stain, ×400.)**

DIFFERENTIAL DIAGNOSIS. Aspirate immune activation may be observed in other circumstances. In viral infections, the TCI and blast count are increased, with additional elevation of the numbers of large granular lymphocytes in the aspirate and peripheral blood, as described later in the section on viral infection. In acute rejection, however, it is only in the aspirate that there are increased numbers of large granular lymphocytes. In the first few days after transplantation, mononuclear leukocytes may infiltrate the graft in response to surgical manipulation. If aspiration is repeated 1 week after transplantation, the perioperative inflammation is noted to subside. Calcineurin inhibitor use is occasionally associated with focal intragraft lymphocyte collections, which will seem to indicate immune activation if aspirated; however, there is no increase in immunoblasts. Lymphoceles adjacent to the allograft are infrequently aspirated; the fluid appears yellow, as opposed to the clear or blood-tinged normal aspirates, and normal and reactive mesothelial cells may be present. If the needle also passed through the kidney, there may be immunoblasts, lymphocytes, and, rarely, tubular cells. Clinical correlation is required to assess the likelihood of sampling a lymphocele.

In all instances, after the first 2 to 3 postoperative days, elevated tubular cell MHC class II antigen expression is related to acute rejection and can be used to aid in determining the etiology of immune activation.

Infection

Viral Infection

In viral infections, there is aspirate immune activation, with increased numbers of immunoblasts and particularly plasma cells, and a TCI of more than 3. The aspirate and peripheral blood samples often have the elevated numbers and size of large granular lymphocytes, the peripheral blood increase representing a specific host response observed in viral infections. The peripheral blood may also have atypical mononuclear cells and increased numbers of blasts out of proportion to the degree of graft activation. Tubular cell injury is variable, ranging from swelling to necrosis; intracellular inclusions are not observed. CMV infection has been extensively studied with immunostaining for the early CMV nuclear protein; antigen can be demonstrated in more than 35% of tubular cells in the face of active CMV disease. Increased numbers of tubular cells with MHC class II antigen expression are generally not present unless there is a recent prior or concurrent acute rejection episode. *In situ* hybridization techniques may be used to detect viral genomes (including CMV, herpesvirus, and Epstein-Barr virus) in tubular or endothelial cells.

DIFFERENTIAL DIAGNOSIS. As described, the increase in size and number of peripheral blood large granular lymphocytes, the presence of viral genome or protein, and the absence of MHC class II antigen aid in distinguishing viral infection from acute rejection. Increases in immunoblasts and the TCI may accompany tubular injury in the first few postoperative days but then subside.

Bacterial and Fungal Infections

In cases of bacterial or fungal infection, there is typically an increase in the number of intragraft neutrophils relative to the peripheral blood. There is no immune activation, and tubular cell damage is variable, ranging from swelling to necrosis. Organisms may be observed extracellularly and within neutrophil cytoplasm. Because the aspirate is obtained using sterile medium, it may also be used for culture.

If organisms are not evident, if the neutrophil increase is small, and if there is substantial tubular cell injury, it may be impossible to distinguish infection from tubular necrosis. When no organisms are observed and there is modest tubular cell damage, the lack of immune activation may simulate the aspirate from a well-functioning graft.

Acute Tubular Necrosis

In acute tubular necrosis, tubular cells range from swollen and irregularly vacuolated to phagocytic, degenerated, and necrotic (Fig. 13.10). Endothelial cells may be normal or swollen. There is no immune activation, the TCI is less than 3, and there are four or fewer immunoblasts and plasma cells. Mitotic figures, presumably in tubular epithelial cells, may be observed. The degree of tubular cell injury tends to correlate with the clinical course, and serial aspiration demonstrates diminishing tubular cell injury as renal function improves. Acute calcineurin inhibitor toxicity may mimic acute tubular necrosis because the characteristic isometric vacuoles are not always observed.

Acute Calcineurin Inhibitor Nephrotoxicity

In acute calcineurin inhibitor nephrotoxicity, there are small, cytoplasmic isometric vacuoles in more than half of the tubular cell

Neutrophil

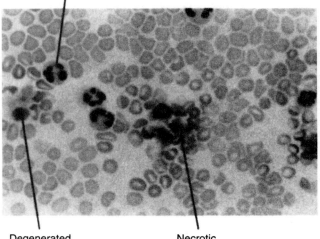

Degenerated   Necrotic
tubular cell   tubular cells

Fig. 13.10.   Fine-needle aspirate demonstrating acute tubular necrosis. There are degenerated and necrotic tubular cells, with occasional neutrophils. No increase in mononuclear leukocytes is evident. (May-Grünwald-Giemsa stain, ×400.)

Isometrically
vascuolated
neutrophil

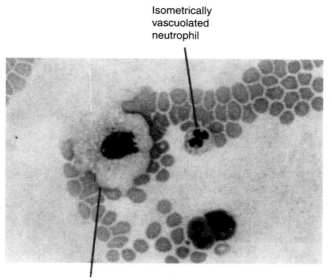

Isometrically
vascuolated
tubular cell

Fig. 13.11. Aspirate preparation from a patient with acute cyclosporine toxicity. Small uniform (isometric) vacuoles are in the cytoplasm of the tubular cell and a neutrophil. (May-Grünwald-Giemsa stain, ×450.)

population (Fig. 13.11). The vacuoles may be somewhat larger with tacrolimus toxicity. Similar vacuoles may be seen in endothelial cells and aspirate leukocytes, particularly neutrophils. Vacuoles are not present in peripheral blood leukocytes. Tubular cells may also display phagocytosis, degeneration, and necrosis. The TCI is less than 3 or may be slightly increased because of elevated numbers of intragraft lymphocytes from the focal interstitial infiltrates that may occur with calcineurin inhibitor use. There is no elevation of the immunoblast or plasma cell count.

Some patients with calcineurin inhibitor nephrotoxicity have tubular degeneration with scant isometric vacuoles, mimicking tubular necrosis. The vacuolated tubular cells occur focally in proximal tubules; hence, repeat aspiration may yield vacuolated cells and a definitive diagnosis. Isometric vacuoles and tubular necrosis are observed in occasional aspirates performed within the first 3 to 4 days after transplantation in the absence of toxicity; they do not persist beyond the first week.

SELECTED READINGS

Bosmans JL, Woestenburg A, Yserbaert DK, et al. Fibrous intimal thickening at implantation as a risk factor for the outcome of cadaveric renal allografts. *Transplantation* 2000;69:2388.

Chung WY, Nast CC, Ettenger RB, et al. Acquired cystic disease in chronically rejected renal transplant. *J Am Soc Nephrol* 1992; 2:1298.

Colvin RB. Renal transplant pathology. In: Jennette JC, Olson JL, Schwartz MM, et al., eds. *Heptinstall's pathology of the Kidney*. New York: Lippincott-Raven, 1998:1409–1540.

Colvin RB, Cohen A, Sianoz C, et al. Evaluation of the pathologic criteria for acute renal allograft rejection: reproducibility, sensitivity and clinical correlation. *J Am Soc Nephrol* 1997;8:1930.

Curtis JJ, Julian BA, Sanders CE. Dilemmas in renal transplantation: when the clinical course and histologic findings differ. *Am J Kidney Dis* 1996;27:435.

Davis CL, Chandler WL. Thromboelastography for the prediction of bleeding after transplant renal biopsy. *J Am Soc Nephrol* 1995; 6:1250.

Gaber LW, Moore LW, Gaber AO, et al. Correlation of histology to clinical reversal: a thymoglobulin multicenter trial report. *Kidney Int* 1999;55:2415.

Gaber LW, Moore LW, Alloway RR, et al. Correlation between Banff classification, acute renal rejection scores and reversal of rejection. *Kidney Int* 1996;49:481.

Gudat F, Mihatsch MJ, Ryffel B, et al. Cyclosporine nephropathy. In: Tisher CC, Brenner BM, eds. *Renal pathology*. Philadelphia: JB Lippincott, 1994.

Habib R, Zurowska A, Hinglais N, et al. A specific glomerular lesion of the graft: allograft glomerulopathy. *Kidney Int* 1993;44(Suppl):104S.

Muruve NA, Steinbeker K, Luger AM. Are wedge biopsies of cadaveric kidneys obtained at procurement reliable? *Transplantation* 2000;69:2384.

Myers BD, Newton L. Cyclosporine-induced chronic nephropathy: an obliterative microvascular renal injury. *J Am Soc Nephrol* 1991; 2:5451.

Nast CC. Fine needle aspiration cytology. In: Racusen LC, Solez K, Burdick JF, eds. *Kidney transplant rejection*. New York: Marcel Dekker, 1998:419–443.

Nast CC, Wilkinson A, Rosenthal T, et al. Differentiation of cytomegalovirus infection from acute rejection using renal allograft fine needle aspirates. *J Am Soc Nephrol* 1991;1:1204.

Neumayer HH, Kienbaum M, Graf S, et al. Prevalence and long-term outcome of glomerulonephritis in renal allografts. *Am J Kidney Dis* 1993;22:320.

Nickeliet V, Klimkait T, Binet IF, et al. Testing for polyomavirus type BK DNA in plasma to identify renal allograft recipients with viral nephropathy. *N Engl J Med* 2000;342:1309.

Nickerson P, Jeffrey J, McKenna R, et al. Identification of clinical and histopathologic risk factors for diminished renal function 2 years post-transplant. *J Am Soc Nephrol* 1998;19:482.

Racusen LC, Solez K, Colvin RB, et al. The Banff 97 working classification of renal allograft pathology. *Kidney Int* 1999;55:713.

Revelo MP, Pauesa Kon P, Weidner M, et al. A 37-year old woman with systemic lupus erythematosus and acute allograft failure. *Am J Kid Dis* 2000;35:1242.

Solez K, Racusen LC, Marcussen N, et al. Morphology of ischemic acute renal failure, normal function, and cyclosporine toxicity in cyclosporine-treated renal allograft recipients. *Kidney Int* 1993; 43:1058.

Kidney and Kidney–Pancreas Transplantation in Diabetic Patients

John D. Pirsch and Hans W. Sollinger

Diabetes mellitus is the leading single cause of end-stage renal disease (ESRD), accounting for one third of new ESRD patients each year. About 40% of the ESRD population has diabetes; 12% of cases are classified as type I and 28% as type II. The incidence of ESRD due to type II diabetes is increasing progressively in all countries with a western lifestyle. Diabetes is second only to glomerular disease as an indication for transplantation, and it is the cause of ESRD in 20% of all transplant recipients each year. Although the incidence of diabetic nephropathy in insulin-dependent diabetes mellitus appears to be falling, this diagnosis remains the one that most commonly leads to kidney transplantation in adult whites, Asians, and Native Americans.

There is little question that kidney transplantation, alone or combined with pancreas transplantation, is the treatment of choice for end-stage diabetic nephropathy. Live donor kidney transplantation in diabetic recipients is associated with a survival advantage compared with cadaveric transplantation; however, both forms of transplantation offer a pronounced survival advantage over chronic dialysis (see Chapter 1). Care must be taken in comparing transplant and dialysis patient groups because, as a whole, they are not strictly comparable. Patients with the least severe morbid manifestations of diabetes are more likely to select, or be selected for, transplantation. When transplanted diabetic patients are compared with diabetics awaiting transplants, the transplanted group has a clear-cut survival advantage. Controlled studies evaluating the quality-of-life benefits of these treatment modalities have clearly illustrated the benefits of transplantation over dialysis for patients with diabetes. Although all forms of kidney replacement therapy can stabilize or slow some of the secondary complications of diabetes, successful transplantation with correction of uremia and control of blood pressure can stabilize or improve complications, such as neuropathy, diabetic gastroparesis, and retinopathy.

This chapter considers the management issues associated with kidney and pancreas transplantation in diabetic patients and the pros and cons of the different forms of pancreas transplantation.

KIDNEY TRANSPLANTATION

Preoperative Assessment

The preoperative evaluation of potential kidney transplant recipients is discussed in Chapter 6. This section considers issues particularly relevant to diabetic patients. The propensity for the premature development of atherosclerosis in diabetic patients mandates careful screening for overt and covert vascular disease.

Coronary Artery Disease

About one third of potential diabetic transplant recipients have significant coronary artery disease. Most of these patients do not suffer typical angina or other cardiac symptoms; hence, the possibility of covert coronary artery disease should be considered in every diabetic transplant candidate. In many transplantation programs, all diabetic patients undergo screening with an exercise stress test to help determine which patients should undergo further evaluation with cardiac catheterization. The stress test is usually supplemented with thallium or sestamibi scintigraphy or echocardiography to increase its specificity. Many diabetic patients with kidney failure, however, have poor functional capacity or are physically unable to exercise adequately to reach a target heart rate. In some centers, these patients undergo an oral or intravenous dipyridamole-thallium stress test or a dobutamine stress echocardiogram designed to simulate the effect of exercise on the heart. The sensitivity and specificity of some standard noninvasive tests are shown in Table 14.1.

Because of the poor sensitivity and specificity of noninvasive testing, recipients with multiple risk factors or a positive or inadequate stress test should undergo cardiac catheterization before transplantation. Patients with coronary lesions amenable to bypass or angioplasty should be treated before transplantation. Patients with significant coronary artery disease who are not candidates for intervention may not be transplant candidates, although centers differ in their approach to such patients.

In an attempt to avoid an expensive and invasive work-up in all diabetic patients, attempts have been made to determine which diabetic candidates are most unlikely to suffer covert coronary artery disease. Patients without cardiac symptoms who are younger than 45 years of age and have had diabetes for fewer than 25 years, who have not smoked for more than 5 pack-years, and who have a totally normal electrocardiogram have a low incidence of covert coronary artery disease; therefore, further work-up may be unnecessary. An algorithm for screening diabetic transplant candidates for coronary artery disease is shown in Fig. 14.1.

Diabetic patients who wait for prolonged periods on the cadaveric transplant waiting list should have their cardiac status reassessed

Table 14.1.   Usefulness of noninvasive screening to detect 75% or greater coronary artery stenosis in symptom-free diabetic patients before transplantation

	Sensitivity (%) (n = 41)	Specificity (%) (n = 35)
Thallium scintigraphy[a]	62	76
Exercise radionuclide ventriculography[a]	50	67
Dobutamine stress echocardiography[b]	75	76

[a] Data from Vandenberg et al., 1996.
[b] Data from Herzog et al., 1999.

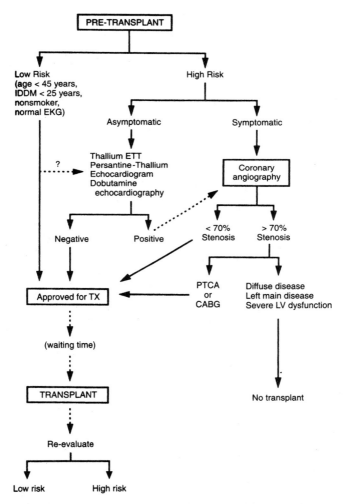

Fig. 14.1. Algorithm for screening of diabetic transplant candidates for coronary artery disease based on data that suggest that non-invasive evaluation of low-risk patients may be unnecessary. (From Williams ME. Management of the diabetic transplant recipient. *Kidney Int* 1995;48:1600, reprinted with permission of Blackwell Science, Inc.)

at intervals of 1 to 2 years, with repetition of noninvasive testing; coronary angiography should be repeated when indicated. Known risk factors for coronary artery disease should be repeatedly reviewed and addressed.

Cerebrovascular and Peripheral Vascular Disease

The increased susceptibility of diabetic transplant recipients for cerebrovascular and peripheral vascular disease mandates particular attention to these issues in the pretransplantation evaluation. A history of cerebrovascular events or intermittent claudication and the finding of carotid bruits or poor peripheral pulses may require further assessment. Noninvasive studies should precede angiography, and consultation with a vascular surgeon may be warranted.

Infections

Patients should be free of significant infections, such as peritonitis, osteomyelitis, or unhealed foot ulcerations at the time of transplantation. If a patient develops these complications while awaiting a transplant, his or her candidacy should be placed on hold until the problem is resolved.

Predialysis Transplantation

For patients with diabetic nephropathy, transplantation should be strongly considered before the initiation of dialysis (glomerular filtration rate of 20 mL/min or less or a serum creatinine level of 4 to 5 mg/dL). Early transplantation can obviate the need for dialysis access, can prevent episodes of congestive heart failure and volume overload, and can correct hypertension, which may contribute to loss of vision. Early transplantation may slow retinopathy and correct neuropathy secondary to uremia, which can exacerbate diabetic neuropathy. The development of diabetic complications on dialysis may impair the rehabilitation potential of transplantation.

Predialysis diabetic transplant candidates who require coronary angiography risk precipitation of dialysis by contrast nephropathy. This risk needs to be carefully weighed against the risks associated with delaying transplantation or leaving coronary artery disease undiagnosed. Predialysis transplantation is also discussed in Chapter 6.

Insulin Requirements

By the time many diabetic patients develop advanced nephropathy or the need for dialysis, their insulin requirements have often diminished, or their diabetes may be controlled by oral agents or diet alone. After transplantation, the carbohydrate intolerance induced by corticosteroids, cyclosporine, and tacrolimus (see Chapter 4) may lead to increased insulin requirements and cause non–insulin-dependent diabetic patients to require insulin. Patients should be forewarned.

Preoperative Preparation

For patients with severe gastroparesis, a nasogastric tube may need to be placed. Poor gastrointestinal function may compromise absorption of immunosuppressive therapies, and intravenous formulations of mycophenolate and corticosteroids should be considered in the early postoperative period. Most centers have abandoned the use of intravenous cyclosporine and tacrolimus, which are usually well absorbed, even from the malfunctioning gastrointestinal tract. Slow resumption of bowel function may follow transplantation, and, occasionally, nasogastric suction may be required in cases of prolonged ileus. In the immediate preoperative period when the patient is receiving nothing by mouth, half the normal dose of insulin should be given. Blood glucose levels should be monitored every 4 hours and a sliding scale used for dosing regular insulin. Patients should undergo dialysis if there is significant evidence of volume overload or congestive heart failure. The immunosuppressive protocol used does not differ in diabetic transplant recipients, although attempts may be made to lessen the reliance on corticosteroids.

Postoperative Complications

Several studies have shown no significant difference in major postoperative complications in diabetic versus nondiabetic patients, especially with regard to wound complications. Postoperative ileus, nausea, and vomiting are more common but are secondary to diabetic enteropathy. Because of the use of high-dose corticosteroids, frequent blood sugar monitoring is essential, and an insulin drip may be necessary in the first 24 to 48 hours after transplantation. All patients should receive instruction in blood sugar self-monitoring and in using sliding-scale administration of regular insulin for the control of episodes of hyperglycemia. Long-acting insulin, such as NPH, should be used on a twice-a-day regimen. Occasionally, dividing the prednisone dose into a morning and afternoon dose helps to control postprednisone hyperglycemia.

Graft Dysfunction

REJECTION.   The incidence of rejection and cyclosporine toxicity in diabetic patients is not different from that in nondiabetic patients. When possible, a kidney biopsy should be employed to determine the cause of graft dysfunction to prevent unnecessary immunosuppression in this high-risk population. Therapy with high-dose corticosteroids is frequently accompanied by poor blood sugar control and requires close monitoring.

PSEUDOREJECTION.   In patients with poor blood sugar control, hypovolemia can cause elevations in the blood urea nitrogen and creatinine levels and mimic a rejection episode. Careful review of the previous blood sugar record and careful assessment of volume status are usually sufficient to make this diagnosis. Occasionally, functional obstruction secondary to neurogenic bladder also simulates rejection. This condition is usually diagnosed by ultrasound or renal scan, which shows a large distended bladder and a prominent renal pelvis. The volume of the postvoid residual may be more than 500 mL, and Foley catheter drainage with a fall in creatinine level confirms the diagnosis.

URINARY TRACT INFECTION.   Urinary tract infections (UTIs) are more common in diabetic recipients because of the higher incidence of neurogenic bladder. Prophylaxis with daily double-strength trimethoprim-sulfamethoxazole is recommended.

Long-Term Complications

Peripheral Vascular Disease

Although successful kidney transplantation is a solution for the nephropathy associated with insulin-dependent diabetes mellitus, many other diabetic manifestations, including peripheral vascular disease, continue to progress. Up to 30% of patients have been reported to have undergone at least one amputation within 3 years of transplantation. Meticulous foot care is essential to help prevent amputations. Although many ischemic ulcers are secondary to microvascular disease, macrovascular occlusion secondary to atherosclerotic plaquing is not uncommon. Angiography should be employed when indicated to identify patients with peripheral vascular lesions that are amenable to bypass grafting.

Retinopathy

Stabilization of retinopathy is common after transplantation, with most patients experiencing no change in visual acuity or showing some improvement. Recipients with severely impaired vision may note some improvement, although some patients progress to blindness.

Neuropathy

Neuropathy shows initial improvement with the correction of uremia; however, there is slow deterioration with the progression of the diabetes.

DIABETIC GASTROPATHY.   Diabetic gastropathy is common, and gastroparesis is best treated with metoclopramide, 10 mg given four times daily, or cisapride, 10 mg given four times daily before meals. Side effects associated with metoclopramide include mental confusion and a Parkinson-like syndrome with cogwheel rigidity, which is an indication to decrease the dose or discontinue the medication. Many patients who require metoclopramide before transplantation may discontinue it afterward. Diabetic diarrhea can be treated with oral or transdermal clonidine.

NEUROGENIC BLADDER.   Neurogenic bladder is a frequent complicating factor after transplantation. Bethanechol chloride, 10 to 25 mg given four times daily, may improve bladder emptying, but cholinergic side effects may limit its use. Intermittent self-catheterization may be necessary in some patients.

ORTHOSTATIC HYPOTENSION.   Orthostatic hypotension with supine hypertension is common secondary to autonomic neuropathy and may be transiently exacerbated after successful transplantation, particularly if the patient was in a fluid-positive state before transplantation. Treatment includes fludrocortisone acetate (Florinef), 0.1 to 0.3 mg daily; midodrine (an alpha-adrenoreceptor agonist) up to 10 mg three times a day; or sodium chloride tablets if the patient is not edematous. Clonidine has been shown to improve orthostatic hypotension, probably by a peripheral venoconstricting effect. Orthostatic hypotension typically resolves as the hematocrit rises; this process can be expedited with erythropoietin injections if necessary.

Hypertension

Hypertension is common after transplantation and may be due to the effects of cyclosporine or tacrolimus, retained native kidneys, or rarely, renal artery stenosis (see Chapter 9). Agents useful in treatment include the spectrum of antihypertensives; however, diuretics and beta-blockers should be used with caution. Diuretics may impair glucose control or increase cholesterol levels; beta-blockers may block the hypoglycemic response to norepinephrine and epinephrine and predispose the patient to severe hypoglycemic episodes. Calcium-channel blockers are effective;

however, verapamil and diltiazem increase cyclosporine levels. Close monitoring of cyclosporine or tacrolimus levels is necessary if these agents are used. Nifedipine, which does not interfere with cyclosporine metabolism, is effective in controlling posttransplantation hypertension. The long-acting preparation is preferred. Alpha-blockers are also effective, but side effects at higher doses may limit their use. Angiotensin-converting enzyme inhibitors or receptor blockers are effective for blood pressure control, and these agents may have additional cardiac and renoprotective benefits. Kidney function may decline during their use, especially in undiagnosed renal artery stenosis or chronic rejection, and hyperkalemia and anemia may occur.

Hyperlipidemia

Hyperlipidemia should be treated aggressively in diabetic transplant recipients, particularly in the presence of coronary artery disease. Dietary treatment alone is usually ineffective; 3-hydroxy-3-methylglutaryl coenzyme A (HMG-CoA) reductase inhibitors, starting at low doses with careful monitoring of muscle and liver enzymes, are the agents most likely to be effective (see Chapter 9).

Bone Disease

Diabetic transplant recipients are particularly susceptible to osteoporosis and its consequences (see Chapter 9), and a fracture rate of up to 40% has been described on long-term follow-up. Ideally, lumbar spine and hip bone mineral density should be measured by dual x-ray absorptiometry at the time of transplantation and at yearly intervals thereafter. The biphosphonates represent the most effective means of prevention and treatment.

Recurrent Diabetic Nephropathy

Pathologic changes in the allograft consistent with diabetic nephropathy are common after transplantation; graft loss secondary to recurrent diabetic nephropathy, however, is unusual. In the future, with longer survival of transplant recipients, recurrent diabetic nephropathy may become a more significant problem.

Pregnancy

Pregnancy in transplant recipients is discussed in Chapter 9. Pregnant diabetic transplant recipients represent a particularly high-risk group; a limited number of successful pregnancies have been reported. Prematurity is universal, and deterioration of graft function is common. These factors, together with the potentially limited maternal life span, should be considered in the decision to proceed with the pregnancy.

KIDNEY–PANCREAS TRANSPLANTATION

Surgical Options

To provide the pancreatic islets needed to produce insulin and cure diabetes, it is necessary to transplant both the exocrine and endocrine pancreas. This situation will change if and when pancreatic islet transplantation becomes a readily available clinical reality (see the section on transplantation of pancreatic islets). Three patient groups can be considered for whole organ pancreas transplantation: *pancreas alone* (PA), for patients who have not yet developed advanced kidney disease; *simultaneous pancreas–kidney* (SPK) transplantation, for patients with renal failure; and *pancreas-after-kidney* (PAK) transplantation, for patients who have previously undergone successful kidney transplantation. Each of these approaches has advantages and disadvantages, which must be considered when determining the indications for pancreas transplantation (Table 14.2). In 1999, in the United States, Medicare approved reimbursement for pancreas transplantation for patients with ESRD (i.e., SPK and PAK), and the procedure has become feasible for a much larger population of patients.

Much of the success of all types of cadaveric pancreas transplantation depends on meticulous attention to the technical aspects of donor selection, organ harvesting, and back-table preparation. Detailed discussion of these issues is beyond the scope of this text, and the reader is referred to the article by Mizrahi and colleagues (see Selected Readings).

Preuremic Pancreas Transplantation

Some centers offer PA transplantation as a therapeutic alternative for recurrently ketotic "brittle" patients and for patients with hypoglycemic unawareness. The number of patients receiving pancreas transplants has increased over the past several years with improving immunosuppression. The prolonged normoglycemia that follows the successful procedure does not, unfortunately,

Table 14.2.   Pancreas transplantation options

	Pro	Con	1-year survival in 1994–1998
Preuremic pancreas alone	Good surgical risk. Complications at early stage.	Major surgical procedure. Side effects of immunosuppressive therapy may outweigh potential benefits. Mediocre results.	Patient 95% Pancreas 64%
Pancreas after kidney transplantation	Patient already immunosuppressed.	Surgical procedure. Advanced diabetic complications. Mediocre results.	Patient 95% Pancreas 71%
Simultaneous kidney and pancreas transplantation	Only one surgical procedure. Same immunosuppression. Good results.	Advanced diabetic complications.	Patient 94% Pancreas 83% Kidney 90%

lead to resolution of established nephropathy or retinopathy. For most diabetic patients, the risk-to-benefit ratio for PA transplantation is unfavorable because a pancreas transplant exposes them both to the risks of surgery and to the long-term side effects of immunosuppressive therapy.

Transplantation of the Pancreas After the Kidney

In PAK transplantation, immunosuppressive therapy is not a major concern. In the long-term, the drug therapy the patients are already receiving for their kidney transplant is not significantly changed after the addition of a pancreas transplant. The significant risks for these patients are the risk of the surgical procedure itself and the short-term risk of a temporary postoperative boost in their immunosuppressive therapy. Unfortunately, these patients have already suffered significant secondary diabetic complications, and it is uncertain whether a well-functioning pancreas transplant will accomplish more than rendering these patients insulin independent. The results of PAK transplantation are worse than those of SPK transplantation but have improved with the availability of the newer immunosuppressive agents (see Chapter 4). PAK transplantation may be a particularly relevant option for patients with a live donor, in which case the kidney is placed on the left side in anticipation of the pancreas transplantation several months later.

Simultaneous Kidney and Pancreas Transplantation

SPK transplantation is the preferred type of pancreas transplantation. It has the advantage that only one surgical procedure is required and there is only one source of foreign histocompatibility antigens. Immunosuppressive therapy is similar to the therapy that these patients would receive with a kidney transplant alone. As in PAK transplantation, however, many patients have already suffered substantial secondary diabetic complications, and the extent to which these complications will reverse or stabilize is uncertain (see the section on the effect of pancreas transplantation on secondary diabetic complications). Nevertheless, SPK transplantation is established as a therapeutic and effective procedure; substantial improvement in the quality of life as compared with kidney transplantation alone has been documented by several centers (see the section on choice of procedure).

Outcome of Pancreas Transplantation

Eighty-six percent of pancreas transplantations performed in the United States between 1994 and 1998 were SPK transplantations. Data reported to the United Network for Organ Sharing for this time period (Table 14.2) show an overall 1-year pancreas graft survival rate of 83% and patient survival rate of at least 94% (the 1-year patient survival for diabetic recipients of a kidney transplantation alone is similar). Pancreas transplantation does not adversely affect 1-year kidney graft survival, which was 90% for SPK procedures. One-year pancreas graft survival for PAK and PA recipients was worse than for SPK recipients. Accurate comparison of survival statistics for SPK versus kidney transplantation alone for diabetics is difficult because the SPK recipients tend to be younger, with less vascular disease. In fact, the mortality rate after SPK transplantation has been reported to increase considerably if patients with heart disease are not excluded as candidates.

Surgical Techniques

Much of the controversy with respect to the optimal surgical technique for pancreas transplantation has been focused on the handling of the exocrine pancreatic secretions. The most commonly used techniques are enteric drainage and bladder drainage. Other management techniques (duct injection and obliteration) account for less than 1% of cases.

Enteric Drainage of Exocrine Secretions

Enteric drainage of exocrine pancreas secretions has become the most popular of the drainage options. The whole pancreas, together with a segment of donor duodenum, is transplanted with side-to-side anastomosis into the recipient small bowel (primary enteric drainage) (Fig. 14.2). Enteric drainage of the pancreas has several advantages over bladder drainage. It is associated with fewer urologic problems, fewer UTIs, a lower incidence of pancreatitis, and less severe metabolic disturbance. The major problem with enteric drainage is an anastomotic leak, which may lead to early graft loss, intraabdominal sepsis, and the inability to monitor urine amylase for rejection.

Bladder Drainage

The number of centers choosing bladder drainage as their procedure of choice is decreasing. Whole pancreatic grafts are used with a side-to-side pancreaticoduodenocystostomy (Fig. 14.3). The advantages of bladder drainage include a lower surgical complication rate and the use of urinary amylase for monitoring rejections (see the section on the diagnosis of rejection). The pancreas is placed contralateral to the simultaneously performed kidney transplan-

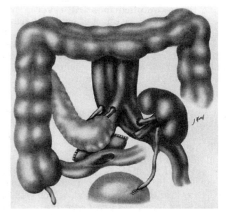

Fig. 14.2.   Enteric drainage (ED) technique. The donor duodenal segment is anastomosed in a side-to-side fashion to the ileum or distal jejunum. (From Pirsch JD, Odorico JS, Sollinger HW: Kidney-pancreas transplantation. In: Schrier RW, Henrich WL, Bennett WM, eds. *Atlas of diseases of the kidney*, vol 5. Philadelphia: Current Medicine, 1999, with permission.)

tation. The disadvantages of bladder drainage are discussed later and are the primary reason for its decreasing popularity.

Systemic Versus Portal Venous Drainage

Carbohydrate metabolism in successful pancreas transplant recipients is similar to that in immunosuppressed nondiabetic kidney transplant recipients. Most transplantation centers use systemic venous drainage of the transplanted pancreas (Figs 14.2 and 14.3). As a result, basal and stimulated peripheral serum insulin levels are two to three times higher than normal because the insulin does not undergo first-pass hepatic uptake and degradation. Patients may be susceptible to postprandial hypoglycemia, and the high ambient insulin levels, insulin resistance, and abnormal lipoprotein metabolism may accelerate atherosclerosis. Portal venous drainage of the transplanted pancreas is preferred in some centers. Portal drainage reduces peripheral hyperinsulinemia and is theoretically more "physiologic." The technique is somewhat more technically challenging, and its relative benefits have not been clearly established.

Complications

Significant surgical complications after pancreas transplantation with bladder drainage occur in about half of patients (Table 14.3), although most are manageable. Even at centers with the best results, the rate of early reoperation and the length of hospital stay are considerably greater for SPK transplantation than for kidney transplantation alone.

For bladder-drained pancreas transplants, urologic complications are common (Table 14.4). About 24% of bladder-drained pan-

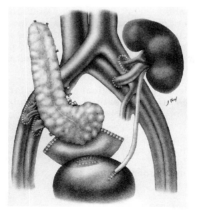

Fig. 14.3. Schematic diagram of the bladder drainage technique for simultaneous kidney and pancreas transplantation. Note side-to-side pancreaticoduodenocystostomy. (In: Schrier RW, Henrich WL, Bennett WM, eds. *Atlas of diseases of the kidney,* vol 5. Philadelphia: Current Medicine, 1999, with permission.)

Table 14.3.   Technical complications in the first year after transplantation in 500 SPK transplants

Complication	Number of Patients[a](%)
Enzymatic leak after bladder drainage	60/388 (15.5)
Enzymatic leak after primary enteric drainage	9/112 (8)
Pancreas thrombosis	5 (1)
Kidney thrombosis	4 (0.8)
Ureteral leak/stricture	7 (1.4)
Intraabdominal abscess	15 (3.0)
Peritonitis and fluid collections	58 (11.6)
Wound infection/dehiscence	60 (12.0)
Other	4 (0.8)

[a] Denominator of 500 transplant unless otherwise stated.
From Sollinger HW, Odorico JS, Knechtle SJ, et al. Experience with 500 simultaneously pancreas-kidney transplants. *Ann Surg* 1998;228:284, with permission.

creas transplants eventually need enteric conversion by removing the pancreas with its duodenal segment from the bladder and reanastomosing it to a loop of small bowel. If possible, the conversion is delayed until at least 6 months after transplantation, at which time the risk for acute rejection is small and the doses of immunosuppressants are relatively low.

Enzyme and Urine Leaks

A leakage from the duodenal segment is most often encountered within the first 3 months after transplantation and is the most frequent serious postoperative complication. For bladder-drained pancreas transplants, leaks occur in about 15% of patients. Enteric-drained pancreas transplants have a lower frequency of leak (8%), but the complication more often leads to graft loss. Patients present with sudden onset of abdominal pain, which may be agonizing, and the serum amylase level is often elevated. For

Table 14.4.   Urological complications in 388 bladder-drained SPK transplants

Complication	Number of Patients (%)
Urinary track infection	242 (62.5)
Hematuria	69 (17.7)
Duodenal segment/bladder leak	60 (15.4)
Urethral stricture	11 (2.8)
Urethral disruption	10 (2.5)
Ureteral stricture	4 (1.03)
Ureteral leak	3 (0.77)

From Sollinger HW, Odorico JS, Knechtle SJ, et al. Experience with 500 simultaneously pancreas-kidney transplants. *Ann Surg* 1998;228:284, with permission.

bladder-drained pancreas transplants, the diagnosis of urine leak is most often made with a cystogram or radionuclide scan (see Chapter 12). Re-exploration is usually required, with closure of the leak or enteric conversion. In some patients with very small leaks, conservative therapy, consisting of placement of a Foley catheter for several weeks, is adequate. Small leaks may be difficult to detect radiologically and are suggested by recurrence of pain after removal of the Foley catheter.

Leaks from enteric-drained pancreas transplants are heralded by the sudden onset of severe abdominal pain, rising amylase and creatinine levels, and fever. They are particularly dangerous because of the intraperitoneal spillage of enteric succus. Diagnosis must not be delayed. Urgent operative intervention is usually required, although contained leaks can sometimes be managed successfully by percutaneous drainage.

Graft Pancreatitis

Pancreatitis of the allograft is a common postoperative complication and can occur in a variety of settings. In the immediate postoperative period, the effects of preservation and handling of the pancreas may induce a transient mild hyperamylasemia without significant clinical consequence. Pancreas rejection may also be heralded by an increase in serum amylase levels, which may be an important marker of rejection in PAK or PA transplantation. Enzymatic leaks may also cause hyperamylasemia.

For bladder-drained pancreas transplants, reflux pancreatitis has been described and is believed to be due to the irritant effects of refluxing urine on the pancreas. It is most common in patients with distended neurogenic bladders. It is managed by Foley drainage, often followed by self-catheterization to avoid high urinary residuals; $alpha_1$-adrenergic receptor blocking agents such as terazosin (Hytrin) may be useful. Enteric conversion may be required.

Vascular Thrombosis

Vascular thrombosis is a well-recognized complication after pancreas transplantation. Systemic anticoagulation with low-dose heparin or dextran infusions is routinely employed at many centers for several days after transplantation. Dextran infusion occasionally causes acute renal failure with tubular vacuolization—an occurrence that may cause diagnostic confusion. Vascular thrombosis of the pancreas can be caused by either arterial or venous thrombosis. In the case of arterial thrombosis, which is rare, the pancreas on reexploration appears soft and pale. In contrast, venous thrombosis is characterized by a large, engorged, dark-blue discolored pancreatic graft.

Pancreatic vascular thrombosis usually presents as abdominal pain with persistent elevation of blood sugar levels and hyperamylasemia. It may be difficult to differentiate from other causes of postoperative pain and graft dysfunction. Diagnosis is usually made radiologically, but exploration is required if the results of diagnostic tests are equivocal or if the clinical situation deteriorates. The thrombosed pancreatic graft must be removed immediately because it constitutes a life-threatening focus of infection and toxemia.

Intraabdominal Abscess

Serious infections are more common after pancreas transplantation than after kidney transplantation alone, and in most series, they are the most common cause of death. The most feared complication is the formation of intraabdominal abscesses or infected peripancreatic fluid collections. In most instances, conservative therapy with antibiotics and percutaneously inserted drains is adequate; if the patient does not respond or infection persists, however, abdominal exploration and possible pancreatectomy should be considered early on. A late complication of peripancreatic infection is the development of a mycotic aneurysm at the site of the arterial anastomosis, resulting in life-threatening bleeding. If the diagnosis of a mycotic aneurysm is suspected, it must be confirmed by angiography, and the pancreas must be removed.

Complications Specific to Bladder-Drained Pancreas Transplants

Urinary Tract Infections

UTIs occur with a high frequency after pancreas transplantation with bladder drainage. In some cases, persistent UTIs are caused by sutures protruding from the anastomotic site; these sutures have to be removed through a cystoscope. In some cases, stone formation around retained sutures is noted. Use of absorbable sutures may prevent this problem.

Recurrent UTIs are a troublesome clinical problem. They are likely a result of the altered physiologic milieu of the bladder due to pancreatic exocrine secretions. Multiple recurrent UTIs are best treated by enteric conversion.

Hematuria

Hematuria after pancreas transplantation with bladder drainage may occur in the acute postoperative period or chronically. Whereas acute postoperative hematuria is usually due to a bleeding vessel, either from the suture line or from the duodenal segment, chronic hematuria may be due to an ulcer in the duodenal segment, granulation tissue at the suture line, or persistent cystitis. In acute cases, cystoscopy, clot evacuation, and cauterization of the bleeding point are usually sufficient. Chronic hematuria is usually treated by excision of the inflammatory focus, removal of sutures, or enteric conversion.

Urethritis

Sterile urethritis with dysuria and balanitis occurs after bladder-drained pancreas transplantation because of the irritant effect of pancreatic enzymes on the lower urinary tract mucosa; urethral strictures sometimes result. They can usually be treated conservatively by Foley drainage or suprapubic cystostomy; enteric conversion is sometimes required.

Metabolic Abnormalities

Complications can arise in bladder-drained pancreas transplantation as a consequence of the loss of large quantities of alkaline, enzyme-rich pancreatic fluid through the urinary tract. Metabolic acidosis, hyponatremia, and extracellular fluid volume depletion may develop, and oral and sometimes intravenous sodium chloride and bicarbonate supplementation are required. If patients are receiving tacrolimus (see the section on immunosuppressive therapy), the bicarbonate should be administered at least 2 hours before or after the dose to avoid impaired tacrolimus absorption.

Immunosuppressive Therapy

Immunosuppressive therapy for all forms of whole organ pancreas transplantation is the same in principle as for kidney transplantation alone and is discussed in detail in Chapter 4. Because of the frequency of acute rejection episodes in SPK transplantation, there is a tendency to use more aggressive immunosuppressive protocols with antibody induction and tacrolimus maintenance therapy often in combination with mycophenolate mofetil. It may be wise to maintain somewhat higher than usual cyclosporine or tacrolimus levels.

Diagnosis of Rejection

The diagnosis of rejection after pancreas transplantation may be extremely difficult. This difficulty can be explained by the histologic sequence of events, which is characterized by a cellular infiltrate first involving the exocrine pancreatic tissues. In the initial phases of the rejection process, the islets are spared, and serum glucose remains normal. Only at the later stages of rejection, when fibrosis, inflammation, and destruction of the islets occur, does the patient become hyperglycemic. At this stage, rejection is usually irreversible. Rejection must be recognized early, before the development of hyperglycemia, to prevent complete destruction of islet tissues.

In SPK transplantation, the kidney allograft is usually involved first in the rejection process, and a significant elevation of serum creatinine levels or a kidney biopsy permits the diagnosis of rejection to be made. Treating the kidney allograft rejection usually adequately treats the concomitant pancreas rejection.

The timely diagnosis of pancreas rejection in PAK and PA transplantation is much more difficult, which may explain their inferior results. Markers of pancreas injury include levels of serum amylase, lipase, and human anodal trypsinogen. Timed urine collections for amylase (expressed as units per hour, typically in a 4-hour collection) are useful in bladder-drained pancreas transplants; the excretion decreases in the early phase of rejection when only the exocrine gland is involved. The definitive diagnosis of pancreas rejection requires invasive techniques, such as transcystoscopic biopsy of the head of the pancreas or percutaneous biopsy using an 18-gauge disposable automatic needle (see Chapter 13), both of which carry a small risk for bleeding and fistula formation. A classification system has been proposed for the pathologic diagnosis of rejection and as a guide to therapy (see Papadimitriou et al. in Selected Readings).

Effect of Pancreas Transplantation on Secondary Diabetic Complications

The purpose of pancreas transplantation is to improve the quality of life of patients with end-stage diabetic nephropathy over and above that which can be achieved by kidney transplantation alone. This is achieved by normalization of carbohydrate metabolism, which frees the patients from years of insulin therapy and dietary constraint, and by arresting, preventing, and even reversing secondary diabetic complications. Although there is no question that a successful procedure makes the patient insulin independent, the effect on secondary manifestations of diabetes is less clear-cut and is the subject of ongoing research and controversy.

Nephropathy

When renal allografts from nondiabetic donors are placed into a diabetic recipient, morphologic signs of diabetic nephropathy in the form of thickening of the glomerular basement membrane appear as early as 2 years after transplantation. No microscopic evidence of diabetic nephropathy is seen up to 4 years after SPK transplantation. Mesangial and glomerular volume and basement membrane thickness are less after SPK transplantation than after kidney transplantation alone. Whereas changes of diabetic nephropathy can often be seen on biopsy specimens of kidneys transplanted alone into diabetic patients, loss of grafts to diabetic nephropathy is unusual, although renal function is better maintained in recipients of SPK transplants. Within the time frame of follow-up presently available, the benefit of SPK transplantation with respect to diabetic nephropathy is usually more evident histologically than clinically.

Neuropathy

Pancreas transplantation alone in preuremic patients has been shown to result in significant improvement in motor and sensory nerve conduction velocity. Subjective and objective improvement of established neuropathy occurs after both SPK and kidney transplantation alone, although a variety of markers of autonomic function have been shown to improve more after SPK transplantation. It is difficult to differentiate between improvement in the uremic and diabetic components of neuropathy, and the added benefit of SPK transplantation may take months or years to manifest clinically.

Retinopathy

Initial studies reported that neither PTA nor SPK transplantation produced a greater improvement in retinopathy than kidney transplantation alone. It is possible that this disappointing failure to show benefit may relate to the relatively short period of follow-up. Long-term studies have observed a trend in favor of pancreas transplantation during follow-up of at least 3 to 4 years.

Microcirculation

Using thermography, muscle oxygen tension measurements, and laser Doppler determination, SPK transplantation has been shown to have a beneficial effect on the microcirculation that is greater than with kidney transplantation alone. This objective determination is strengthened by the clinical observation that SPK transplant recipients suffer fewer amputations and diabetic ulcers of the lower extremities than diabetic patients receiving kidney transplantation alone.

Coronary Artery Disease

Many centers apply more stringent criteria to exclude significant coronary artery disease in candidates for SPK transplantation than in candidates for kidney transplantation alone. Such a policy prevents comparative evaluation of the effect of the pancreas transplantation on the progress of the coronary artery disease. As greater confidence with SPK transplantation has developed, some centers are accepting patients at greater cardiac risk, and comparative groups have shown that the risk for early cardiac-related mortality is equal or greater in the SPK transplant recipients.

Quality of Life

After the first few months following a successful SPK transplantation, patients generally report a better quality of life than that of recipients of kidney transplants alone. SPK transplant recipients have been reported to require less sickness pension, have more full-time employment, and have fewer lost workdays. It is difficult to quantitate the sense of liberation felt by lifetime diabetic patients who no longer must self-inject insulin and monitor every morsel they eat.

Patient Survival

Randomized, controlled trials comparing the survival benefit of kidney alone versus SPK transplantation for diabetics have not been performed.

Uncontrolled data, however, suggest that SPK recipients have improved patient survival rates over diabetic patients transplanted with a kidney alone. The observed survival advantage may be due to patient selection but is reassuring in that the higher morbidity of pancreas transplantation does not appear to be reflected in a survival disadvantage.

Choice of Procedure

Patients and their physician advocates may be faced with a difficult dilemma when choosing between a kidney transplantation alone and an SPK transplantation. This dilemma is reflected in the ongoing discussions on this topic in the medical and transplantation literature. SPK transplantation is associated with increased early morbidity but may offer better long-term quality of life and the greater potential for stabilization or improvement of diabetic complications. Most centers recommend kidney transplantation alone when a live donor is available because this option offers the best long-term patient and graft survival; a PAK transplantation may follow. Patients choosing between SPK and cadaveric kidney transplantation must be thoroughly informed regarding the comparative risks and benefits of the two procedures and, in particular, must have realistic expectations regarding the effect of pancreas transplantation on secondary complications. Patients should also be aware of the fact that, in most regions of the United States, the waiting time for an SPK transplant is about one third of that for a cadaveric transplant alone and that a prolonged period of dialysis may expose them to additional risk.

TRANSPLANTATION OF PANCREATIC ISLETS

The capacity to transplant pancreatic islets successfully and consistently would represent a quantum leap in the management of diabetes mellitus and would relegate our present efforts at whole organ transplantation to the history books. The main appeal of islet transplantation, either as a purified graft or in the form of dispersed pancreatic tissue, is that morbidity of the procedure is very low compared with whole organ transplantation. The goal will be to transplant nonimmunogenic or immunoprotected islets soon after presentation of insulin-dependent diabetes, before the development of diabetic complications.

A normal human pancreas contains about 1 million islets; it has been estimated that more than half a million (about 10,000/kg) are required for normal carbohydrate tolerance. Isolation of sufficient islets from a single cadaveric donor has proved difficult, and multiple pancreases may be required. The results of islet transplantation have generally been disappointing. The islet transplant registry reports that of 305 recipients receiving islet transplantation from cadaver donors, insulin independence was achieved in 13 recipients at 1 year, 7 at 2 years, 4 at 3 years, and 1 at 4 years. In most of these cases, the islets have been injected intraportally to simulate the normal release of insulin into the portal circulation, and all of the patients have required standard immunosuppression.

The problems preventing the stable engraftment of a sufficient number of islets to achieve a state of insulin independence can be broadly classified into four categories: (1) transplantation of an insufficient mass of viable islets, (2) immune-mediated destruction of transplanted islet tissue, (3) drug toxicity (corticosteroids, cyclosporine and tacrolimus are all islet toxic), and (4) metabolic exhaustion due to the foreign microenvironment.

Transplantation of an insufficient mass of islets can be overcome by the use of multiple donors. The disadvantage of this approach is that several donor pancreases are required that could otherwise have been used for whole organ transplantation. Because of the isolated nature of the foreign antigen, immune-mediated destruction of the transplanted islet tissue is vigorous; multiple donors may also make the pancreas even more immunogenic. There are no reliable markers of early islet rejection, and institution of antirejection therapy is often delayed.

Preliminary data suggest that these factors can be largely overcome, and high success rates can be achieved, by minimizing the cold ischemic injury to the islets and by employing a steroid-free immunosuppressive regimen based on low-dose tacrolimus, and sirolimus with anti-CD25 induction (see Chapter 4). Validation of this data may lead to a radical change in the way pancreas transplantation is practiced.

Even well-functioning islets may deteriorate with time, even in the absence of immune attack, a phenomenon ascribed to metabolic exhaustion. Islets removed by separation procedures from their natural environment in the exocrine pancreas may lack growth factors necessary for vascularization and growth. It is possible that the addition of growth factors may overcome this problem, but preliminary attempts have not been encouraging.

Attempts are also being made to make islets less immunogenic by culturing them before transplantation or by immunoprotecting them with membranes or capsules. Successful islet transplantation in monkey models has been reported with selective blockade of the CD40–CD154 costimulatory pathway (see Chapters 2 and 4). If pancreatic islet transplantation is to become a therapeutic reality for all diabetic patients rather than the minority that reach

ESRD, nonhuman sources will be required, and the barriers of xenotransplantation will need to be crossed.

SELECTED READINGS

Gross CR, Limwattananon C, Matthees BJ. Quality of life after pancreas transplantation: a review. *Clin Transplant* 1998;12:351.

Gruessner AC, Sutherland DER. Analysis of United States (US) and non-US pancreas transplants as reported to the International Pancreas Transplant Registry (IPTR) and to the United Network for Organ Sharing (UNOS). In: Cecka JM, Terasaki PI, eds. *Clinical transplants 1998.* Los Angeles: UCLA Tissue Typing Laboratory, 1999:53–71.

Hering BJ, Ricordi C. Islet transplantation for patients with type 1 diabetes. *Graft* 1999;2:12.

Herzog CA, Marwick TH, Pheley AM, et al. Dobutamine stress echocardiography for the detection of significant coronary artery disease in renal transplant candidates. *Am J Kidney Dis* 1999;33:1080.

Hricik DE. Combined kidney-pancreas transplantation. *Kidney Int* 1998;53:1091.

Lederes E. Pancreas transplants for diabetic nephropathy: a time for reassessment. *Amer J Kidney Dis* 2000;35:1238.

Manske CL, Wang Y, Thomas W. Mortality of cadaveric kidney transplantation versus combined kidney pancreas transplantation in diabetic patients. *Lancet* 1995;346:1658.

Manske CL, Thomas W, Wang W, et al. Screening diabetic transplant candidates for coronary artery disease: identification of a low risk subgroup. *Kidney Int* 1993;44:617.

Mizrahi SS, Jones JW, Bentley FR. Preparing for pancreas transplantation: donor selection, retrieval technique, preservation, and basic table preparation. *Transplant Rev* 1996;10:1.

Navarro X, Sutherland DE, Kennedy WR. Long-term effects of pancreatic transplantation on diabetic neuropathy. *Ann Neurol* 1997;42:727.

Papadmitriou JC, Drachenberg CB, Wiland A, et al. Histologic grading of acute allograft rejection in pancreas needle biopsy. *Transplantation* 1998;66:1741.

Pirsch JD, Andrews C, Hricik DE, et al. Pancreas transplantation for diabetes mellitus. *Am J Kidney Dis* 1996;27:444.

Pirsch JD, Odorico JS, D'Alessandro AM, et al. Posttransplant infection in enteric versus bladder-drained simultaneous pancreas-kidney transplant recipients. *Transplantation* 1998;66:1746.

Shapiro AM, Lakey JR, Ryan EA, et al. Islet transplantation in seven patients with type 1 diabetes mellitus using a glucocorticoid-free immunosuppressive regimen. *N Engl J Med* 2000;243:230.

Smets YFC, Westendorp RGJ, van der Pijl JW, et al. Effect of simultaneous pancreas-kidney transplantation on mortality of patients with type-1 diabetes mellitus and end-stage renal failure. *Lancet* 1999;353:1915.

Stratta RJ. Review of immunosuppressive usage in pancreas transplantation. *Clin Transplant* 1999;13:1.

Vandenberg BF, Rossen JD, Grover-McKay M, et al. Evaluation of diabetic patients for renal and pancreas transplantation: noninvasive screening for coronary artery disease using radionuclide methods. *Transplantation* 1996;62:1230.

15

Kidney Transplantation in Children

Samhar I. Al-Akash and Robert B. Ettenger

Kidney transplantation is universally accepted as the therapy of choice for children with end-stage renal disease (ESRD). Successful transplantation in children and adolescents not only ameliorates uremic symptoms but also allows for significant improvement, and often correction, of delayed skeletal growth, sexual maturation, cognitive performance, and psychosocial functioning. The child with a well-functioning kidney can lead a quality of life that cannot be achieved by any dialysis therapy.

Current success in pediatric renal transplantation is attributed to improvements in immunosuppressive therapy, histocompatibility matching, and the provision of age-appropriate clinical care. For pediatric patients of all ages, transplantation results in better survival than dialysis. Nevertheless, success in pediatric kidney transplantation is still a challenging undertaking. Children and adolescents are constantly growing, developing, and changing. Each developmental stage produces a series of medical, biologic, and psychological challenges that must be appropriately addressed if truly successful graft outcome and rehabilitation are to be realized.

Much of the statistical data reviewed in this chapter comes from databases that have provided an invaluable resource for the advancement of pediatric transplantation. These databases have permitted the evaluation and extrapolation of data from multiple pediatric renal transplant programs that tend to be small compared with their adult counterparts. Major databases referred to are the *North America Pediatric Renal Transplant Cooperative Study* (NAPRTCS) and the *United States Renal Data System* (USRDS) annual report.

EPIDEMIOLOGY OF END-STAGE RENAL DISEASE IN CHILDREN

Incidence

The incidence and prevalence of treated pediatric ESRD have been increasing since 1989. As of 1999, the incidence rate of new cases of ESRD in children 0 to 19 years of age was 15 per million U.S. child population per year. The point prevalence of ESRD in this population is 70 per million child population. The incidence of ESRD increases with age, with the highest incidence observed in children between 15 and 19 years of age (28 per million). Adolescents compose about 50% of treated pediatric ESRD patients.

There is a wide variation by race in the incidence rates of treated ESRD. Black children have the highest incidence rate of 27 per million, compared with 12 per million whites, 15 per million Asians and Pacific Islanders, and 17 per million Native Americans for the period between 1995 and 1997. The incidence is higher in blacks across all age groups but is most prominent in the 15- to 19-year-old age group (60 per million blacks compared with 20 per million whites). Boys have higher incidence of treated ESRD than girls in all age groups because of a higher incidence of congenital disorders.

Etiology

Glomerular diseases account for about 30% and congenital, hereditary, and cystic diseases for 26% of cases of pediatric ESRD (Table 15.1). In contrast to adults, ESRD due to diabetes mellitus or hypertension is rare in children.

The etiology of ESRD varies significantly by age. Congenital, hereditary, and cystic diseases cause ESRD in more than 52% of children 0 to 4 years of age, whereas glomerulonephritis and focal segmental glomerulosclerosis account for 38% of cases of ESRD in patients 10 to 19 years of age. The most common diagnosis in transplanted children is structural disease (49%), followed by various forms of glomerulonephritis (14%) and focal segmental glomerulosclerosis (12%) (Table 15.2).

Access to Transplantation

The NAPRTCS registry reports that 5,958 children received 6,534 transplants between 1987 and 1998. At the time of transplantation, about 46% of pediatric recipients of kidney transplants are older than 12 years of age, 34% are 6 to 12 years of age, 15% are between the ages of 2 and 5 years, and only about 5% are younger than 2 years of age. The mean age of pediatric patients receiving a kidney transplant is 10.9 years. Sixty percent are male, 62% are white, 16% are black, and 16% are Hispanic.

Pediatric transplants constitute 4% to 6% of all transplants in the United States. The absolute numbers of pediatric kidney transplants have remained relatively constant. Because of the increasing popularity of transplantation in the entire ESRD community, however, the percentage of pediatric transplantations is decreasing. In 1990, patients younger than 18 years of age composed 4.9% of cadaver donor transplant recipients, whereas in 1998, they represented only 3.6%. Similarly, in 1990, pediatric patients received 13.6% of all live donor transplants, whereas in 1998, they received only 8.6% of such transplants.

Nevertheless, according to the USRDS, the rates for both living-related and cadaver renal transplantation are higher in children than in adults. For children 0 to 19 years of age, there were 29 live donor transplants and 27 cadaver donor transplants per 100 dialysis patient years. These figures are more than double the corresponding rates for adults 20 to 44 years of age. The highest rates of transplantation are in the 5- to 9-year-old group, with 40 live donor transplants and 46 cadaver donor transplants performed per 100 dialysis patient years.

Nearly half of all pediatric kidney transplants come from living donors. In pediatric renal transplantation, living donation has been on the rise in the past few years; since 1995, about 55% of transplants have come from living donors, compared with 42% in the period from 1987 to 1991. This trend is undoubtedly a result of the awareness that transplantation is the best therapeutic option for children with ESRD combined with the increased waiting times for cadaver donor organs (see Chapter 1).

Table 15.1.   Incidence of treated end-stage renal disease in pediatric patients[a] according to primary disease, 1993–1997

Primary Renal Disease	Incidence (%)
Glomerulonephritis (GN)	**29.8**
Focal segmental glomerulosclerosis	10.0
Membranoproliferative GN	2.5
Rapidly progressive GN	2.1
IgA nephropathy	1.6
Goodpasture's syndrome	0.7
Membranous nephropathy	0.5
Other proliferative GN	1.5
Unspecified GN	10.3
Cystic, hereditary, and congenital disease	**26.0**
Renal hypoplasia, dysplasia	8.9
Congenital obstructive uropathy	6.7
Alport's syndrome, other familial disease	2.7
Autosomal dominant polycystic disease	2.0
Autosomal recessive polycystic disease	1.0
Prune belly syndrome	1.1
Congenital nephrotic syndrome	1.2
Medullary cystic disease (nephronophthisis)	1.1
Cystinosis	0.7
Other	0.3
Interstitial nephritis, pyelonephritis	**9.1**
Nephrolithiasis, obstruction, gout	3.2
Chronic interstitial nephritis	2.0
Chronic pyelonephritis, reflux nephropathy	2.7
Nephropathy caused by other agents	0.9
Secondary GN, vasculitis	**8.9**
Systemic lupus erythematosus	4.6
Hemolytic-uremic syndrome	1.9
Henoch-Schönlein purpura	0.9
Wegener's granulomatosis	0.7
Hypertension	**4.8**
Hypertension, no primary renal disease	4.5
Renal artery stenosis or occlusion	0.3
Miscellaneous conditions	**3.8**
Diabetes mellitus	1.6
Neoplasms	0.6
Tubular necrosis (no recovery)	1.0
Uncertain etiology	**7.1**

[a] Patients younger than 20 years of age.
Modified from the USRDS 1999 annual report.

**Table 15.2.   Causes of end-stage renal disease
in pediatric transplant recipients, 1987–1998**

Primary Disease	Percentage of Patients
Structural disease	48.7
Glomerulonephritis	14.5
Focal segmental glomerulosclerosis	11.8
Hemolytic-uremic syndrome	2.6
Congenital nephrotic syndrome	2.6
Familial nephritis (Alport's syndrome)	2.4
Cystinosis	2.2
Renal infarct	1.8
Other	13.4

Children continue to represent an ever-decreasing percentage of the waiting list for cadaver donors. In 1990, patients younger than 18 years of age composed 3.6% of the waiting list, whereas in 1998, they represented only 2.9%, despite the absolute number of such patients increasing by 13%. Median waiting times continue to lengthen for potential pediatric recipients of cadaver donor transplants. In 1998, the median waiting times for children 1 to 5, 6 to 10, and 11 to 18 years of age were 236, 339, and 561 days, respectively.

Timing of Transplantation

Renal transplantation is considered when renal replacement therapy is indicated. In children, dialysis may be required before transplantation to optimize nutritional and metabolic conditions, to achieve an appropriate size in small children, or to keep a patient stable until a suitable donor is available. Many centers want a recipient to weigh at least 8 to 10 kg, both to minimize the risk for vascular thrombosis and to accommodate an adult-sized kidney. In infants with ESRD, a target weight of 10 kg may not be achieved until 12 to 24 months of age. At experienced centers, however, transplantation has been successful in children who weighed less than 10 kg or were less than 6 months of age.

Preemptive transplantation (i.e. transplantation without prior dialysis) accounts for 24% of all pediatric renal transplantations. The major reason cited by patients and families for the decision to undertake preemptive transplantation is the desire to avoid dialysis. Candidates for preemptive transplantation should have careful psychological assessment before transplantation because there may be a tendency for noncompliance in this group of recipients. Nevertheless, there appears to be no impairment in graft outcome in pediatric recipients who have undergone preemptive transplantation when compared with those who have undergone dialysis before transplantation, and some data suggest a small improvement in allograft outcome. The reasons for the improved graft survival are unknown. Because of the prolonged waiting time for cadaveric donors, most kidneys for preemptive transplants are from living donors.

Patient and Graft Survival

Patient survival after transplantation is superior to that achieved by dialysis for all pediatric age groups. The 1-, 2-, and 5-year survival rates are 97%, 96%, and 94%, respectively, for all primary transplants. Survival rates for recipients of primary transplants are excellent for both cadaveric and living donor groups: the 1-, 2-, and 5-year rates for recipients of living donor kidneys are 98%, 97%, and 95%, respectively; they are 97%, 95%, and 92%, respectively, for recipients of cadaveric kidneys. Patients younger than 2 years of age have the lowest graft survival rates: 90% and 79% at 3 years for recipients of living and cadaver donor kidneys, respectively. Infection accounts for 35% of deaths. Other causes include cardiopulmonary disease (16%), malignancy (11%), and dialysis-related complications following graft failure (2.4%). About 45% of patients who die do so with a functioning graft.

Of the more than 6,500 pediatric kidney transplantations reported to NAPRTCS since 1987, about 25% have failed. Chronic rejection is the leading cause of graft failure and accounts for 31% of failures. Other causes include acute rejection (16%), vascular thrombosis (12%), recurrence of original disease (6%), patient noncompliance (3.6%), primary nonfunction (2.6%), infection (2.2%), malignancy (1.2%), and death due to other causes (10%). Although some causes of graft failure, such as graft thrombosis and recurrence of the original disease, have remained constant during the past 10 years, loss from acute rejection has decreased dramatically. On the other hand, loss from chronic rejection has increased and now accounts for 41% of graft failure.

PROGNOSTIC FACTORS INFLUENCING GRAFT SURVIVAL

Dramatic improvements have been made in short- and long-term graft survival rates. Graft survival is 92% at 1 year and 74% at 7 years for live donor transplant recipients and 83% and 59% for cadaveric graft recipients. The following factors are important determinants of the improving graft survival in pediatric patients.

Donor Source

Short- and long-term graft and patient survival rates are better in recipients of live donor transplants in all pediatric age groups. Registry data show that recipients of kidneys from living donors have a 10% to 20% advantage in graft survival at 1, 3, and 5 years. Younger transplant recipients benefit the most from live donor transplantation and enjoy a 20% to 30% better graft survival rate 5 years after transplantation. Shorter cold ischemia time, better human leukocyte antigen (HLA) matches, lower acute rejection rates, and better preoperative preparation help account for the better outcome in recipients of live donor kidneys.

Recipient Age

Children younger than 6 years of age, especially those younger than 2 years of age, have lower graft survival rates than older children, especially with cadaver donor kidneys (Table 15.3). The 5-year graft survival rates in recipients younger than 2 years of age are 80% and 52% for live and cadaver donor transplants, respectively. This is primarily due to early graft losses within

Table 15.3.   Recipient age and graft survival

Recipient age (yr)	Graft Survival (%) in Living Donor Recipients at Follow-up		Graft Survival (%) in Cadaver Donor Recipients at Follow-up	
	6 mo	5 yr	6 mo	5 yr
<2	87	80	67	52
2–5	92	80	82	69
6–12	95	82	86	69
>12	95	77	88	61

the first 6 months after transplantation. Higher rates of vascular thrombosis and irreversible acute rejection help account for this early graft loss.

Young renal transplant recipients tend to have more severe outcomes from acute rejection. In infants with a cadaver donor graft, 14% of acute rejection episodes result in transplant failure or death, compared with rates of 6% to 7% in older children. In recipients of live donor transplants, the results are not as extreme: 8% of acute rejections in infants eventuate in graft loss or death, compared with 4% to 5% in older children.

The 5-year graft survival rates in recipients older than 12 years of age are 5% to 10% lower than those in recipients between 2 and 12 years of age. Higher rates of medication noncompliance have been cited as one cause for these outcomes.

Donor Age

Kidneys from donors aged 16 to 40 years provide optimal graft survival and function. Although transplanted kidneys grow in size with the growth of the recipient, transplantation with cadaver kidneys from donors younger than 6 years old is associated with markedly decreased graft survival, with a relative risk for graft loss of 1.22. The 5-year graft survival rate for recipients of cadaver kidneys from donors younger than 1 year of age is only about 50%, compared with 60% and 70% for recipients of grafts from donors 2 to 5 years of age and older than 6 years of age, respectively. Children younger than 5 years old receiving a kidney from a donor younger than 6 years old have the highest relative risk of graft failure (2.01).

Cadaver kidneys from donors older than 50 years of age are more likely to result in suboptimal long-term outcome (see Chapter 1). The older the donor, the greater is the decline of renal function with time. This is an important consideration in pediatric renal transplantation because graft function has an important effect on posttransplantation growth.

Race

In recipients of live donor kidneys, black race is the most significant factor associated with poor outcome. Black race is second only to young recipient age (less than 2 years) as a predictor of graft failure in recipients of cadaver donor kidneys. Compared with rates in white children, graft survival rates in black children are lower by 10% and 25% 1 and 5 years after transplantation, respectively, for recipients of live donor kidneys. For cadaver donor transplants, the 5-year graft survival in black recipients is lower than that in white recipients by about 20%.

Human Leukocyte Antigen Matching in Children

Long-term graft survival is best when the donor is an HLA-identical sibling. Transplants from HLA haploidentical sibling donors have a half-life (time to failure of 50% of grafts) of 12 to 14 years, compared with 25 years in transplant recipients from HLA-identical siblings. The excellent results of living-unrelated donor transplantation and the importance of HLA matching in cadaveric transplantation are discussed in Chapter 3.

Presensitization

Repeated blood transfusions expose the recipient to a wide range of HLA antigens and may result in sensitization to these antigens, leading to higher rates of rejection and graft failures. The graft failure rate almost doubles in live donor transplant recipients with more than five blood transfusions before transplantation compared with those who had five or fewer transfusions (30% versus 15%, respectively, 5 years after transplantation). The figures for cadaveric transplant recipients are 45% in those with prior history of more than five blood transfusions and 30% in those who had five or fewer transfusions. Fortunately, blood transfusions have become less common since human recombinant erythropoietin became an integral part of ESRD therapy. Similarly, sensitization may result from rejection of a previous transplant, and the 5-year graft survival for repeat cadaveric transplantations is about 20% lower.

Immunologic Factors

Immunologic parameters in younger children are different from those in adults and older children. Such differences include higher numbers of T and B cells, higher CD4+-to-CD8+ T-cell ratio, and increased blastogenic responses. These differences may account for increased immune responsiveness to HLA antigens and may be partly responsible for the higher rates of rejection observed in children.

Technical Factors and Delayed Graft Function

Small children present a difficult challenge in the operating room. The relatively large size of the graft may result in longer anastomosis times, longer ischemia time, and subsequently higher rates of early graft dysfunction. Delayed graft function (DGF; see Chapter 8) occurs in about 5% of live donor and 20% of cadaver donor transplantations and is associated with a reduced graft survival. In children with DGF (defined by the requirement for dialysis within the first week of transplantation), the 3-year graft survival rates are reduced by about 20% and 30% in recipients of cadaver and live donor kidneys, respectively. Risk factors for DGF are more than five prior transfusions, prior transplantation, native nephrectomy, and black race.

The transplanted kidney is usually placed in an extraperitoneal location when possible to allow easier clinical monitoring and access to the graft. Occasionally, native kidney nephrectomy is necessary at the time of transplantation to make room for the transplanted kidney, especially in a very small child. The aorta and inferior vena cava are usually used for anastomosis to ensure adequate blood flow, but smaller vessels may be used. Vascular anastomosis may be problematic in a child with previous hemodialysis accesses placed in the lower extremities. Children should be evaluated thoroughly before transplantation to identify any potential anastomotic difficulties. Unidentified vascular anomalies may lead to prolonged anastomosis times and subsequently higher rates of DGF and graft thrombosis.

Antibody Induction

Antibody induction with polyclonal antibodies or OKT3 is used either for prophylaxis against rejection or in a sequential manner to avoid nephrotoxicity resulting from early use of calcineurin inhibitors (see Chapter 4). In cadaveric transplantation, antibody induction is associated with about a 10% advantage in the 5-year graft survival rate. First acute rejection episodes tend to be more frequent and to occur earlier in patients not treated with an antilymphocyte preparation.

Transplantation Center Volume

Transplant outcome in high-volume pediatric renal transplant centers has been reported to be superior to that found in lower-volume centers. High-volume centers (defined by the performance of more than 100 pediatric transplants between 1987 and 1995) reported a lower incidence of graft thrombosis and DGF, improved long-term graft survival, and more frequent use of antibody induction.

Cohort Year

The results of pediatric renal transplantation have been dramatically improving. Cadaver donor transplants performed in 1987 to 1988 had a 1-year graft survival rate of 71.7%, whereas live donor transplants had a 1-year survival rate of 88%. In 1997 to 1998, the 1-year graft survival rates for live and cadaveric donor transplants were 92.6% and 94.1%, respectively.

Recurrence of Original Disease

Recurrent disease in the renal graft accounts for graft loss in about 6% of primary transplantations and 10% in repeat transplantations. Both glomerular and metabolic diseases can recur after transplantation, with most recurrences caused by glomerular disease. The most common causes of recurrence in children are discussed next. Recurrent disease in adults is discussed in Chapters 6 and 9.

Glomerular Diseases

Focal segmental glomerulosclerosis (FSGS) is the most common cause of graft loss due to recurrent disease. It recurs in 30% to 40% of patients undergoing primary transplantation and in 50% to 80% of those undergoing subsequent transplantation and leads to graft failure in about half of these patients. Recurrence is usually characterized by massive proteinuria, hypoalbuminemia, and often the full-blown picture of nephrotic syndrome with edema or anasarca and hypercholesterolemia. It may present immediately or weeks to months after transplantation. Predictors of recurrence include rapid progression to ESRD from the time of initial diagnosis (less than 3 years), poor response to therapy, younger age at diagnosis (but older than 6 years of age), black race, and presence of mesangial proliferation in the native kidney. In recent years, a protein permeability factor has been isolated from sera of patients with FSGS, and its concentration was found to correlate with recurrence and severity of disease in the transplanted kidney. The precise nature of this factor remains unclear, and there is no clinically approved assay.

Early posttransplant recognition of recurrent FSGS is important because plasmapheresis (which may lower the serum levels of protein permeability factor), and high-dose cyclosporine, may lead to significant reduction in graft losses due to recurrent FSGS. Cyclosporine is used in doses that maintain trough levels between 500 and 700 ng/mL or higher and is tapered slowly after achieving remission of the nephrotic syndrome and as cholesterol concentration decreases, or if significant toxicity develops. Rapid tapering of cyclosporine may induce relapse. Plasmapheresis is generally used with a frequency that matches disease severity and is occasionally required on a weekly basis for prolonged periods. Cyclophosphamide has been found to induce remission by some investigators. Live donor transplant recipients have a higher rate of recurrence; however, the controlled settings of live donor transplantation allow for preoperative and early postoperative plasmapheresis. This approach may prevent or decrease the severity of recurrent disease. The potential for recurrence of FSGS is not generally regarded as a contraindication to live donor transplantation, although if a primary transplant has been lost to rapid recurrence, it may not be wise to use a living donor for a repeat transplantation.

ALPORT'S SYNDROME. Alport's syndrome itself does not recur; however, anti-glomerular basement membrane (anti-GBM) glomerulonephritis may occur after transplantation and often leads to graft loss. This usually occurs in hemizygous males with Alport's syndrome because of complete absence of the alpha$_5$ noncollagenous portion of type IV collagen in the GBM; the entity has also been reported in heterozygous females with Alport's syndrome. Anti-GBM glomerulonephritis presents as rapidly progressive crescentic glomerulonephritis with linear deposits of IgG along the basement membrane and most commonly leads to graft loss. Asymptomatic cases with linear IgG deposits have also been reported. Fortunately, this complication is rare and probably affects less than 5% of recipients with Alport's syndrome.

MEMBRANOPROLIFERATIVE GLOMERULONEPHRITIS. Histologic evidence of recurrence of membranoproliferative glomerulonephritis type I varies widely, with reported rates from 20% to 70%. Graft loss occurs in up to 30% of cases. Histologic recurrence of type II disease occurs in virtually all cases; however, most of these recurrences are benign without causing graft dysfunction or loss. Presence of crescents in the native kidney may predict severe recurrence that often leads to graft loss. Plasmapheresis and high-dose corticosteroids have been reported to be beneficial in a few cases of recurrent type II disease.

IGA NEPHROPATHY AND HENOCH-SCHÖNLEIN PURPURA. Histologic recurrence with mesangial IgA deposits is common and occurs in about half of patients with IgA nephropathy and in about 30% of patients with Henoch-Schönlein purpura. Most of the recurrences are asymptomatic, but graft loss may occur, often associated with crescent formation.

HEMOLYTIC-UREMIC SYNDROME. Transplantation should be performed at least after 1 year of quiescent disease to lessen the chances of recurrence. Recurrent hemolytic-uremic syndrome has been reported in up to half of cases in some series; however, rates as low as 1% to 4% have been observed in large series. The diarrhea-associated, or "typical," form does not usually recur after transplantation. Recurrence of the "atypical" form has been linked to the use of cyclosporine and antithymocyte globin, and more recently to tacrolimus use. Recurrence is localized to the kidney without evidence of hemolysis or thrombocytopenia in more than half of cases. It typically presents shortly after starting treatment with cyclosporine or tacrolimus, with a decline in urine output, a decrease in the rate of decline in serum creatinine, or an elevated serum creatinine level, with or without hematuria or proteinuria. Doppler or nuclear perfusion studies typically show evidence of acute tubular necrosis with no impairment in perfusion except in severe cases. Because of the nonspecific clinical course, a renal biopsy should be performed as soon as possible to confirm the diagnosis. The most important aspects of therapy are stopping the calcineurin inhibitor and starting plasmapheresis, in addition to augmenting the rejection prophylaxis regimen. Restarting cyclosporine or tacrolimus after recovery of the graft function has been reported to be successful, but with recurrence rates of 20% to 30%. In some series, substitution of cyclosporine for tacrolimus (or *vice versa*) has been successful, and there is anecdotal experience of sirolimus use in this situation.

ANTI-GLOMERULAR BASEMENT MEMBRANE DISEASE. Anti-GBM disease is rare in children. A high level of circulating anti-GBM antibody before transplantation is thought to be associated with higher rate of recurrence. Therefore, a waiting period of 6 to 12 months with an undetectable titer of anti-GBM antibody is recommended before transplantation to prevent recurrence. Reappearance of anti-GBM antibody in the serum may be associated with histologic recurrence. Histologic recurrence has been reported in up to half of cases, with clinical manifestations of nephritis in only 25% of these cases. Graft loss is rare, and spontaneous resolution may occur.

CONGENITAL NEPHROTIC SYNDROME. The Finnish type of congenital nephrotic syndrome is an autosomal recessive disease that manifests as heavy proteinuria, edema, and ascites in the neonatal period. It does not recur after transplantation; however, *de novo* steroid-resistant nephrotic syndrome has been reported in up to 24% of cases. It presents with proteinuria, hypoalbuminemia, and edema that may start immediately or as late as 3 years after transplantation. Precedent infection with cytomegalovirus (CMV) or Epstein-Barr virus (EBV) occurs in most cases. The histologic lesion in these cases is that of minimal-change disease, although some patients have glomerular endothelial cell swelling. Response to therapy with steroids and cyclophosphamide is poor, and graft loss occurs in more than 60% of cases. Within the NAPRTCS database, vascular thrombosis and death with a functioning graft (mostly due to infectious complications) occur in 26% and 23% of cases, respectively, and account for higher rate of graft failure in this particular group.

MEMBRANOUS NEPHROPATHY.   Recurrence of membranous nephropathy is rare in children. *De novo* membranous nephropathy occurs more frequently and affects less than 10% of transplanted children. It usually presents later (4 months to 6 years after transplantation) than recurrent membranous nephropathy, which usually becomes apparent within the first 2 years (the mean follow-up at the time of diagnosis is 10 months in de novo disease, compared with 22 months in recurrent disease). The occurrence of either form of membranous nephropathy does not appear to affect graft outcome in the absence of rejection.

OTHER GLOMERULAR DISEASES.   Recurrence of systemic lupus erythematosus is rare, and recurrent disease does not cause significant clinical disease and is often responsive to immunosuppressive therapy. Wegener's granulomatosis recurs in a small number of patients and rarely causes graft loss. Cyclophosphamide appears to be beneficial in the treatment of recurrent Wegener's granulomatosis.

Metabolic Diseases

PRIMARY HYPEROXALURIA TYPE I.   Oxalosis results from deficiency of hepatic peroxisomal alanine glyoxylate aminotransferase (AGT). Deficiency of this enzyme leads to deposition of oxalate in all body tissues, including the kidneys, myocardium, and bone. Renal transplantation alone does not correct the enzymatic deficiency, and therefore, graft loss is inevitable in these cases because of oxalate deposition in the graft. More recently, therapy with a combined or two-stage liver and kidney transplantation has led to higher rates of success. The transplanted liver corrects the enzymatic deficiency and helps to mobilize tissue oxalate, whereas the transplanted well-functioning kidney excretes the mobilized plasma oxalate.

Success of this approach is greatly facilitated by immediate graft function with a good diuresis. This goal can be accomplished with the use of a large live donor kidney, avoidance of early use of cyclosporine or tacrolimus, and the use of antibody induction. Aggressive perioperative hemodialysis serves to decrease the oxalate load to safe levels and prevent nephrocalcinosis (aim for plasma oxalate level of less than 50 mg/mL). Aggressive long-term dialysis before transplantation may serve to decrease tissue deposition of oxalate. Posttransplant treatment includes pyridoxine, neutral phosphate, citrate, and noncalciuric diuretics. Prevention and early treatment of infections and dehydration are also crucial to maintain good graft function. Finally, combined transplantation early in the course of renal disease, preferably before the glomerular filtration rate (GFR) decreases below 20 to 25 mL/min per 1.73 m^2, serves to optimize outcome and prevent severe complications of the disease that may lead to irreversible morbidity and handicap.

NEPHROPATHIC CYSTINOSIS.   Transplantation in children with cystinosis corrects the transport defect in the kidney but not other organs affected by the disease. Hypothyroidism, visual abnormalities, and central nervous system manifestations are not corrected by transplantation and require ongoing therapy with cysteamine and thyroid hormone. Cystine crystals can be found in the renal graft interstitium within macrophages of host origin. This does not result in recurrence of Fanconi's syndrome or graft dysfunction.

SICKLE CELL ANEMIA. The graft survival rate in patients with sickle cell disease is low, with only about 25% of grafts functioning beyond 1 year after transplantation. The improvement in the hematocrit results in higher numbers of abnormal red blood cells, leading to sickling episodes in the renal graft.

PRETRANSPLANTATION EVALUATION

Evaluation of the Potential Living Donor

The evaluation and preparation of a living donor for a child is essentially the same as for an adult (see Chapter 5). As a general rule, it is possible to consider an adult donor of almost any size for a child, no matter how young. Live donation from siblings is usually restricted to donors who have reached their 18th birthday, although the courts have given permission for younger children to donate under extraordinary circumstances.

Histocompatibility matching considerations are not different for pediatric recipients of kidneys from live donors. HLA-identical transplants are optimal and enable the lowest amount of immunosuppression to be used, thereby minimizing steroid and other side effects. The first living donor for a child is most frequently a one-haplotype–matched parent. There are some theoretical reasons why maternal live donor transplants may fare better than paternal ones (see Chapter 3), but differences in outcome, if any, are small. Second-degree relatives and zero-haplotype–matched siblings may also be considered as donors. The excellent results of nonbiologically related live donor transplants are not dependent on high degrees of HLA matching. Siblings may become donors as they reach the age of consent.

Evaluation of the Recipient

The evaluation of the potential pediatric transplant recipient is similar to that performed in adults (see Chapter 6), but because certain problems occur with more frequency in children, the emphasis may be different. It is important to establish the precise cause of ESRD in children whenever possible. Surgical correction may be required for certain structural abnormalities before transplantation (see Urologic Problems). The precise cause of metabolic or glomerular disease should also be established if possible, because of the possibility of posttransplantation recurrence. Discussions of some common medical, surgical, and psychiatric issues in pediatric transplant candidates follow.

Neuropsychiatric Development

INFANTS. Infants with ESRD during the first year of life frequently suffer neurologic abnormalities. These include alterations in mental function, microcephaly, and involuntary motor phenomena, such as myoclonus, cerebellar ataxia, tremors, seizures, and hypotonia. The pathogenesis is unclear, although aluminum toxicity has been incriminated. Preemptive kidney transplantation or institution of dialysis at the earliest sign of head-circumference growth rate reduction or developmental delay may ameliorate the problem. Some studies describe an improvement in psychomotor delay in some infants with successful transplantation, with a significant percentage of infants regaining normal developmental milestones. Tests of global intelligence show increased rates of improvement after successful transplantation.

OLDER CHILDREN.   It is often difficult to assess to what extent uremia contributes to cognitive delay and impairment in older children. Uremia has an adverse, but often reversible, effect on a child's mental functioning, and it may often cause psychological depression. It may be necessary to institute dialysis and improve the uremic symptomatology before making a precise assessment of the child's mental function. Initiation of dialysis often clarifies the picture and permits progression to transplantation in situations in which it might otherwise have not seemed feasible. On the other hand, severely retarded children respond poorly to the constraints of ESRD care. A child with a very low IQ cannot comprehend the need for procedures that are often confusing and uncomfortable. In this situation, the family must be involved and supported in the decision to embark on a treatment course that does not include chronic dialysis or transplantation.

SEIZURES.   A seizure disorder requiring anticonvulsant medication may be present in up to 10% of young pediatric transplant candidates. Before transplantation, seizures should be controlled, whenever possible, with drugs that do not interfere with calcineurin inhibitor or prednisone metabolism (see Chapter 4). Benzodiazepines are a good choice when circumstances permit. Carbamazepine does reduce calcineurin inhibitor and prednisone levels, but its effect is not as strong as that of phenytoin (Dilantin) or barbiturates. Should it prove to be necessary to use one of the latter drugs for seizure control, a moderately augmented dose of prednisone should be given twice daily. The calcineurin inhibitor may need to be administered 3 times per day or the dose adjusted upward to achieve the desired trough levels, which should be monitored closely.

Psychoemotional Status

Psychiatric and emotional disorders are not by themselves contraindications to dialysis and transplantation; however, the involvement of health care professionals skilled in the care of affected children is mandatory. Primary psychiatric problems may be amenable to therapy and should not exclude children from consideration for transplantation.

Noncompliance is a particularly prevalent problem in adolescent transplant recipients. Patterns of medication and dialysis compliance should be established as part of the transplant evaluation. Psychiatric evaluation should be performed in high-risk cases. If noncompliance is identified or anticipated, behavioral modification programs or other interventions should be in place before transplantation.

Cardiovascular Disease

Children and adolescents are unlikely to have overt cardiovascular disease that requires invasive diagnostic work-up. Hypertension and chronic fluid overload during dialysis may predispose to left ventricular hypertrophy, and severe hypertensive cardiomyopathy and congestive heart failure may supervene. Even at this relatively late stage, kidney transplantation may be beneficial to cardiac function. The importance of hypertension control in children with ESRD cannot be overemphasized, and bilateral nephrectomy is occasionally required. Premature cardiovascular disease is a common feature of adults who have suffered childhood ESRD, and attention to "adult" cardiovascular disease risk factors in childhood may serve to minimize long-term morbidity and mortality.

Infection

COMMON BACTERIAL PATHOGENS. Urinary tract infections and infections related to peritoneal dialysis are the most common sources of bacterial infection in children with ESRD. Aggressive antibiotic therapy and prophylaxis of urinary tract infections in children may effectively suppress infection, although pretransplantation nephrectomy is occasionally required for recalcitrant infections in children with reflux. Peritonitis and related infections with peritoneal dialysis are discussed later.

CYTOMEGALOVIRUS. The incidence of CMV infection increases with age, and young children are unlikely to have developed CMV seropositivity. This should be considered when planning posttransplantation CMV prophylaxis (see Chapter 10).

EPSTEIN-BARR VIRUS. It is important to establish the EBV antibody status of the child. As with CMV, EBV infections and resultant seropositivity increase with age. Primary EBV infection, in the context of potent immunosuppression, may predispose to a particularly aggressive form of posttransplantation lymphoproliferative disorder (PTLD) (see Chapter 9).

IMMUNIZATION STATUS. Immunizations should be brought up to date whenever possible. Live viral vaccines are contraindicated in the immunosuppressed patient; therefore, every effort should be made to complete these vaccinations before transplantation, varicella vaccination included. Vaccination of the immunosuppressed host may fail to induce an adequate immune response, especially with the use of agents, such as mycophenolate mofetil (MMF), that suppress antibody production.

Diphtheria and tetanus vaccine, as well as hepatitis B, can be given safely after transplantation, although pretransplantation administration is preferred. *Haemophilus influenzae* type vaccine is also safe, but data regarding its use after transplantation are not available. Influenza and pneumococcal vaccines are recommended for the pediatric transplant recipient. Most of the available data on their effectiveness come from transplant recipients treated with cyclosporine or azathioprine. Studies are needed to address the immune responsiveness to vaccines under immunosuppression with newer agents.

Urologic Problems

Urologic problems are best addressed before transplantation. Children with urologic disease and renal dysplasia often require multiple operations to normalize urinary tract anatomy and function. Such procedures include ureteric reimplantation to correct vesicoureteric reflux, bladder augmentation or reconstruction, creation of a vesicocutaneous fistula using the appendix to provide a simple and cosmetically acceptable way for intermittent catheterization (Mitrofanoff's procedure), and excision of duplicated systems or ectopic ureteroceles that may cause recurrent infections. Intractable urinary tract infection, in the presence of hydronephrosis or severe reflux, may require nephrectomy before transplantation. Nephrectomy should be avoided if possible because leaving the kidneys *in situ* may facilitate fluid management during dialysis, an important consideration for small children in whom fluid balance may be tenuous.

The presence of an abnormal lower urinary tract is not a contraindication to transplantation. If the bladder has been defunctioned because of a prior urinary diversion, attempts to prepare it for use after transplantation are warranted. Malformations and voiding abnormalities (e.g., neurogenic bladder, bladder dyssynergia, remnant posterior urethral valves, urethral strictures) should be identified and repaired if possible. Excellent results have been reported using a previously defunctioned bladder for transplantation. In recipients with an abnormal bladder, there is an increased incidence of posttransplantation urologic complications and urinary tract infection. In some studies, graft outcome is inferior to that in patients with normal lower urinary tracts.

Bladders that have not been used for extended periods can be hydrodilated and assessed for adequacy. If the bladder is not usable, an ileal loop or similar diversion or augmentation can be created before transplantation. If a child has a neurogenic bladder or other voiding abnormality, it may be possible to teach self-catheterization safely and successfully. Urinary tract infection may occur when catheterization technique is poor, and noncompliance may lead to partial obstruction.

Renal Osteodystrophy

Aggressive diagnosis and treatment of hyperparathyroidism, osteomalacia, and aluminum bone disease are important in the pretransplantation period. Control of hyperparathyroidism with vitamin D analogues, or even parathyroidectomy, may be required. Failure to do so may predispose to posttransplantation hypercalcemia and limit the growth potential of a successful transplant recipient.

Children Receiving Peritoneal Dialysis

Children being treated with peritoneal dialysis have graft and patient survival rates that are similar to those of children receiving hemodialysis. The extraperitoneal placement of the transplant may allow for continued peritoneal dialysis after transplantation in the event of DGF. Intraperitoneal graft placement is not an absolute contraindication to peritoneal dialysis. A recent episode of peritonitis or exit-site infection in a child awaiting a transplant does not preclude transplantation. Potential transplant recipients should be appropriately treated for 10 to 14 days and have a negative peritoneal fluid culture off antibiotic treatment before contemplating transplantation. In addition, the preoperative peritoneal cell count should not suggest peritonitis.

If a chronic exit-site infection is present at the time of surgery, the catheter should be removed and appropriate parenteral antibiotics administered. An overt tunnel infection should be treated before transplantation. The incidence of posttransplantation peritoneal dialysis-related infections is low. Such infections typically respond to appropriate antibiotic therapy, although catheter removal may be necessary for recurrent infections. In the absence of infections, the peritoneal catheter may be left in place until good graft function has been established for 2 to 3 weeks.

Nephrotic Syndrome

In children with glomerular diseases, proteinuria usually diminishes as kidney function deteriorates and ESRD ensues. Occasionally, florid nephrotic syndrome may persist, particularly in children with focal glomerulosclerosis. Control of heavy proteinuria prior to transplantation is important and can sometimes be achieved with prostaglandin inhibitors such as meclofenamate, although renal embolization or bilateral nephrectomy may be required. In the child with congenital nephrotic syndrome of the Finnish type, unilateral or bilateral nephrectomy is usually performed early in the course of the disease to allow for better skeletal growth while on dialysis. The best approach in these children is debated. Congenital nephrotic syndrome due to diffuse mesangial sclerosis usually requires early bilateral nephrectomy as part of the treatment of Wilms' tumor or its precursor commonly present at the time of diagnosis (Drash syndrome).

Portal Hypertension

Portal hypertension may occur in certain forms of ESRD common in children, such as that resulting from autosomal recessive polycystic liver disease. Its manifestations must be controlled; esophageal varices require portosystemic shunting, and, if neutropenia and thrombocytopenia are present as a result of hypersplenism, partial splenectomy or splenic embolization may be required before transplantation.

Prior Malignancy

Wilms' tumor is the principal malignancy producing ESRD in children. A disease-free period of 1–2 years should be observed before considering transplantation because earlier transplantation has been associated with development of recurrent or metastatic disease in nearly half of reported cases. Premature transplantation in this setting has also been associated with overwhelming sepsis, which may be related to chemotherapy for the tumor. The presence of a primary nonrenal malignancy is not an absolute contraindication to transplantation, although an appropriate waiting time must be observed between tumor extirpation and transplantation (see Chapter 6).

Preemptive Transplantation

Nearly 25% of all pediatric transplantations performed between 1987 and 1999 preceded institution of dialysis. Most of these transplants were from living donors (33%, compared with 13% cadaveric donors). A preemptive transplantation protects a child from the physical and emotional stress of dialysis and the need for dialysis access, although there is some evidence that medication noncompliance may be more common when a child has not received prior dialysis. The 1-year graft survival statistics are not impaired by pretransplantation dialysis.

Nutrition

Poor feeding is a prominent feature of uremia in children. Aggressive nutritional support is essential. Early tube feeding is often employed to improve caloric intake and promote growth, especially in children started on dialysis therapy at a young age. Because of technical difficulty, a target weight of 8 to 10 kg should be reached before the child undergoes transplantation. This weight may not be reached until 2 years of age, even with the most aggressive nutritional regimens. Transplantation in children weighing less than 5 kg has been successfully performed at some centers.

PERIOPERATIVE MANAGEMENT OF THE PEDIATRIC RENAL TRANSPLANT RECIPIENT

Preparation for Transplantation

Live donor transplantation permits commencement of an immune-conditioning regimen (e.g., with MMF and prednisone) 1 week before the transplantation date. A final crossmatch is performed within 1 week of transplantation. All recipients are admitted within 24 hours of transplantation. A detailed history and physical examination are performed to identify any risk factors, especially the presence of active or recent infection. A final set of laboratory tests is obtained to detect any metabolic abnormalities that require correction by dialysis. Aggressive fluid removal is discouraged in the immediate preoperative period to reduce the risk for DGF (see Chapter 8). Plasmapheresis is done when recurrent FSGS is anticipated. The current (i.e., mid-2000) immediate preoperative immunosuppressive regimen for cadaver donor transplant recipients at the UCLA pediatric renal transplantation program combines daclizumab, 1 mg/kg by intravenous infusion; one dose of MMF 600, mg/m² given orally; and one oral dose of cyclosporine, 5 mg/kg.

Intraoperative Management

Immunosuppression is continued intraoperatively with methylprednisolone sodium succinate (Solu-Medrol), 10 mg/kg given intravenously at the beginning of the operation. Close attention is paid to blood pressure and hydration status to reduce the incidence of DGF. Typically, a central venous catheter is inserted to monitor the central venous pressure (CVP) throughout the operation. Hydration should be optimized to achieve adequate renal perfusion. A CVP of 12 to 15 cm H_2O should be achieved before removal of the vascular clamps, but higher CVP is desirable in the case of a small infant receiving an adult-sized kidney. Additionally, the mean arterial blood pressure is kept above 65 or 70 mm Hg by adequate hydration with a crystalloid solution or 5% albumin, and if necessary, the use of dopamine. Dopamine is usually started at 2 to 3 µg/kg/min and increased as required and is continued for 24 to 48 hours postoperatively to assure adequate renal perfusion. Blood transfusion with packed red blood cells is often required in very small recipients because the hemoglobin may drop as a result of sequestration of about 150 to 250 mL of blood in the transplanted kidney. Mannitol and furosemide are given before removal of the vascular clamps to increase the effective circulatory volume and facilitate diuresis. After the transplanted kidney starts to produce urine, volume replacement should be commenced immediately with $\frac{1}{2}$ normal saline. Occasionally, an intraarterial vasodilator, such as verapamil, is used to overcome vasospasm that may impair renal perfusion.

Postoperative Management

Urine output replacement with $\frac{1}{2}$ normal saline is started in the recovery room and continued in the intensive care unit for 24 to 48 hours, in addition to replacement of insensible water losses. Dextrose is not added to the replacement solution to prevent osmotic diuresis and is only used as part of the insensible water loss replacement solution. The lack of concentrating ability of the newly transplanted kidney accounts for the obligatory high urine output that may be observed in the first few posttransplantation days. As the kidney function improves and the serum creatinine levels fall close to normal values, urinary-concentrating ability recovers, and urine output decreases from several liters per day to amounts that match daily fluid intake. At this time, urine output replacement can be stopped, and daily fluid intake is usually set to provide about 150% to 200% the normal daily intake, preferably administered orally.

Hypertension is commonly observed but rarely aggressively corrected in the immediate postoperative period to avoid sudden swings in blood pressure that may impair renal perfusion. If hypertension persists, a calcium-channel blocker is usually the first drug of choice, especially when cyclosporine is used as part of the immunosuppressive regimen. Electrolyte disorders encountered early in the postoperative course are discussed in Chapter 8. Prophylaxis against CMV infection is outlined in Table 15.4 and Chapter 10. Immunosuppression is begun the first postoperative day.

Immunosuppressive Drugs and Protocols

Immunosuppressive protocols for pediatric renal transplant recipients are based on the same principles as those for adults (see Chapter 4, Part IV). The UCLA pediatric renal transplant program immunosuppressive protocol, as of mid-2000, is detailed in Tables 15.5 through 15.7. Central to all current immunosuppressive

Table 15.4. Cytomegalovirus (CMV) prophylaxis protocol at the UCLA Children's Hospital pediatric renal transplant program

Donor Status	Recipient Status	Ganciclovir[a]	CMV Hyperimmune Globulin (Cytogam)[b]
Positive	Positive	Yes	No
Positive	Negative	Yes	Yes
Negative	Positive	Yes	No
Negative	Negative	No	No

[a] Ganciclovir is given intravenously initially (2.5 mg/kg daily) until oral intake is tolerated; oral ganciclovir dose = 20–30 mg/kg/dose orally t.i.d. for 10–12 weeks.
[b] Cytogam dose = 100 mg/kg/dose IV. The first dose is given immediately postoperatively; doses are then given every 2 weeks thereafter for a total of five doses.

Table 15.5.   Immunosuppressive protocol for pediatric kidney transplantation at the UCLA Children's Hospital

Pretransplantation (1 wk in living donor recipients only)
- Prednisone: 0.5 mg/kg daily (minimum dose = 20 mg/day)
- MMF: 600 mg/m^2/dose b.i.d.
  + Famotidine: 1 mg/kg/dose b.i.d. (maximum = 20 mg b.i.d.) is added to minimize gastrointestinal side effects of prednisone and MMF (other H_2 blockers, except cimetidine, or H^+ pump blockers may be used)

Pretransplantation (6–24 hr)
- Daclizumab: 1 mg/kg in 50 mL of normal saline IV over 30 min
- Cyclosporine: 5 mg/kg PO between 6–12 hr pretreatment
  Note: If tacrolimus is to be used, a dose of 0.1 mg/kg PO is given within 6–12 hours
- MMF: 600 mg/m^2 PO within 6 hr

Intraoperatively
- Solumedrol: 10 mg/kg IV at the beginning of surgery (maximum dose of 1 g)

Immediate postoperative period
- Solumedrol: 0.5 mg/kg/day IV (minimum dose = 20 mg/day)[a]
- MMF: 600 mg/m^2/dose IV q 12 hr[a]
- Cyclosporine: 10–15 mg/kg/day PO divided b.i.d. For children who weigh less than 10 kg or are younger than 6 yr of age, give 400–500 mg/m^2/day divided t.i.d.[b] The dose is adjusted to achieve trough levels of 250–350 ng/mL.
  + Famotidine or H_2 blocker

Maintenance therapy
- Daclizumab: 1 mg/kg in 50 mL normal saline IV over 30 min at 2, 4, 6, and 8 wk after transplantation
- Prednisone: Dose tapering is started 2 wk after transplantation and continued to reach a maintenance dose 0.07–0.1 mg/kg/day by 3–4 months.
- MMF: 600 mg/kg/dose PO b.i.d.[c]
- Cyclosporine: Dose is adjusted to achieve the desired trough levels (see Table 15.4)
  + Famotidine or H_2 blocker

MMF, mycophenolate mofetil; H_2, histamine-2
[a] The drug is given orally when the patient tolerates oral intake.
[b] Cyclosporine is started once urine output has been established and the serum creatinine level is below 2.5–3 mg/dL or less than 50% of its baseline value before transplantation.
[c] The dose can be spread to a three-times-daily schedule if gastrointestinal symptoms develop early.

Table 15.6. Therapeutic cyclosporine trough levels and prednisone doses in pediatric transplant recipients at UCLA Children's Hospital

Time After Transplantation (wk)	12-hr Cyclosporine[a] Whole-blood Trough Levels, (ng/mL)	Prednisone Dose (mg/kg/day)
0–4	250–350	0.33
4–8	200–250	0.25
8–12	175–225	0.20
12–16	150–200	0.14–0.18
>16	125–175	0.12–0.15 (0.07–0.10 by 3–4 months)

[a] If tacrolimus is used, target levels of 10–15 ng/mL should be maintained for the first 3–4 wk after transplantation. Afterward, levels of 5–10 ng/mL are targeted.

regimens is a calcineurin inhibitor (cyclosporine or tacrolimus) in combination with steroids and an adjunctive antiproliferative agent (azathioprine or MMF). According to the 1999 NAPRTCS annual report, cyclosporine is used in about 74% and tacrolimus in 22% of pediatric transplant recipients. Azathioprine has been replaced by MMF for most patients. Pediatric experience with sirolimus is limited. Corticosteroids continue to be used in more than 95% of transplant recipients 1 year after transplantation, although there has been a steady increase in the percentage of patients treated with alternate-day steroids regimens. Antibody induction therapy (see Chapter 4, Part II) is used in about half of pediatric transplant recipients.

The choice of the immunosuppressive regimen employed is mostly center specific, but modifications are often made to address the clinical circumstances. For example, when transplantation is contemplated in a child with prior malignancy, a two-drug regimen or even monotherapy may be considered, the use of antibody induction is generally avoided, and living donation is encouraged to provide the best HLA matches. Children with prior transplants that failed because of repeated episodes of acute rejection may be highly sensitized and therefore may require a more intensified immunosuppressive regimen. Tacrolimus may be preferred to cyclosporine when there is particular concern about noncompliance because of the cosmetic side effects of cyclosporine (see later).

Corticosteroids

Corticosteroids remain an integral part of most immunosuppressive protocols despite their toxicity. Fortunately, the emergence of more powerful immunosuppressive agents has led to a dramatic improvement in acute rejection rates and has allowed the use of lower daily doses of steroids. Concerns remain about familiar side effects, such as hypertension, obesity, diabetes mellitus, hyperlipidemia, and osteopenia; in children, retarded skeletal growth, aseptic necrosis of the femoral head, and cosmetic side effects are

**Table 15.7.   Guidelines for drug dose tapering
in pediatric renal transplant recipients**

---

1. Cyclosporine

Minimal or no change in the first 4 weeks to allow for faster tapering
of prednisone

Dose reduction should not exceed 10–20% at any time.

Cyclosporine and prednisone doses should not be lowered on the
same day (risk of precipitating an acute rejection).

Serum creatinine and cyclosporine levels should be checked 2–3 days
after each change and before the next change is made.

(The same guidelines are applied to patients treated with
tacrolimus.)

---

2. Prednisone

Start tapering the dose 2–3 weeks after transplantation if stable
and cyclosporine level is within the desired range.

Initial dose tapering is by 2.5 mg each time, about 10% (may reduce
by 5 mg if total dose is > 2 mg/kg). Once a 10-mg dose is reached,
dose reduction is by 1 mg each time.

Longer periods of time should elapse before further tapering at the
lower dose range.

Cyclosporine and prednisone doses should not be lowered on the
same day.

Serum creatinine and cyclosporine levels should be checked 2–3 days
after each change and before the next change is made.

---

3. Mycophenolate Mofetil

Dose reduction is only indicated if hematologic or GI side effects
develop.

Dose reduction is done in 30–50% increments.

It can be safely withheld for a few days up to 2–3 weeks for severe
side effects.

---

significant additional problems associated with chronic steroid
use. Steroid withdrawal trials in children have been conducted
with variable degrees of success. Improvement in blood pressure
and lipid profiles has been overshadowed by high rates of acute
rejection occurring in up to 70% of children in some series. Graft
loss due to rejection has occurred in some patients. Acute rejection in pediatric transplant recipients further impairs skeletal
growth as a result of renal insufficiency and the high doses of corticosteroids used for treatment. Steroids, therefore, continue to be
used in most regimens, with an increased tendency toward using
lower daily maintenance or alternate-day dosing (discussed later
in the section on growth). There are currently no reliable immunologic or clinical indicators to predict in which pediatric transplant
recipients steroids can be safely withdrawn.

Newer, less toxic steroid preparations have been used success-fully in the treatment of pediatric nephrotic syndrome and in renal transplantation. Preliminary studies with deflazacort (DFZ, an oxazoline derivative of prednisolone) in combination with a stan-dard immunosuppressive regimen suggest that it is an effective immunosuppressive agent with fewer side effects than other commonly used corticosteroid preparations. Growth velocity and growth hormone secretion were found to be improved in patients who received DFZ as part of their therapy. DFZ also improved the cushingoid features and significantly decreased the weight-to-height ratio of pediatric recipients.

Calcineurin Inhibitors

CYCLOSPORINE.   There are some important differences in the use of cyclosporine between adults and children. Children require higher doses than adults when calculated on a milligram per kilo-gram of body weight basis, particularly when the original Sand-immune formulation is used. This is especially true when cyclo-sporine is used in children younger than 2 years of age, particularly in the early postoperative period. The requirement for higher doses is believed to be due to a higher rate of metabolism by the hepatic cytochrome P450, resulting in faster clearance. Dosing based on surface area, or thrice-daily dosing, appears to provide better ther-apeutic levels in smaller children and in children in whom metab-olism is accelerated (e.g., patients receiving certain anticonvulsant medications). In children, a daily dose of less than 5 mg/kg/day has been found to be associated with higher risk for acute and, subse-quently, chronic rejection. The reduced variability in drug levels and enhanced bioavailability seen with the Neoral preparation of cyclosporine may be particularly beneficial in children by permit-ting easier dose reduction and monitoring, which may reflect in a reduced incidence of rejection episodes.

The side-effect profile of cyclosporine in children is similar to that seen in adults (see Chapter 4, Part I). Hirsutism, gingival hyper-plasia, and coarsening facial features may be particularly trouble-some in children. Hispanic and black children appear to be at higher risk. In the adolescent population, especially girls, these side effects may be devastating, causing severe emotional distress and possibly leading to dangerous noncompliance. Close attention must be paid to these complications because they may predict non-compliance; switching to tacrolimus may be helpful. Seizures are observed more commonly in children treated with cyclosporine than in adults. Children, like adults, are likely to develop hyper-cholesterolemia and hypertrygliceridemia and may be candidates for lipid-lowering agents. Hyperglycemia is less common in chil-dren than in adults and occurs in less than 5% of children (less than 1% in some series) treated with cyclosporine. Overt diabetes melli-tus may occasionally occur.

TACROLIMUS.   There appears to be no long-term difference in transplantation outcome for children immunosuppressed with cyclosporine or tacrolimus. Hypertension, gingival hypertrophy, and hirsutism are less prevalent and less severe with tacrolimus; PTLD and posttransplantation glucose intolerance are more com-mon. The nephrotoxicity profiles of tacrolimus and cyclosporine are indistinguishable in children, as they are in adults. Neurotoxicity with tacrolimus is more serious, with more marked tremor and a higher incidence of seizures.

Adjunctive Immunosuppressive Agents

The adjunctive agents are immunosuppressants that are generally used in combination with a calcineurin inhibitor and prednisone to reduce the incidence of acute rejection episodes. MMF is used in about 70% of U.S. pediatric renal transplant recipients and has largely replaced azathioprine. The capacity of MMF to reduce the incidence of acute rejection episodes relative to azathioprine is similar to that described in adults (see Chapter 4, Part I and Fig. 4.6). In the NAPRTCS database, cadaveric transplant recipients appeared to benefit the most from MMF, with acute rejection rates of 18%, compared with 60% for historical controls taking azathioprine. For living donor transplant recipients, the relative benefits of MMF were small. In children, as in adults, gastrointestinal and hematologic side effects can be troublesome and may respond to dose reduction. Dosing guidelines in children are outlined in Tables 15.5 to 15.7. MMF has been used successfully in children for the treatment of steroid-resistant acute rejection. There are currently no reported clinical studies on the safety and efficacy of sirolimus (rapamycin) in children. The results from the adult clinical trials are promising and suggest that sirolimus may have an important place in pediatric transplantation.

Biologic Immunosuppressive Agents

The indications for the use of antibody-induction therapy with OKT3 or the antithymocyte globulins (Atgam and Thymoglobulin) are discussed in Chapter 4 and do not differ between adults and children. The side-effect profiles of these agents are also similar. In pediatric cadaveric transplantation, there is close to a 10% advantage in the 5-year graft survival rate when antibody induction is used. Acute rejection episodes are about 30% less frequent and tend to occur later.

The anti-CD25 monoclonal antibodies (daclizumab and basiliximab) may be of particular benefit in children because of their effectiveness, ease of administration, and absence of side effects. In an open-label multicenter pediatric study with daclizumab used in addition to a triple-drug regimen with either cyclosporine or tacrolimus together with MMF and prednisone, the rate of acute rejection was found to be only 7% at 6 months and 16% at 1 year after transplantation. All rejections were mild and steroid responsive. No first-dose or cytokine-release effect or anaphylactic reactions were observed. Rates of opportunistic infections were not increased.

Acute Rejection in Pediatric Transplantation

Acute rejection episodes in pediatric renal transplantation account for about 15% of graft failures. With standard immunosuppressive therapy, an acute rejection episode is experienced in about 26% of recipients of live donor transplants and 30% of cadaveric transplant recipients. The first rejection episode occurs within the first 3 months after transplantation in about half of patients, with higher frequency and earlier recurrence in recipients of cadaveric transplants. Black race, DGF, and poor HLA matching may predispose to rejection episodes. In children, as in adults, acute rejection is the single most important predictor of chronic rejection. It precedes graft failure from chronic rejection in more than 90% of cases. Chronic rejection is the most common cause of graft loss in children.

Diagnosis of acute rejection in the very young transplant recipient is not always straightforward and requires a high index of suspicion. Because most small children are transplanted with adult-sized kidneys, the elevation in serum creatinine may be a late sign of rejection as a result of the large renal reserve compared with the body mass. Significant allograft dysfunction may be present with little or no increase in the serum creatinine level. One of the earliest and most sensitive signs of rejection is the development of hypertension along with low-grade fever. In children, any increase in serum creatinine, especially if accompanied by hypertension, should be considered a result of acute rejection until proved otherwise. Late diagnosis and treatment of rejection are associated with higher incidence of resistant rejections and graft loss.

The differential diagnosis of acute allograft dysfunction in children is similar to that in adults (see Chapter 8). Renal biopsy is the gold standard for diagnosis. Urinalysis and culture, viral cultures, and ultrasound and radionuclide imaging studies (see Chapter 14) are used to diagnose other causes of graft dysfunction and should be performed without delay before allograft biopsy.

Treatment of Acute Rejection

The techniques used to treat acute rejection are similar in children to those used in adults (see Chapter 4, Part IV). Complete reversal of acute rejection, as judged by a return of the serum creatinine level to baseline, is achieved in about half of children; 40% to 45% achieve partial reversal, and graft loss occurs in the remainder. Complete reversal from acute rejection is even less likely with subsequent rejection episodes. Younger transplant recipients are at higher risk for graft loss from acute rejection.

CORTICOSTEROIDS. In children, as in adults, high-dose corticosteroid pulses are the first line of treatment of acute rejection, and about 75% of episodes are responsive to treatment. After the diagnosis is made, intravenous methylprednisolone is given in doses that range from 5 to 10 mg/kg/day for 3 to 5 days. After completing therapy, the maintenance corticosteroid is resumed at the prerejection level or is increased and then tapered to baseline levels over a few days. The serum creatinine level may rise slightly during therapy and may not go back to baseline until 3 to 5 days after therapy is completed.

OKT3.   OKT3 reverses up to 90% of the acute rejection episodes that do not respond to steroids. The pediatric protocol for OKT3 administration is shown in Table 15.8. In children, as in adults, OKT3 can be administered on an outpatient basis after the first few doses. Before completion of the OKT3 course, the calcineurin inhibitor dose should be increased so that at completion of the course, blood levels are somewhat higher than they were before treatment; this may reduce the incidence of rebound rejections. When rebound rejections do occur, they may be amenable to high-dose steroid treatment.

Table 15.8.   OKT3 protocol for treatment of acute rejection

Before Initiating Therapy

Careful examination of the patient for signs of fluid overload
Chest radiograph to confirm absence of signs of fluid overload,
    especially pulmonary edema
If weight is >3% above dry weight, use diuretics or dialyze vigorously
    to attain dry weight

Before First and Second Doses of OKT3

Acetaminophin, 250–500 mg PO
Diphenhydramine hydrochloride (Benadryl), 1–2 mg/kg IV
Methylprednisolone, 10 mg/kg IV 1–3 hours before OKT3 (dose may
    be divided to be given before and after OKT3)

OKT3 Dose

Body weight < 30 kg = 2.5 mg OKT3[a]
Body weight > 30 kg = 5 mg OKT3[a]
Cyclosporine, hold during 1st and 2nd doses to assure adequate
    diuresis and balanced fluid status, continue at half dose during
    remainder of OKT3 therapy, and increase dose by 15–25% after
    conclusion of OKT3.
Prednisone, return to maintenance dose after second dose of OKT3

[a] May use lower 1st and 2nd doses of 1 or 1.5 mg.

Some programs routinely monitor the effectiveness of OKT3 by
following the levels of CD3+ T cells. Immunologic monitoring is
mandatory during a second course of OKT3 because the development of OKT3 antibodies may abrogate the effectiveness of the
drug. Children may regenerate the CD3–T-cell receptor complex
more rapidly than adults, and twice-daily dosing of OKT3 is occasionally necessary to effect successful rejection reversal. After a
first course of OKT3, up to 35% of children may develop anti-
OKT3 antibodies. The titer of antibodies is usually low and can
be overcome by increasing the OKT3 dose; however, about 15% of
children develop high titers of antibody, which prevent further
use. The side effects of OKT3 are similar in children and adults.
Children must be euvolemic before administration of the first
dose to prevent pulmonary edema. Fever is nearly universal, and
diarrhea and vomiting occur in nearly half of children treated.
Severe headache is common and may represent a mild form of
aseptic meningitis. There have been occasional fatalities associated with OKT3-mediated cerebral edema.

Refractory Rejection
Refractory rejection usually refers to those episodes of acute rejection that do not respond to, or reoccur after, treatment with steroid
and OKT3. About 75% of cases can be reversed by switching to
tacrolimus or adding MMF, if this drug had not been part of the

immunosuppressive protocol. Relatively high doses and trough levels are required. Sirolimus is a potential treatment option, although experience with this drug for refractory rejection is limited. Whenever such aggressive immunosuppressive therapy is employed, the risk for opportunistic infections and PTLD increases. Viral prophylaxis and infection surveillance are critical.

Noncompliance in Pediatric Transplantation

At least half of pediatric cadaveric transplant recipients demonstrate significant noncompliance in the posttransplantation period. This figure exceeds 60% in adolescents. Noncompliance is the principal cause of graft loss in 10% to 15% of all pediatric kidney transplant recipients; for retransplanted patients, this figure may exceed 25%. Reversible and irreversible episodes of graft dysfunction related to noncompliance occur in up to 40% of adolescents and are somewhat less frequent in younger children. Patterns of noncompliance vary from partial compliance to complete noncompliance. Partial compliance ranges from the occasional missed dose to an occasional extra dose. It is most commonly the result of forgetfulness, misunderstanding of a dose change or modification, or the presence of events that lead to the belief that medications are not helping. In children, complete noncompliance is often the result of underlying emotional or psychosocial stress.

Measuring Compliance

Methods to measure compliance are crude and provide only a general estimate at best. The easiest method is asking patients directly about their compliance; patients, however, tend to tell physicians what they want to hear! Assessments made by patients of failure to take medications are often accurate, whereas denials of noncompliance are not. Serum drug level monitoring is only helpful when the drug level is either inexplicably low or high. Other methods to measure noncompliance include pill counts and assessment of prescription refill rates. A continuous microelectronic device, usually attached to the cap of the medication bottle, records each opening of the bottle as a presumptive dose and records the time and frequency of taking the medication. Recorded data can then be retrieved and an assessment of compliance made.

Predicting Compliance

Pretransplantation prediction of posttransplantation noncompliance is difficult. Risk factors include a disorganized family structure, female sex, adolescence, and a history of previous graft loss due to noncompliance. Personality problems related to low self-esteem and poor social adjustment are found with higher frequency in noncompliant patients. Studies indicate that compliance has no correlation with intelligence, memory, education, or the number of drugs that a patient takes, although the daily frequency of taking medications may affect compliance greatly. A linear decline in compliance rates has been demonstrated with increasing number of doses per day. Frequent clinic visits may improve compliance. Noncompliance in children must be suspected when there is unexplained diminution in cushingoid features, sudden weight loss, or unexplained swings in graft function or trough blood levels of the calcineurin inhibitors.

Strategies to Improve Compliance

Education, planning dose regimens, clinic scheduling, communication, and getting patients involved in the medical management are the main strategies. The child should know that the physician is their advocate and is interested in how they take their medications. Providing patients with specific reminders or cues to which the medication can be tied can be of great help. These cues should be simple and preferably part of the patient's daily activities, such as meal times, daily rituals, specific clock times, a certain television program, tooth brushing, shaving, and so forth. Contracting with pediatric patients and rewarding them is another strategy to enhance compliance. Finally, asking the same questions about compliance each visit and explaining the consequences of noncompliance repeatedly reinforces the compliance message and physician interest.

Psychological Intervention

Behavior modification programs and other means of psychological intervention may be beneficial in some patients. In the pretransplantation period, an ongoing program of counseling should be undertaken in high-risk patients. Clearly defined therapeutic goals should be set while the patient is receiving dialysis, and family problems that are recognized in the pretransplantation period should be addressed before activation on the transplant list. The presence of at least one highly motivated caretaker is a helpful factor in long-term graft success.

Adolescence brings with it rapid behavioral and bodily changes. The adolescent's strong desire to be normal conflicts with the continued reminder of chronic disease that the taking of medication engenders; this tendency is particularly true when medications are taken many times a day and alter the physical appearance. Ambivalence between the desire for parental protection and autonomy, combined with a magical belief in his or her invulnerability, sets the stage for experimentation with noncompliance. Adolescents with psychological or developmental problems may use impulsive noncompliance during self-destructive episodes. The transplantation teams must be aware of these developmental issues so that they can initiate appropriate psychological intervention before the onset of significant noncompliant behavior.

Growth

Retarded skeletal growth is a constant feature in children with chronic renal failure and ESRD. The severity of growth retardation is directly related to the age of onset of renal failure; the earlier the onset, the more severe. Renal osteodystrophy, metabolic acidosis, electrolyte disturbances, anemia, protein and calorie malnutrition, delayed sexual maturation, and accumulation of uremic toxins have all been implicated in the development of growth retardation.

Growth retardation is typically assessed by the *standard deviation score* (SDS) or height deficit score (also known as the *Z score*). These measure the patient's height compared with that of unaffected children of similar age.

Determinants of Posttransplantation Growth

Growth improves after transplantation; however, catch-up growth is not realized in most patients. The following factors have a major influence on posttransplantation growth.

AGE AT TRANSPLANTATION.   Children younger than 6 years of age have the lowest standard deviation scores before transplantation, and these exhibit the best improvement in their SDS after transplantation. Two years after transplantation, infants younger than 1 year of age have an improvement in their SDS by 1 full standard deviation (SD), compared with an improvement of only 0.5 SD for those between 2 and 5 years of age, and 0.1 SD in those between the ages of 6 and 12 years. Children older than 12 years of age tend to have minimal or no growth after transplantation. Older children occasionally continue to grow into puberty; however, the growth spurt experienced by most growing children at this age may be blunted or lost.

The fact that youngest children benefit the most in statural growth from early transplantation provides a strong argument for expedited transplantation in an attempt to optimize and perhaps normalize stature. In addition, earlier transplantation allows less time for growth failure while receiving dialysis and therefore less requirement for catch-up growth.

CORTICOSTEROID DOSE.   The precise mechanism by which steroids impair skeletal growth is unknown. They may reduce the release of growth hormone, reduce insulin-like growth factor (IGF) activity, directly impair growth cartilage, decrease calcium absorption, or increase renal phosphate wasting. Strategies to improve growth include the use of lower daily doses of steroids, the use of alternate-day dosing, or dose tapering to complete withdrawal.

Alternate-day steroid dosing continues to gain acceptance in pediatric renal transplantation and, at 4 years after transplantation, is the regimen used in 26% of all patients. This dosing schedule has been shown to improve linear growth significantly without increased rates of rejection or graft loss. Conversion to alternate-day dosing should be considered in selected, stable patients in whom compliance can be assured.

Ideally, steroids are withdrawn completely. In tacrolimus-based immunosuppressive regimens, withdrawal of steroids has been successfully performed in more than 70% of patients, usually by 5 months after transplantation. The effect of this approach on growth has been remarkable, with improvement in the SDS at 2 years after transplantation in children younger than 13 years of 3.62 SD in the withdrawn group compared with 1.48 SD in the nonwithdrawn group. The rates of acute rejection in the withdrawn group, however, were high, and this could adversely affect growth by virtue of a decline in graft function and the need for high-dose steroids to treat rejection. In adults in whom steroids were withdrawn, a decline in graft function has been observed (see Chapter 4, Part IV), and long-term follow-up of steroid-withdrawn children is required before this regimen can be adopted on a widespread basis.

GROWTH HORMONE.   The use of recombinant growth hormone (rhGH) in pediatric renal transplant recipients significantly improves growth velocity and SDS. The NAPRTCS reports that growth velocity almost tripled 1 year after starting rhGH therapy, with a slight slowing after 2 and 3 years of therapy. There is some evidence to suggest that rhGH increases allogeneic immune responsiveness, leading to acute rejection and graft loss in addition to direct adverse effects on graft function. These adverse effects were not observed in the NAPRTCS data. Growth hormone therapy is generally started in prepubertal children at least 1 year after transplantation and continued until catch-up growth is achieved or until puberty ensues. Cyclosporine levels may fall after initiation of rhGH therapy, and the dose should be increased by 10% to 15%.

ALLOGRAFT FUNCTION.   An allograft GFR of less than 60 ml/min/1.73 m^2 is associated with poor growth and low IGF levels; optimal growth occurs with a GFR greater than 90 mL/min/1.73 m^2. Graft function is the most important factor after high corticosteroid dosage in the genesis of posttransplantation growth failure. The immunosuppressive properties of corticosteroids needed to control rejection and preserve kidney function must be balanced against the need to minimize steroids to maximize growth. Thus, an excessive steroid dose leads to impairment of growth and an inadequate dose to impairment of graft function. Administration of high-dose recombinant human growth hormone may induce acceleration of growth even in the presence of chronic graft dysfunction.

Posttransplantation Sexual Maturation

Restoration of kidney function by transplantation improves pubertal development. This occurs most likely by normalization of gonadotrophin physiology. Elevated gonadotrophin levels and reduced gonadotrophin pulsatility are observed in chronic renal failure, whereas children with successful kidney transplants demonstrate a higher nocturnal rise and increased amplitude of gonadotrophin pulsatility.

Female patients who are pubertal before transplantation typically become amenorrheic during the course of chronic renal failure. Menses with ovulatory cycles usually return within 6 months to 1 year after transplantation; hence, potentially sexually active adolescents should be given appropriate contraceptive information.

Adolescent female transplant recipients have successfully borne children; the only consistently reported neonatal abnormality has been an increased incidence of prematurity. Adolescent boys should be made aware that they can successfully father children. No consistent pattern of abnormalities has been reported in their offspring.

Posttransplantation Infections

The spectrum of infections and their presentation may differ somewhat between children and adults (see Chapter 10). Infection in the immunocompromised child remains the major cause of morbidity and mortality after transplantation.

Bacterial Infections

Pneumonia and urinary tract infections are the most common posttransplantation bacterial infections. Urinary tract infection can progress rapidly to urosepsis and may be confused with episodes of acute rejection. Opportunistic infections with unusual organisms usually do not occur until after the first posttransplantation month.

Viral Infections

The herpesviruses (CMV, herpesvirus, varicella zoster, and EBV) pose a special problem in view of their common occurrence in children. Many young children have not yet been exposed to these viruses, and because they lack protective immunity, their predisposition to serious primary infection is high. The incidence of these infections is higher in children who receive antibody induction therapy and after treatment of acute rejection, and prophylactic therapy is advisable.

CYTOMEGALOVIRUS. The incidence of CMV seropositivity is about 30% in children older than 5 years of age and rises to about 60% in teenagers; thus, the younger the child, the greater the potential for serious infection when a CMV-positive donor kidney is transplanted. CMV infection may have the same devastating effect on the course of pediatric transplantation as on adult transplantation, and various strategies have been proposed to minimize its impact. It has been suggested that seronegative children receive only kidneys from seronegative donors; however, given the frequency of seropositivity in the adult population, this restriction would penalize seronegative children with a prolonged wait for a transplant at a critical growing period. CMV hyperimmune globulin, high-dose standard immune globulin, high-dose oral acyclovir, and oral ganciclovir are all potentially valuable therapeutic options. Ganciclovir is effective therapy for proven CMV infection in children, as in adults.

VARICELLA ZOSTER VIRUS. The most commonly seen manifestation of varicella zoster virus infection in older pediatric transplant recipients is localized disease along a dermatomal distribution. In younger children, however, primary varicella infection (chickenpox) can result in a rapidly progressive and overwhelming infection with encephalitis, pneumonitis, hepatic failure, pancreatitis, and disseminated intravascular coagulation. It is important to know a child's varicella zoster antibody status because seronegative children require prophylactic varicella zoster immune globulin (VZIG) within 72 hours of accidental exposure. VZIG is effective in favorably modifying the disease in 75% of cases. With the development of a new varicella vaccine, it is likely that all seronegative children with ESRD will be appropriately vaccinated.

A child with a kidney transplant who develops chickenpox should begin receiving parenteral acyclovir without delay; with zoster infection, there is less of a threat for dissemination, although acyclovir should also be used. In both situations, it is wise to discontinue azathioprine or MMF until 2 days after the last new crop of vesicles has dried. The dose of other immunosuppressive agents will depend on the clinical situation and response to therapy.

EPSTEIN-BARR VIRUS. About half of children are seronegative for EBV, and infection will occur in about 75% of these patients. Most EBV infections are clinically silent. PTLD in children, as in adults, may be related to EBV infection in the presence of vigorous immunosuppression (see Chapter 9).

HERPES SIMPLEX VIRUS.   The typical perioral herpetic ulcerations are common in immunosuppressed children and usually respond to oral acyclovir therapy. Disseminated herpes infection is rare.

Posttransplantation Antibiotic Prophylaxis

Protocols for posttransplantation antibiotic prophylaxis in children vary from center to center. Most centers use an intravenous cephalosporin for the first 48 hours after transplantation to reduce infection from graft contamination and the transplant incision. The use of nightly trimethoprim-sulfamethoxazole for the first 3 to 6 months after transplantation serves as prophylaxis against *Pneumocystis carinii* pneumonia and urinary tract infections. Prophylactic oral myconazole (nystatin) minimizes oral and gastrointestinal fungal infections. CMV prophylaxis has been discussed. Children who have undergone splenectomy should be immunized with pneumococcal vaccine and should receive postoperative prophylaxis for both gram-positive and gram-negative organisms, both of which may cause overwhelming sepsis.

Posttransplantation Hypertension and Cardiovascular Disease

Persistent posttransplantation hypertension is a serious problem in children, as it is in adults. More than two thirds of transplanted children treated with cyclosporine are hypertensive, and many require multiple medications for blood pressure control. The differential diagnosis is the same as that for adults. It should be emphasized, however, that late-onset hypertension, especially when accompanied by low-grade fever, is commonly the first sign of acute rejection and may be present before any change in the serum creatinine level. Calcium-channel blockers are generally well tolerated in children and are the agents of choice for blood pressure management.

Concern regarding long-term posttransplantation cardiovascular morbidity and mortality has generally been directed toward the adult posttransplantation population. Risk factors should also be addressed in children who will hopefully grow to adulthood with their transplants. Serum cholesterol levels are frequently higher than the 185-mg/dL "at-risk" level for children with transplants. Dietary measures are appropriate to reduce hyperlipidemia. There are currently insufficient data to make firm recommendations for the use of pharmacologic measures in children, but the HMGCoase reductase inhibitors are generally effective and safe.

Rehabilitation of Transplanted Children

Successful reentry into school after transplantation requires coordinated preparation of the child, family or caregivers, classmates, and school personnel. Treatment side effects, social and emotional difficulties, academic difficulties, school resources, and caregiver attitudes all play a role and should be addressed.

Within a year of successful transplantation, the social and emotional functioning of the child and the child's family appears to return to pre-illness levels. Pretransplantation personality disorders, however, continue to manifest themselves. Within 1 year after transplantation, more than 90% of children attend school, and less than 10% are not involved in any vocational or education programs. Three-year follow-up shows that nearly 90% of children are in appropriate school or job placement. Surveys of 10-year survivors of pediatric kidney transplants report that most patients consider their health to be good; engage in appropriate social, educational, and sexual activities; and experience a very good or excellent quality of life.

SELECTED READINGS

Al-Uzri A, Sullivan EK, Fine RN, et al. Living-unrelated renal transplantation in children: a report of the North American Pediatric Renal Transplantation Study (NAPRTCS). *Pediatr Transplant* 1998;2:139.

Benfield MR, McDonald R, Sullivan EK, et al. The 1997 annual renal transplantation in children report of the North American Pediatric Renal Transplant Cooperative Study (NAPRTCS). *Pediatr Transplant* 1999;3:152.

Birkeland SA, Larsen KE, Rohr N. Pediatric renal transplantation without steroids. *Pediatr Nephrol* 1998;12:87.

Burd RS, Gillingham KJ, Farber MS, et al. Diagnosis and treatment of cytomegalovirus disease in pediatric renal transplant recipients. *J Pediatr Surg* 1994;29:1049.

Cramer JA. Practical issues in medication compliance. *Transplant Proc* 1999;31(Suppl 4A):7S.

David-Neto E, Lemos F, Furosawa E, et al. Impact of cyclosporin A phosmacokinetics on the presence of side effects in pediatric renal transplantation. *J Am Soc Nephrol* 2000;11:343.

Davis ID. Pediatric renal transplantation: back to school issues. *Transplant Proc* 1999;31(Suppl 4A):61S.

Enke BU, Bokenkamp A, Offner G, et al. Response to diphtheria and tetanus booster vaccination in pediatric renal transplant recipients. *Transplantation* 1997;64:237.

Ferraris JR, Tambutti ML, Redal M, et al. Immunosuppressive activity of deflazacort in pediatric renal transplantation. *Transplantation* 1996;62:417.

Fivush BA, Neu AM. immunization guidelines for pediatric renal disease. *Semin Nephrol* 1998;18:256.

Gagnadoux M-F, Niaudet P, Najarian JS, et al. Renal transplantation in the first 5 years of life. *Kidney Int* 1993;44(Suppl 43):S40.

Hariharan S, Peddi VR, Savin V, et al. Recurrent and de novo renal diseases after renal transplantation: a report of the renal allograft disease registry. *Am J Kidney Dis* 1998;31:928.

Hokken-Koelega A, Stinjen T, De Jong R, et al. A placebo-controlled, double-blind trial of growth hormone treatment in prepubertal children after renal transplant. *Kidney Int* 1996;49(Suppl 53):S128.

Jabs K, Sullivan EK, Avner ED, et al. Alternate-day steroid dosing improves growth without adversely affecting graft survival or long-term graft function: a report of the North American Pediatric Renal Transplantation Cooperative Study (NAPRTCS). *Transplantation* 1996;61:31.

Matas AJ, Chavers BM, Nevins TE, et al. Recipient evaluation, preparation, and care in pediatric transplantation: the University of Minnesota protocols. *Kidney Int* 1996;49(Suppl 53):S99.

Muller T, Sikora P, Offner G, et al. Recurrence of renal disease after kidney transplantation in children: 24 years of experience in a single center. *Clin Nephrol* 1998;49:82.

Osorio AV, Sullivan EK, Alexander SR, et al. ABO-mismatched renal transplantation in children: a report of the North American Pediatric Renal Transplantation Cooperative Study (NAPRTCS) and Midwest Organ Bank. *Pediatr Transplant* 1998;2:26.

Schurman SJ, McEnry PT. Factors influencing short-term and long-term pediatric renal transplant survival. *J Pediatr* 1997;130:455.

Shapiro R. Tacrolimus in pediatric renal transplantation: a review. *Pediatr Transplant* 1998;2:270.

Tejani AH, Stablein DM, Sullivan EK, et al. The impact of donor source, recipient age, pre-operative immunotherapy and induction therapy on early and late acute rejections in children: a report of the North American Pediatric Renal Transplantation Cooperative Study (NAPRTCS). *Pediatr Transplant* 1998;2:318.

Tejani A, Cortes L, Stablein D. Clinical correlates of chronic rejection in pediatric renal transplantation: a report of the North American Pediatric Renal Transplantation Cooperative Study. *Transplantation* 1996;61:1054.

Tyden G, Berg U, Bohlin A-B, et al. Renal transplantation in children less than two years old. *Transplantation* 1997;63:554.

Vats AN, Donaldson L, Fine RN, et al. Pretransplant dialysis status and outcome of renal transplantation in North American children: a NAPRTCS study. *Transplantation* 2000;69:1414.

Psychiatric Aspects of Kidney Transplantation

Kirk Murphy

Patients who are candidates for renal or pancreatic transplantation present numerous challenging and clinically relevant psychiatric issues. Within academic medicine, the mental health needs of transplant recipients and donors lie within the scope of transplantation psychiatry—a subsection of consultation-liaison psychiatry, which is, in turn, a subspecialty within psychiatry. In the face of such quaternary subspecialization, clinicians seeking to meet the mental health needs of transplant patients may mistakenly conclude that they require arcane and esoteric knowledge to care for these patients. Fortunately, the task is a manageable one. The focus of this discussion is therefore to identify the conceptual, diagnostic, and clinical issues most likely to confront psychiatrists, physicians, and other health professionals with responsibility for the mental health needs of renal transplantation patients.

GENERAL CONSIDERATIONS

Whereas the formal roles assumed in the transplant process by psychiatrists, psychologists, and social workers may vary from center to center, the clinical needs of transplantation patients are similar. Although many of the clinical details involved in the provision of psychiatric care for transplantation patients are unique, the so-called *biopsychosocial* model provides a robust framework on which to organize clinical impressions and plans. This model encourages the integration of diverse symptomatology and presentation within a heterogeneous group along three primary axes: the *biologic, psychological,* and *social* characteristics of individual patients. The following general discussion explores the model in the context of clinical issues arising in the psychiatric care of transplant recipients.

With respect to biology, the most obvious delineation is that between donors and recipients. For this reason, the special issues pertinent to donors are covered separately. Among recipients as a group, the most salient biologic issue common to the group is that of immunologic rejection of the transplanted organ. With the exception of recipients receiving allografts from identical twins, all transplant recipients require immunosuppressive medications as long as they have a functioning transplant. Because optimal graft function is currently associated with the use of corticosteroids, transplant recipients are invariably at risk for their psychiatric side effects. Moreover, because most other immunosuppressants are associated with central (and often peripheral) neurotoxicity, patients are at significantly elevated risk for a variety of psychiatric symptoms.

Yet another important biologic consideration is the etiology of the condition that led to end-stage renal disease (ESRD). From a psychiatric perspective, the most significant etiologic distinction is between conditions that are known to be causally associated with central nervous system disease or dysfunction and those that are not. Among the former group, diabetes mellitus, hypertension, and systemic lupus erythematosus are the most significant, although Alport's syndrome (and any other diagnoses associated with impairment of visual or auditory acuity) may be of potential significance.

The psychological issues facing transplantation patients may be divided along multiple planes. The most fundamental distinction is that between donor and recipient. Within the latter group, the psychiatric issues confronting patients before transplantation differ in many ways from those that may arise after transplantation. Among transplant recipients, the issues of acute medication side effects, surgical complications, and questions of acute rejection or delayed graft function are most relevant in the immediate post-transplantation period. Whereas issues such as quality of life, medication compliance, the risk for chronic rejection, and long-term sequelae of immunosuppression become more relevant as the post-transplantation time interval lengthens. Moreover, the psychiatric issues confronting patients with a history of multiple complications or severe rejection after transplantation differ from those confronting patients whose course has been relatively uneventful.

The extent to which a patient became accustomed to medical treatment before the onset of ESRD is an important variable affecting their psychological response to transplantation. The helplessness and loss of control that transplantation may incur may be far more intrusive for patients with no experience of dependence on medical care before ESRD than for patients who have become familiar with medical care as a result of their own chronic illness or that of their relatives. The nature of these previous experiences is an additional variable, which may positively or negatively affect their expectations of transplantation and the physicians and other providers caring for them. Finally, the extent to which a patient does or does not tolerate dialysis treatments (or insulin maintenance therapy for potential pancreas transplant recipients) may have a substantial effect on their reaction to the prospect of transplant failure.

Social issues have substantial implications for assessment and management of psychiatric issues in transplant recipients. The most obvious social variable is the extent to which illness may have affected the patient's available social and emotional support system. The unanticipated onset of ESRD may pose a significant challenge to the emotional capacities and defense mechanisms of the patient, spouse, other individuals, or the larger social unit. Conversely, some patients may have suffered the vicissitudes of chronic disease in childhood and early adult life. The result of the early onset of chronic disease may significantly affect developmental milestones of young adulthood, such as differentiation from the family of origin and the establishment of outside support networks. In this context, health professionals must be mindful of the prospect that such alternatives to putative norms of psychosocial development are, in fact, creative adaptations by family systems. Another potential consequence of early-onset ESRD is that the cosmetic and social consequences of posttransplantation immunosuppression may lead some young recipients to forego adherence to medication regimens to facilitate acceptance by their peers. This specific example serves to illustrate the fact that psychiatrists and other health professionals who maintain curiosity about the social and emotional matrices of their patients' lives are more likely to succeed in communicating with them regarding potentially deleterious behaviors.

The fortuitous fact that within the United States all individuals with ESRD become eligible for health insurance by Medicare serves to maximize the demographic diversity of the patient pool with potential access to renal transplantation. The association of increased risk for both hypertension and diabetes with various specific ethnic groups also plays a role in determining the extent to which patients of varying ethnicity constitute the total pool of candidates for renal transplantation at various centers. Particularly among first-generation immigrants, ethnicity may be a covariant with cultural values, linguistic fluency, and economic status. Psychiatrists and other health care professionals must be cognizant of the role of these variables in the patient's capacity to navigate the complexities of the tertiary health care setting.

Regardless of national origin, the availability or absence of economic resources for a given patient can also be of critical importance to health professionals working with the emotional needs of transplant recipients. In most health care systems, economic resources are one—and often the primary—factor determining access to transportation, lodging (at health care centers distant from patients' residences), child or elder care permitting clinic attendance, and long-term access to immunosuppressant medications. Stressors arising directly from these issues or indirectly (from their very tangible implications for graft survival) have substantial psychological effects on transplant recipients. The presence or absence of financial resources can also determine whether a transplant recipient experiences substantial economic burdens resulting from ESRD and may affect their expectation and emotions regarding the consequences of success or failure of the transplant.

Educational experience is another relevant demographic variable. It is of particular importance to the success or failure of attempts to inform patients about immunosuppressant regimens and the potential risks and benefits of the transplantation procedure. Mental health professionals can have a direct role in optimizing long-term transplant function by insuring successful communication between transplant team members and transplant patients of all educational backgrounds.

PRETRANSPLANTATION ASSESSMENT

In broad terms, the purpose of the pretransplantation psychosocial assessment of both transplant recipients and their potential donors is to afford both parties an opportunity to acquire sufficient information to maximize the probability of a successful outcome. For donors, this information must include a thorough and comprehensible discussion of the nature of the risks of renal donation and of the precise extent and limits of potential benefits to both the recipient and donor. For the recipients, the information must include a clear and accessible discussion of the potential risks arising from immunosuppression and the transplant surgery itself as well as the extent and limits of potential benefits arising from transplantation.

The conduct of the evaluation must afford the opportunity to obtain a longitudinal history of psychiatric symptomatology (including psychoactive substance use). It should assess the patient's capacity to comprehend and thus give informed consent and adhere to the immunosuppressive regimen. It should also provide a cross-sectional evaluation of the presence or absence of symptomatology consistent with active psychiatric diagnoses of relevance to transplantation.

Although corticosteroids and other immunosuppressants may induce neuropsychiatric symptoms in patients with no prior psychiatric history, such symptoms are most commonly observed in patients with a preexisting history of thought disorder, mood disorder, anxiety disorder, or cognitive disorder. Although schizophrenia and other thought disorders are relatively uncommon (estimated lifetime prevalence between 1% and 2%), the disorders tend to be chronic and hence are more likely to be active during a single clinical visit. In contrast, the episodic nature of many mood and anxiety disorders may minimize the likelihood of symptoms being present at the time of examination. Moreover, the symptoms associated with anxiety and mood disorders are generally less obvious to general clinical observers than are the presentations associated with chronic thought disorders. The more subtle presentation of anxiety and mood disorders has perhaps served to obscure the fact that such diagnoses are relatively common. Estimates of lifetime prevalence rates of mood and anxiety disorders in the general population vary between 12% and 20%; in the population of individuals with diabetes mellitus, the lifetime prevalence rates are closer to 30% to 40%.

The symptoms of thought, anxiety, and mood disorders are clearly the manifestations of biologic perturbations in the central nervous system. Available evidence strongly suggests that as the number of episodes of mood or severe anxiety disorder increases over an individual's lifetime, so too does the likely severity and frequency of future episodes. Additional evidence also suggests associations between the presence of symptomatic mood and anxiety disorders, and increased probability and severity of chronic medical illnesses (including diabetes, coronary artery disease, and possibly hypertension) and morbidity and mortality from major surgical procedures. The obvious pertinence of such findings for the reduction of transplant morbidity mandates careful assessment of the longitudinal history of psychiatric symptoms in transplant candidates. The fact that such a history is necessary for the expeditious diagnosis and management of acute psychiatric symptoms (especially those associated with corticosteroids) in the immediate posttransplantation period further underscores the importance of such information for the transplant team as a whole.

The fundamental importance of this clinical information for the management of conditions that may contribute to posttransplantation morbidity and mortality mandates the use of thorough and valid techniques to elicit the presence or absence of psychiatric symptoms. The use of structured clinical interviews employing diagnostic instruments of demonstrated validity allows the clinician conducting the pretransplantation psychosocial assessment the maximal opportunity to detect accurately the presence of psychiatric diagnoses relevant to transplantation. The use of casual, unstructured questioning that places on the patient the responsibility of defining and recognizing medical diagnoses ("Do you have depression? Do you have any psychiatric disorders?") is inadequate and may lead to the failure to recognize episodic conditions (particularly mood or anxiety disorders) relevant to the posttransplantation management of psychiatric symptoms. Although a detailed discussion of diagnostic instruments used in psychiatric assessment falls outside the scope of this chapter, the *Anxiety Disorders Interview Scale—Revised* (ADIS-R) is a convenient method to facilitate rapid and thorough evaluation of transplant candidates. The ADIS-R focuses on anxiety and, to a lesser extent, mood disorders. For reasons discussed previously, accurate diagnosis of anxiety and mood disorders is of cardinal importance in anticipating the effects of high-dose corticosteroid therapy associated with immunosuppression.

Assessment of the history of psychiatric symptoms is best prefaced with an explanation of the reason for seeking such information. The psychiatrist should explain that the brain, like many other organs in the body, is susceptible to disruption by immunosuppressants and other transplant-related events. The patient should appreciate that information obtained from the psychiatric history will allow for appropriate pretransplantation prophylactic measures to optimize posttransplantation comfort and function. Patients who are reluctant to discuss their psychiatric history should be reassured that the mere presence of such a history is not, in and of itself, a reason to deny access to transplantation and that few psychiatric diagnoses are absolute barriers to transplantation. In the United States, the *Americans With Disabilities Act* forbids any attempt to restrict access to transplantation or other medical services merely because of the presence of psychiatric symptoms or history.

Evaluation of Transplant Donors

Living kidney donation is an act of profound human generosity, and when appropriate consideration is given to all its medical and psychosocial aspects, it can be a source of much gratification for all the parties involved. The psychosocial assessment of potential transplant donors must focus wholly on the needs and issues relevant to the donor's well-being. Given the highly asymmetric nature of the physical benefits arising from renal donation, few if any circumstances in medical or psychiatric practice demand a more rigorous application of the ancient principle of *primum non nocere* (first, do no harm) than does the evaluation of potential organ donors.

The increasing shortage of cadaveric donors has been a stimulus to broaden the traditional range of individuals who are being considered as living donors (see Chapter 5). Whereas living donors were typically first-degree relatives for whom the nature of the relationship with the recipient and the motivation for donation was usually clear-cut, donors are increasingly individuals who are not biologically related. The psychosocial evaluation of unrelated, or "emotionally related," living donors requires particular attention to insure that their psychiatric well-being is protected.

Most individuals undergoing assessment for renal donation have made a free, informed, and autonomous decision to participate in the process. The evaluating psychiatrist, however, can never take this fact for granted. For this reason, it must be emphasized that the purpose of the interview is to elicit and implement the donor's desires regarding transplantation. Potential donors should be explicitly informed of the option to elect not to proceed. They should be able to trust that they can exercise this option without fear that the motives for their decision will become known to the prospective recipient or any other parties, without their approval. Some potential donors actually do not wish to serve as donors yet find themselves unable or unwilling to communicate their wishes to the prospective recipient or other emotionally relevant parties. Others, when informed of the existence of cadaveric donation as an alternative, elect not to proceed as a donor. Donors may have been led to understand the recipient's life may be at stake, a situation that is rare in kidney transplantation. The fact that donor nephrectomy is not wholly devoid of risk is sufficient to cause some to reconsider their participation. A more subtle, and hence more difficult to evaluate, situation is that of donors who do not directly report a desire to forego participation in transplantation but who provide information suggestive of strong ambivalence or emotional conflict regarding their participation.

The psychiatrist, therefore, is obliged to ensure that the prospective donor is acting in the absence of coercion and in the presence of accurate information regarding the consequences of his or her decision for the health of the recipient. In this context, the psychiatrist's sole ethical and clinical obligation is to the prospective donor. The psychiatrist (or other mental health professional) conducting the psychosocial evaluation of the donor must have no previous clinical relationship with the potential recipient. Only by maintaining rigorous boundaries can psychiatrists be experienced and perceived as pursuing the interests of their patient: the potential donor.

For donors to enjoy a truly free choice regarding their participation, the transplantation team must respect the donor's ethical and legal right to reach an independent decision within the context of strict medical confidentiality. A corollary to the requirement for adamant delineation of boundaries surrounding psychosocial assessment of the donor is that absolute confidentiality must be maintained during and after the donor's evaluation. Rigorous protection of the donor's privacy requires that information arising from this clinical encounter must be obtained and maintained in a fashion that prevents all possibility of disclosure to potential recipients, the recipients' family members and associates, and any health care providers extrinsic to the donor's transplantation evaluation. For this reason, the physicians and other health care providers with direct responsibility for providing care for the potential recipient should avoid participating in the evaluation of prospective donors for the recipient. For the same reason, the donor and psychiatrist must meet in the absence of family members, significant others, friends, or anyone else (with the exception of a professional translator, if required).

Another consequence of the statutory and ethical imperative to protect donors' confidentiality is that when translators are required, the translator must be unknown to the donor or recipient. The use of professional health care translators free of any relationship to donor or recipient is most feasible in large medical care centers in areas with substantial linguistic diversity; even in these settings, however, arranging such translation services for health care may require some effort. In circumstances or localities in which the appropriate professional medical translators are unavailable, arranging donor psychosocial evaluations at other centers where such services are available is a potential option. The use of remote (e.g., telephonic) professional translators at other medical centers, when appropriate, provides an alternative to physical travel by the donor to such locations. Because of the specialized vocabulary and information required for medical translation, any of the foregoing arrangements is infinitely preferable to the use of general-purpose translation services provided (in the United States) by commercial long-distance telephone services.

Although creation of such rigorous privacy standards is irrelevant to many donors and thus may potentially be regarded as excessive, the unwilling donors who arrive for pretransplantation psychosocial evaluation after multiple encounters with other components of the transplantation service offer convincing refutation of the hypothesis that such stringent confidentiality measures are unnecessary.

Evaluation of prospective donors must include consideration of the possibility of direct financial incentive to the donor in the form of payment or other remuneration by the recipient or third parties acting on the recipient's behalf. Financial inducements for solid organ donation are a violation of federal law in the United States (see Chapter 17). Any suggestion on the part of donors (or other involved parties) of such arrangements must be the focus of intense scrutiny. The presence of financial arrangements as an incentive for renal donation is incompatible with the donor's participation in transplantation.

Evaluation of Transplant Candidates

There has been a steady reduction in the psychiatric diagnoses or findings regarded as absolute contraindications to transplantation. Psychiatric and general medical evaluation of candidates (see Chapter 5) have in common the purpose of considering those issues that are of predictive value for the survival of the allograft itself and for the overall health of the transplant recipient.

Adherence (Compliance)

The most critical psychiatric issue influencing graft survival is whether the patient has the capacity to comply with the various components of a complex immunosuppressive protocol and to the associated regimen of intense medical surveillance. (*Compliance* is the term most commonly used for this capacity, although many prefer the term *adherence,* which implies greater autonomy on the patient's part.) There are surprisingly few variables with predictive value for compliance. Adolescence is robustly associated with noncompliance, although a history of florid noncompliance with immunosuppression as a teenager is often not predictive of noncompliance as an adult. Patients who, irrespective of age, display a relatively stable pattern of conflict with medical care recommendations despite deleterious consequences are at great risk for noncompliance with posttransplantation immunosuppression. Patients with severe thought disorder, extremely severe personality disorder (especially borderline personality), severe mood disorder (especially bipolar disorder), or psychoactive substance disorder (excluding tobacco) are at extremely high risk for noncompliance unless their primary psychiatric disorders can be successfully mitigated by treatment or other interventions before transplantation (such as the creation of a conservatorship or other such external locus of responsibility).

Regardless of circumstance or etiology, the presence of substantial medication noncompliance in transplant candidates at the time of evaluation does correlate with increased risk for posttransplantation noncompliance. In these candidates, it may be wise to require a period of some months of documented adherence to a medication regimen or dialysis schedule to assess whether the candidate currently possesses the capacity to tolerate the highly structured medication and clinical regimen that follows transplantation. Some candidates who display an incapacity to tolerate such a structured regimen can subsequently be assisted in gaining that ability through cognitive or interpersonal psychotherapies.

Cognitive Disorders

For patients with cognitive disorders or other psychiatric conditions unrelieved by or unamenable to treatment, transplant candidacy can only be meaningfully assessed in the context of the patient's external environment. The extent to which the caregivers in that environment can reliably compensate for aspects of the patient's condition that serve as barriers to compliance needs to be individually assessed. Even patients with severe cognitive impairment can comply with the posttransplantation regimen if their family and caregivers are committed to the success of transplantation.

From a psychiatric perspective, the detrimental effects of transplantation on the overall function of recipients arise chiefly from either cognitive impairment or the provocation or exacerbation of psychiatric symptoms. For transplant recipients whose social life and emotional support are derived solely from their dialysis center, the result of successful renal transplantation may be to exacerbate isolation and loneliness, both of which can exacerbate or even engender cognitive and psychiatric dysfunction.

In the selection of transplant candidates, the presence of cognitive dysfunction raises at least two questions for evaluating psychiatrists: (1) Can transplantation be expected to ameliorate or exacerbate the cognitive dysfunction? (2) Will any probable or possible exacerbation of cognitive impairment result in functional restrictions for the recipient? As a rule, answering the first question requires a putative or differential diagnosis of the cognitive impairment. Such a diagnosis inevitably requires the longitudinal history of psychiatric symptoms discussed previously and almost always requires neurocognitive testing to assess the precise deficit that may underlie the observed cognitive impairment. In general, cognitive impairments associated with impaired attention that arises from mood disorders, anxiety disorders, endocrine abnormalities, or perturbations of sleep or metabolic disorders associated with ESRD may be expected to improve after transplantation. In contrast, cognitive impairments associated with irreversible neuronal loss arising from severe hypoglycemia, poorly controlled hypertension, cerebral infarct, or primary dementias such as Alzheimer's disease are unlikely to demonstrate significant improvement. For these patients, the crucial question of whether neurotoxicity arising from immunosuppressant agents will lead to further functional impairments can be answered only, if at all, on an individual basis.

Substance Abuse

Depending on the practices and values of an individual transplantation center, the question of optimizing allograft and recipient survival may or may not extend to consideration of individual behaviors regarding dietary choices, exercise, or tobacco dependence. Psychiatrists who are cognizant of the risks, benefits, and efficacy of various forms of medical and nonmedical management of obesity and nicotine dependence are best able to serve the needs of both transplant candidates and the transplantation teams.

The presence of active substance abuse or dependence is generally regarded as a contraindication to renal transplantation. In contrast, a past history of substance abuse that has been followed by successful abstinence for 6 months or greater is seldom, if ever, a valid contraindication. Among transplant candidates who present with active substance abuse or dependence, the most appropriate course is generally to defer acceptance for transplantation pending successful completion of substance abuse treatment and a specified period of abstinence verified through random serum qualitative checks for substances of abuse. The possibility of false-positive test results or other factors that diminish the validity of qualitative testing for patients with ESRD must be considered. For this reason, transplantation teams should obtain confirmation of qualitative "drug screen" results through assays of the highest possible accuracy and specificity before making clinical assessments or decisions.

Among transplant candidates with current or previous substance abuse or dependence, the probability of comorbid psychiatric diagnoses is significantly greater than among candidates without such diagnoses. For this reason, careful assessment of psychiatric history and symptomatology is of particular importance in candidates with substance abuse diagnoses.

Psychiatric History

The extent to which the posttransplantation medication regimen may itself lead to psychiatric symptoms that decrease overall function is largely determined by the patient's previous psychiatric history. For the purposes of candidate selection, patients with a history of moderate to severe symptoms of thought, mood, or anxiety disorder that have proven refractory to adequate medication trials are at greatest risk for compromised function arising from uncontrolled symptoms after transplantation. This group of candidates, as well as those candidates with a history of thought disorder, recurrent mood disorder, or longstanding anxiety disorder who are unwilling to accept maintenance treatment, poses a difficult challenge. Fortunately, of all transplant candidates with a history of significant psychiatric symptoms, the proportion of those with either symptoms refractory to adequate treatment or a refractory refusal to allow treatment is extremely small. Far more common is the patient with a history of moderate to severe psychiatric symptoms that have gone undiagnosed or have received inadequate treatment. If these patients are willing and able to receive effective psychiatric treatment before transplantation, their history of symptoms should not be regarded as a contraindication to transplantation.

TREATMENT OF POSTTRANSPLANTATION PSYCHIATRIC SYMPTOMS

Medication Withdrawal

With the possible exception of hallucinogens, almost any psychotropic agent administered or used on a chronic or frequent basis can lead to withdrawal symptoms mediated through the central nervous system. One of the most common and most easily avoided psychiatric conditions arising in the immediate posttransplantation period is the result of inadvertent discontinuation of psychoactive medications on admission to the hospital for transplantation. Psychoactive substance withdrawal in the posttransplantation period is complicated by the fact that most immunosuppressants can act to increase neuronal excitability and thereby decrease seizure threshold.

This condition is most likely present when a patient has been using benzodiazepines (especially short-acting agents such as alprazolam or triazolam) or other sedative-hypnotics for the management of insomnia, anxiety disorders, or other conditions before transplantation. In these patients, the clinical picture usually progresses along a continuum of hyperarousal ranging from nervousness and anxiety to disinhibition, delirium, and withdrawal seizures. Prompt treatment of the symptoms of benzodiazepine withdrawal is mandatory. For moderate withdrawal symptoms, a starting dose of 0.5 to 1 mg of intravenous lorazepam can be carefully titrated upward, with an end point of reversing significant tachycardia and systolic hypertension arising from the withdrawal. Significant reductions in respiratory rate or falling oxygen saturation are suggestive of respiratory depression arising from benzodiazepine administration. In the event of incorrect identification of benzodiazepine withdrawal or overly enthusiastic management of a correctly identified episode of withdrawal, the benzodiazepine receptor antagonist flumazenil and the equipment and capacity for emergent intubation must be available. Avoiding abrupt or rapid discontinuation of benzodiazepines and other sedative-hypnotics is the safest way to prevent this potentially lethal complication from arising during transplantation.

Symptomatic withdrawal syndromes that include mental status changes have been associated with the discontinuation of a variety of psychotropic medications. The most frequent are the following:

1. Diphenhydramine (which many dialysis patients receive in high oral or parenteral dosages)
2. Serotonin-specific reuptake inhibitors (SSRIs; the withdrawal symptoms may be delayed by up to 36 hours)
3. Postsynaptic serotonin receptor agonists (nefazodone and trazodone)
4. Dopamine receptor antagonists (commonly used to treat dysregulation of gastrointestinal motility in dialysis patients)

Resumption of the discontinued medication is the most effective short-term intervention to control withdrawal symptoms as long as potential drug interactions with immunosuppressants are considered. In the event of withdrawal symptoms arising from the discontinuation of nonpharmaceutical substances such as ethanol or nicotine, provision of an agent with cross-tolerance properties (benzodiazepines for ethanol) or by an alternative route of administration (transdermal nicotine) may also be useful.

Delirium

The central nervous system makes exacting demands of the body to maintain functional homeostasis. Delirium is an acute manifestation of failure to maintain such homeostasis. Delirium is a clinical diagnosis characterized by (1) a disturbance in consciousness manifest in reduced capacity to focus, sustain, or shift attention; (2) change in cognition or development of perceptual disturbance; (3) development and fluctuation of symptoms over a course of hours to days. Delirium is relatively familiar in acute care hospitals in general and in posttransplantation patients in particular, and its development is always a cause for concern. Delirium is robustly associated with increased risk for morbidity and mortality. Medication withdrawal, narcotic analgesia, infection, immunosuppressant neurotoxicity, and protracted sleep disturbance can cause delirium. Given the diversity of causal factors associated with delirium, effective management, even in the absence of certainty regarding etiology, is essential for clinicians responsible for the care of transplant recipients.

Oral or parenteral haloperidol is commonly used in the management of delirium, although more rapid control of both behavioral dysinhibition and agitation may be attained with parenteral droperidol. Droperidol offers the dual advantage of more rapid onset and a lesser chance of akathisia (a subjective sense of restlessness arising from extrapyramidal dopamine receptor blockade), thus minimizing the possibility of a positive feedback loop in which greater amounts of dopamine receptor antagonist are administered to manage apparent restlessness. Droperidol should be administered initially in test doses of 0.625 to 1.25 mg every 5 minutes, with monitoring for the extremely rare reported side effects of hypotension and bradycardia; if neither condition becomes manifest, the dosage may be titrated upward to 2.5 to 10 mg over 10 to 15 minutes until control of acute agitation is attained. In patients with clinically significant hypotension or bradycardia arising from cardiac dysfunction, parenteral haloperidol may be used as a substitute for droperidol. Given the fact that the duration of onset of haloperidol in this context is generally 20 to 30 minutes, the frequency of repeat dose administrations must be reduced accordingly. As with any delirium, the use of "low-potency" agents (of which chlorpromazine may be regarded as a prototypical example) is contraindicated secondary to anticholinergic side effects, which exacerbate cognitive impairment.

Insomnia

Insomnia is the most common subjective neuropsychiatric symptom in the posttransplantation period. Although acute or intensive care hospital settings are intrinsically capable of engendering insomnia, corticosteroids are the most powerful and most common cause of insomnia in the first days and weeks after transplantation. Management of insomnia can generally be attained with the use of temazepam, with a dose of 15 to 30 mg sufficing for most patients. The use of the hypnotic triazolam (Halcion) or other short-acting triazolobenzodiazepines such as alprazolam (Xanax) and midazolam (Versed) is inappropriate. In the posttransplantation period, short-acting benzodiazepines are associated with an increased risk for both rebound insomnia and cognitive or perceptual disturbances that can progress to frank delirium, profound affective lability, or overt hallucinations.

Anxiety

In the acute posttransplantation period, as many as one fifth of all patients complain of the affective state of anxiety or the subjective experience of restlessness. These symptoms are most typically associated with corticosteroids but may also occur with nonsteroidal immunosuppressants. Patients with a preexisting history of anxiety disorders (panic disorder, agoraphobia and other phobias, obsessive-compulsive disorder, and posttraumatic stress disorder) are at highest risk for this complication. Initial management of anxiety should include careful attention to the possibility of inadvertent medication withdrawal as well as the possibility of akathisia arising from the use of dopamine receptor antagonists used most frequently to treat nausea. In these cases, relief of anxiety is best attained by resumption of the discontinued psychotropic agent or discontinuing the dopamine receptor antagonists. In most transplant recipients who manifest anxiety, neither of the aforementioned etiologies is present, and anxiety can be treated with clonazepam, 0.25 to 0.5 mg as needed every 8 to 12 hours, with titration of dosage and frequency of administration upward as required for symptomatic relief. For patients who require parenteral administration or develop sad mood or overt depression in the context of clonazepam administration, anxiety may be managed with lorazepam, 0.25 to 0.5 mg orally or intravenously every 4 to 6 hours. As in the management of insomnia, alprazolam (Xanax) and other short-acting benzodiazepines should be avoided. Barbiturates, because of their low therapeutic index and immunosuppressant drug interactions, have no place in the management of posttransplantation anxiety.

Mood Disorders

Broadly speaking, mood disorders manifest as insufficient cerebral activation (depression) or excessive cerebral activation (mania). Transplant recipients may also develop a mixed state characterized by affective lability, pressured speech, or behavioral dysinhibition in the presence of intact sensorium and maintenance of orientation. Patients exhibiting behavioral dysinhibition should be acutely stabilized with parenteral droperidol, in doses equal to or greater than those discussed previously in the management of delirium, while awaiting psychiatric consultation.

Depression is characterized by a persistent (greater than 2 weeks) state of sad mood or anhedonia, together with changes in thought content (hopeless or suicidal ideation), thought process (rumination), attention (decreased concentration), social relatedness (withdrawal), and somatic function (diminished energy and perturbations in sleep or appetite). The diagnosis of a first episode of depression in the posttransplantation period is complicated by the fact that corticosteroids and other immunosuppressants may produce diminished concentration as a function of disruption in attention. Corticosteroids also commonly increase appetite and cause insomnia. For these reasons, the onset of persistent sad mood or anhedonia, hopeless or negative ideation, and suicidal ideation are the most reliable indicators of depressive episodes in the posttransplantation period.

Patients with a previous history of major depression or other affective disorders are at greatest risk for depression in the posttransplantation period. Pretransplantation identification of a history of recurrent (two or more episodes) major depression should trigger prophylactic therapy. SSRIs of moderate half-life, such as sertraline (Zoloft) or paroxetine (Paxil), are generally the best choices. The capacity of paroxetine to enhance sleep quality is an added advantage for patients troubled by sleep disturbance associated with ESRD. In patients experiencing a first episode of depression and in those in whom the diagnosis of recurrent major depression was missed before transplantation, either sertraline (50 to 150 mg every morning) or paroxetine (10 to 40 mg at bedtime) generally ameliorates the symptoms within several days to a few weeks. Use of temazepam for insomnia or low-dose clonazepam (0.25 to 0.5 mg every 8 to 12 hours) for anxiety engendered by depressive ideation or related symptoms can be of great relief to patients awaiting the onset of antidepressants.

Mania is characterized by persistently elevated mood, which may be of an ego-syntonic (euphoric), or ego-dystonic (irritable) nature. It occurs together with alterations in concentration (diminished attention), thought process (flight of ideas or loosening of associations), speech process (rapid or pressured speech), somatic function (insomnia, restlessness, or hypersexuality), judgment (diminished impulse control or grandiosity), or behavioral dysinhibition. Mania may range from mildly intrusive to catastrophically disruptive. Incorrectly managed mania can cause allograft loss (due to noncompliance with immunosuppression or follow-up appointments), severe disruption of clinical or domestic settings, and behavioral dysinhibition, which can engender lethal events for the recipient or others. Psychiatric consultation for suspected mania is imperative. While awaiting psychiatric consultation, acute dysinhibition requires environmental (constant observation) and pharmacologic (parenteral droperidol as used in delirium, with the addition of parenteral lorazepam for more rapid onset of sedation if needed) management. Less severe symptoms of mania may be managed by clonazepam (0.5 to 2 mg every 4 to 6 hours, with careful titration to avoid excessive sedation progressing to respiratory depression in patients without tolerance to benzodiazepines). Gabapentin in an initial dosage of 100 to 200 mg given three times daily, with titration up to 400 to 600 mg four times daily, is also effective in the management of mania associated with transplantation. Exacerbation of preexistent bipolar affective (manic-depressive) disorder with high-dose corticosteroids is the rule, rather than the exception, and transplant recipients should receive mood stabilizers (valproic acid or gabapentin) before transplantation. As in the case of recurrent major depression, the safest and most effective way to manage mania after transplantation is for candidates with a preexisting history to be started on prophylactic medications before transplantation.

Hallucinations and Delusions

In most patients, the presence of hallucinations (perturbations of perception) and delusions (perturbations of cognition) in the posttransplantation period are manifestations of delirium. Appropriate management includes both palliative treatment of the distressing symptoms and efforts to identify and treat correctable causes.

Occasionally, hallucinations and delusions may arise without disturbance or fluctuation in consciousness. This picture is most likely to arise in patients with auditory or visual impairment before transplantation but may also occur without sensory impairment. In recipients with no other psychiatric symptoms who are unconcerned by occasional visual hallucinations in the form of small dots or streaks of light, pharmacologic intervention may be unnecessary. When pharmacologic intervention is desired either because of patient preference or because of more overt symptoms, low doses of risperidone (0.25 to 0.5 mg at bedtime or twice daily) are generally sufficient.

IMMUNOSUPPRESSANT AND PSYCHOTROPIC DRUG INTERACTIONS

Careful choice of psychotropic medications for transplant candidates and recipients can minimize the risk for deleterious interactions with immunosuppressants and hence minimize the risk for avoidable allograft dysfunction or rejection. Ideally, the choice of psychotropic agents in transplant recipients is informed by knowledge of the relevant metabolic pathways for psychotropic medications, immunosuppressants, and the adjunctive medications commonly used in transplantation. Although a detailed discussion of these matters exceeds the scope of this chapter, awareness of general principles promotes informed application of specific recommendations.

Most significant drug interactions with psychotropic medications arise from alterations in the rate of oxidative metabolism carried out by the cytochrome P450 hepatic enzyme system, which is particularly important for the metabolism of the calcineurin inhibitors and sirolimus (see Chapter 4). Psychotropics that perturb the baseline activity of the IID6 and IIIA3/4 isoenzymes have the greatest propensity for deleterious changes in immunosuppressant levels.

Specific Recommendations

1. Among "serotonergic" antidepressants, the capacity to raise calcineurin inhibitor levels is in the following order: fluvoxamine → nefazodone → fluoxetine → trazodone → paroxetine → sertraline → citralopram. Sertraline doses that equal or exceed 200 mg/day result in increased isoenzyme inhibition and thus disproportionately increased serum levels. The dose of reboxetine may need to be reduced when it is coadministered with azole antifungal agents.

2. Among anxiolytics and hypnotics, serum levels and half-lives of the triazolobenzodiazepines (alprazolam, midazolam, and triazolam), propofol, buspirone, and zolpidem are potentially increased by azole antifungals, macrolide antibiotics, and cimetidine.

3. Among anticonvulsants used in mood stabilization, carbamazepine may lead to decreases in immunosuppressant levels as a result of isoenzyme induction. Valproate is chiefly metabolized by phase II (conjugative) pathways and thus poses far less risk for untoward interactions. Gabapentin, which is excreted unchanged, appears to carry no risk of altered immunosuppressant levels arising from altered metabolism.

4. Among atypical antipsychotics, sertindole and olanzapine levels are increased by interaction with posttransplantation medications to a greater extent than are levels of risperidone. With appropriate dosage modifications, all may be used successfully in transplant recipients.

5. Among typical antipsychotics, low-potency agents such as chlorpromazine are subject to alterations in serum levels resulting from changes in hepatic enzyme activity. High-potency agents such as haloperidol and droperidol appear to be less liable to such changes. For this reason (as well as anticholinergic properties, which can exacerbate cognitive dysfunction), low-potency agents are a suboptimal choice for most transplant recipients.

6. St. John's Wort, a popular over-the-counter herbal remedy for depression, has been associated with graft loss as a result of isoenzyme induction and accelerated metabolism of immunosuppressants. Its use is contraindicated in transplant recipients.

7. Fluvoxamine and nefazodone may cause increases in cisapride levels, resulting in lethal cardiac arrhythmias.

8. Coadministration of mirtazapine and clonidine has been reported to induce severe hypertension due to action of these agents at central alpha-2 inhibitory noradrenergic receptors. The coadministration of these agents in transplant recipients is contraindicated.

SELECTED READINGS

Benedetti E, Asolati M, Dunn T, et al. Kidney transplantation in recipients with mental retardation. *Am J Kidney Dis* 1998;31:509.

Burn DJ, Bates D. Neurology and the kidney. *J Neurol Neurosurg Psychiatry* 1998;65:810.

Fugh-Berman A. Herb-drug interactions. *Lancet* 2000;355:134.

Greenstein S, Siegal B. Compliance and noncompliance in patients with a functioning renal transplant: a multicenter study. *Transplantation* 1998;66:1718.

Klapheke MM. The role of the psychiatrist in organ transplantation. *Bulletin of the Menninger Clinic* 1999;63:13.

Nemeroff CB, DeVane CL, Pollock BG. Newer antidepressants and the cytochrome P450 system. *Am J Psychiatry* 1996;153:311.

Rodin G, Abbey S. Kidney transplantation. In: Craven J, Rodin G, eds. *Psychiatric aspects of organ transplantation*. Oxford, UK: Oxford University Press, 1992:145–163.

Schlitt HJ, Brunkhorst R, Schmidt HH, et al. Attitudes of patients before and after transplantation towards various allografts. *Transplantation* 1999;68:510.

Trzepacz PT, DiMartini A, Tringali R. Psychosomatic issues in organ transplantation. Part I. Pharmacokinetics in organ failure and psychiatric aspects of immunosuppressants and anti-infectious agents. *Psychosomatics* 1993;34:1991.

17

Ethical and Legal Issues in Kidney Transplantation

Leslie Steven Rothenberg

Medicine and surgery in the 21st century are filled with ethical dilemmas; the field of kidney transplantation is no exception. Questions inevitably involve the underlying ethical principles of respecting the self-determination of patients with decision-making capacity (sometimes called *autonomy*), acting to protect the patient's well-being (sometimes called *beneficence*), and acting in a manner that promotes fairness and equity to all involved (sometimes called *justice*).

The applications of these principles with regard to kidney transplantation are explored in this chapter with reference to the donation and procurement of organs, the selection of patients for transplantation, and the place of kidney transplantation in the allocation of health care resources and the development of national priorities.

DONATION AND PROCUREMENT OF ORGANS

Current Shortage of Cadaveric Organs

The United Network for Organ Sharing (UNOS) reported that as of June 17, 2000, 45,521 people on its national patient list were waiting for a kidney. Kidney transplantations are currently being performed in the United States at a rate of about 12,000 per year; the extent of the scarcity of donor kidneys for transplantation is so great that it would take almost the entire combined total of transplantation performed in a recent 4-year period to meet the need of patients waiting. Furthermore, in recent years, the kidney donor supply has remained fairly constant despite national and local efforts to increase donations. The reported average waiting time for a cadaveric kidney transplant is approaching 2 years, and there are thousands of patients who, using hemodialysis as a back-up, have been waiting longer than 3 years for such a transplant.

The existing kidney organ supply, therefore, is clearly inadequate to meet the current and future needs in this country. Donor kidneys are a genuinely scarce resource, and questions of fairness in their procurement and distribution are inevitable. It is speculative to presume that increased educational programs, new legal approaches, or financial or other incentives can increase the supply of cadaveric organs.

Determination of Death

Acceptance of organ procurement and transplantation depends, in large part, on public confidence that cadaveric organs, including kidneys, are being taken from people who are truly dead in the public's understanding of that term. In other words, the often-quoted truism that the determination of death is a medical decision hides the reality that the concept of death, although given both a medical and legal rationale, is fundamentally a social and not a scientific concept, informed by cultural and religious beliefs.

The medical criteria for whole brain death (see Chapter 5) were authoritatively defined by a U.S. presidential commission in 1981. The major principles are the following:

1. Both cerebral and brain-stem functions must be absent.
2. The cause of this total lack of brain functioning must have been identified and determined to be irreversible.
3. The absence of all brain function must have persisted during a period of treatment and observation.

The Uniform Determination of Death Act (1981) provided the legal framework by stating that "an individual is dead if there is irreversible cessation of circulatory and respiratory functions or if there is irreversible cessation of all brain functions of the entire brain, including the brain stem." This statutory definition has been adopted by most U.S. state legislatures. In other states, courts have upheld these brain-death criteria in judicial rulings.

Yet difficulties persist. The very phrase *brain death* connotes to some the existence of two types of death, regular death and brain death. This distinction is aided by the perception that the death of patients who lose cardiac and respiratory functions and who are not on ventilator support is different from the death of patients on ventilators.

It might be helpful to stop using the phrase brain death and to use only the single word death for people on or off the ventilator, no matter how the determination of that death was made. Yet the phrase brain death is used precisely to explain how this breathing person with a heartbeat could be said to be dead.

Efforts to broaden the category of what constitutes death in humans, including suggestions that babies with anencephaly and patients in persistent vegetative states be treated as though dead for purposes of organ donation, have met with significant public and professional resistance. In the late 1990s, protocols were developed to retrieve organs from patients after they had been declared dead on the basis of cardiopulmonary criteria, even though they did not meet the criteria of whole brain death (so-called non–heart-beating donors; see Chapter 5). Arguments in favor of using organs from executed prisoners have been advanced, some in response to reports of the practice occurring in China.

Altruism Versus Duty or Payment for Organs

Use of Live Donors

About 25% of the kidney transplantations performed in the United States involve living donors. Living donors are usually defined in three categories:

1. *Living-related donors* (such as parents, siblings, or children), who are genetically related to the recipient
2. *Living emotionally related donors* (such as spouses, "significant others," and close friends), who are genetically unrelated
3. *Living-unrelated,* or *altruistic, donors,* who are strangers to the recipient and who may or may not be compensated for their donated kidney

Although living donors do well after donating a single kidney, there was initial resistance in some circles to using such donors in kidney transplantation. The rare death of a living kidney donor, the potential morbidity risks for those who survive, and the uncertainty about the degree of improvement in recipient and graft survival compared with cadaveric donor organs has seemed to militate against their use. The continuing shortage of cadaveric organs, however, has pushed in the other direction.

Organ donation by living donors brings into focus perplexing ethical problems because of the dangers of coercion and external as well as self-generated pressures on the donor. While wishing to respect the freely made decisions of prospective donors with decision-making capacity, and while valuing the life-saving potential of this gift to the recipients and the satisfaction of donors, transplantation teams have been forced to evaluate the motives, capacities, and emotional feelings of prospective donors in a variety of factual contexts. They have also struggled with the question of the level of informed consent that can be obtained in such situations and the level of altruism in such decisions.

The following three clinical vignettes illustrate some of the ethical dilemmas that using such donors may generate:

Susan, a 30-year-old divorcee, suffered from chronic nephritis and hypertension, as well as systemic lupus erythematosus. She was evaluated as a kidney transplant candidate. Susan's parents, ages 63 and 56 years, and four of her adult siblings were tested as possible donors, and the best match was her 23-year-old brother, Marvin. Marvin is healthy but has a severe developmental disability, Down's syndrome, and the mental age of a 3- or 4-year-old. Thus, Marvin does not have the capacity to make the decision to donate his organ, although he states that he wants to help his sister. His sister, in turn, has offered to take care of Marvin after their parents' deaths. The family has agreed that Marvin should be the donor. How should the risks and benefits to Marvin and Susan be evaluated?

Diane and Dione are identical twins born 12 years ago. Dione is now suffering from hemolytic-uremic syndrome and needs a kidney transplantation. Both parents were ruled out as donors on medical grounds. No other related donors are available, leaving her sister, Diane, who, because she is an identical twin, would be an ideal donor. Diane is fond of her sister and says she would like to help her. How should the risks and benefits to Diane and Dione be evaluated?

Mrs. P., a middle-aged woman with diabetic nephropathy and progressive retinopathy, is doing poorly on dialysis. She has 70% panel-reactive antibodies and has been on a cadaveric waiting list for 2 years. She is a patient of a nephrologist, Dr. N., who has encouraged her to discuss the possibility of living-related donation with her siblings. She tells Dr. N. that her sister has volunteered to donate a kidney to her. Dr. N. arranges for testing but then receives a call from the potential donor's husband, who relates that his wife has a strong ambivalence about being a donor, coupled with a fear of having to face her sister with a negative decision. Dr. N. next meets with the potential donor, who repeatedly asks him about the risks involved in the donation, is very tense throughout the conversation, and says at one point, "Is the kidney machine really that bad for her?" The tissue typing shows that the patient's sister is a two-haplotype match to her, and all crossmatching is negative. Dr. N. has real doubts about her willingness to give the kidney freely, yet he realizes that Mrs. P. has a poor prognosis on dialysis and may have to wait a long time for a cadaveric kidney. How should he handle this situation?

These scenarios highlight but a few of the ethical questions. Can families, such as Marvin's, be trusted in making gifts of one child's kidney to save the life of (or remove from hemodialysis) another child, such as Susan? Should Marvin's developmental disability be viewed as an absolute contraindication to his being considered as a donor? How does one weigh the potential for coercion or feelings of obligation implicit in the offer of a potential recipient to take future care of the would-be donor?

Courts hearing such cases have often permitted parents to donate kidneys or bone marrow from their minor children as long as an argument could be made that the donor children will "benefit" from the donation. The concept of benefit here is usually the satisfaction that the donor has helped, or saved the life of, a relative. This judicial standard clearly favors such donations because this abstract concept of a positive benefit, especially if voiced by the would-be donor, is far easier to grasp and endorse than is an understanding of the more negative medical risks for living donors.

The duty or obligation to make a gift of a kidney can also be present in the mind of the donor, even if never articulated. In the examples given previously, Diane may feel such an obligation to her sister, Dione, in addition to her love for her. Mrs. P.'s sister, on the other hand, may be unable to express her opposition to or fear of donating a kidney to Mrs. P. and may resent the pressure to do so.

For these reasons, various national guidelines have emphasized limiting living donation to people who are either genetically or emotionally related to the recipient, whose motives seem altruistic and not based on duty or coercion, and who can make informed decisions with a clear understanding of the risks and benefits involved. It is also required that potential donors not receive any economic reward other than payment of reasonable medical expenses and lost income. This guideline clearly excludes almost all living-unrelated donors (in contrast with living emotionally related donors).

The case of Mrs. P. illustrates the importance of donor advocacy. It must be clear to all parties that donors are not to be sacrificed for recipients. Dr. N. would have been wise to have asked a colleague to evaluate the potential donor (see Chapter 5).

Sale of Organs and Rewarded Gifting

The use of living-unrelated kidney donors may have begun, albeit unwittingly, in 1971 at the Christian Medical College in Vellore, India, when the surgeon, Dr. Mohan Rao, discovered that the donor, introduced to Dr. Rao as the recipient's "cousin," was, in fact, a paid stranger. There is a tradition in India of paying living-related donors. Media advertisements by both kidney donors and would-be recipients have been commonplace, as have efforts to control the brokering of kidneys by carefully monitored programs in individual transplantation centers. The argument is made that that this practice is ethically acceptable given the inability to provide dialysis for more than a small percentage of Indian patients with end-stage renal disease (ESRD) and the social acceptance in India of paid donors as an alternative to the deaths of recipients. Others have said that there is a greater public sympathy in India for kidney donors in need of the money than for the hospitals and medical teams, who are viewed as exploitative.

There is evidence to suggest that wealthy recipients from the Middle East who have gone to India or other underdeveloped countries for living-unrelated transplants have received inferior medical care, have sustained higher than normal complication rates, and have been financially exploited along with their donors. Such commercialized programs may inhibit the development of local transplantation programs involving cadaveric donors because families of prospective donors see no reason to authorize the removal of organs if such organs are available elsewhere for purchase.

Western nations have been quick to condemn such practices. The National Organ Transplantation Act of 1984 in the United States makes the buying and selling of human organs illegal. Britain passed a similar law in 1989 after a scandal was publicized in which four paid Turkish donors were hired by an organ broker. In 1990, three British physicians were disciplined for their role in those transplantations.

Yet, in the United States, donors of sperm and blood plasma are legally paid for their donations. It has been argued that, given the chronic shortage of both cadaveric and even living-related and living emotionally related donors, there should be a program of *rewarded gifting* for kidneys just as there is for sperm and plasma. A pilot program has been introduced in Pennsylvania whereby families of cadaveric donors may receive limited financial compensation to cover burial costs; the effect of this program on cadaveric donation has yet to be assessed.

Those arguing for such a program claim that, even among related donors and recipients, money or some other reward is often secretly exchanged. Moreover, they suggest that people should have the right to sell organs or tissues under controlled circumstances, and the benefit to recipients should be matched by a benefit to donors beyond abstract altruistic joy.

Those who argue most strenuously for a rewarded gifting program would exclude brokers and direct payment from recipients or transplantation programs. They would change the nature of the reward from money to tax rebates or credits, burial grants, insurance policies, future medical coverage, or tuition subsidies for children. They would introduce a carefully regulated system in which both living-related and living-unrelated donors would be evaluated by transplantation centers under uniform medical and ethical guidelines with a third party, such as the government, independently handling the rewards after the transplantation was completed.

Those opposed claim that such programs, even with the limits contemplated, will jeopardize public support for organ transplantation, particularly for cadaveric organ donation. They claim that programs will be costly and are unjustified without greater educational efforts to encourage donation. Some even argue that the use of living donors is increasingly unjustified in the face of improved techniques for cadaveric organ transplantation and a failure to maximize the retrieval of cadaveric organs.

In 1999, numerous U.S. media reports described gifts of kidneys from living-unrelated donors, including an Indiana nurse who offered a kidney to anyone chosen by a Johns Hopkins University transplantation surgeon, a North Carolina middle school teacher who gave a kidney to one of her students, and a Los Angeles woman who donated a kidney to a friend and fellow church member—the latter two involving interracial donations. These reports joined other media coverage of less altruistic situations, including that of an employee of a Japanese consumer finance company who reportedly was told by a "loan shark" to sell one of his kidneys to raise money to pay his debts and that of a pledge by a group of Iranian men to sell one of their kidneys in order to finance an assassination attempt against British author Salman Rushdie.

Anencephalic and Xenograft Organs

Human kidney transplantations using anencephalic organ donors have been reported in the United States, Europe, and Japan. Xenograft organs have also been used, although largely in research on animals. Space does not permit a review of the ethical issues involving anencephalic and xenograft transplantations, but there are concerns about the functional usefulness of the transplanted organs, the application of brain-death standards in the case of anencephalic donors, the animal rights debate in the context of xenograft organs, and the currently unmet need each year of nearly 600 children in the United States who require kidney transplants.

The U.S. center with the greatest experience in seeking anencephalic organ donors, Loma Linda University Medical Center, California, concluded in 1989, after a research effort involving 12 infants and no successful transplantations, that "it is usually not feasible, with the restrictions of current [US] law [regarding the determination of death], to procure solid organs from anencephalic infants."

Allocation of Organs Among Transplantation Centers

In the United States, the national organ procurement and transplantation network is privately operated under governmental supervision. The National Organ Transplant Act (Public Law 98-507), passed by Congress in 1984, called for such a network to be established and administered by a nonprofit entity under contract to the U.S. Department of Health and Human Services. UNOS (see Chapter 3) was created as a legal entity in 1984 as an outgrowth of the South-Eastern Organ Procurement Foundation (SEOPF) of Richmond, Virginia, which had been established in 1975 by several transplantation centers as a means of sharing transplant information and protocols and creating a shared computer registry system. Other U.S. transplantation centers sought to join this computer registry, and, in the late 1970s and early 1980s, a loosely formed national network was created with the SEOPF offices and computers as its center.

UNOS created a system for distributing cadaveric kidneys, based on a scoring approach developed at the University of Pittsburgh by Dr. Thomas Starzl. Beginning in 1987, with refinements in 1995, the UNOS system assigns points to each patient on the transplant waiting list. Three major criteria are used: the quality of the tissue match, the time waiting for the kidney, and the level of preformed antibodies. The system is applied uniformly across the United States. "Zero-antigen mismatch" kidneys, however, must be shared nationally, and less well-matched kidneys are shared on a regional basis with variances approved by UNOS to take into account local needs and circumstances (see Chapter 3).

Family Veto of Organ Donor Cards

The National Kidney Foundation and state motor vehicle departments seeking potential organ donors have sought to portray the decision to donate organs as solely within the control of the would-be donor. Transplantation programs, however, have routinely permitted family members to veto such decisions. Even though properly signed organ donor cards were in the possession of kidney transplantation teams, and although the Uniform Anatomical Gift Act (the model law written in 1968 to provide a legal basis for such gifts in advance of the death of the donor and adopted in all of the states and the District of Columbia) authorized such gifts by any person older than 18 years of age with decision-making capacity, transplantation teams have routinely refused to honor such cards when family members objected, reportedly for public relations reasons.

The mere fact that family members are even asked for their consent in the presence of a properly signed donor card suggests that the donor card process is misleadingly presented as a donor decision process. No warning is given to the donor card signer of the power of the family to veto his or her decision to donate. It is, in fact, a family or next-of-kin decision rather than a donor decision. The ability of the family to veto raises ethical questions about campaigns to obtain signed donor cards.

As of June 2000, 22 states (Arizona, Arkansas, California, Connecticut, Hawaii, Idaho, Indiana, Iowa, Minnesota, Montana, Nevada, New Hampshire, New Mexico, North Dakota, Oregon, Pennsylvania, Rhode Island, Utah, Vermont, Virginia, Washington, and Wisconsin) had adopted a revised Uniform Anatomical Gift Act that specifically provides that next of kin need not consent to organ donations if the document making the gift is given to the donor's attending physician. The new law also removes the previous legal requirements for a witness's signature on the donor card or other document.

Ethical Tensions Within the U.S. Transplantation System

As the 21st century began with an increasing gap between the availability of donor organs and potential recipients, issues related to money, power, and prestige manifested themselves increasingly among the various parties in the transplant system—individual, institutional, and governmental.

The United Network for Organ Sharing Versus the U.S. Department of Health and Human Services

UNOS, historically dominated by the surgeons who direct institutional transplantation programs, adopted a highly adversarial (and publicized) position against the U.S. Department of Health and Human Services (DHHS). As mentioned earlier, the 1984 National Organ Transplant Act authorized DHHS to oversee the national organ network, known technically as the Organ Procurement and Transplantation Network. DHHS, in turn, contracts with UNOS to manage the distribution of organs for transplantation. This relationship soured in 1998 when DHHS Secretary Donna Shalala told Congress that DHHS would issue a regulation requiring the elimination of geography as the primary criterion for determining the allocation of organs. Although UNOS had in 1987 a policy that allowed transfer of organs not critically needed in the community where they were obtained to any patient in the country said to have less than 48 hours to live, this policy was reversed in 1990. The subsequent UNOS policy created 11 regions within the United States and mandated that organs must be offered first to patients on waiting lists within the region before they could be given to patients in other regions. News reports in 1999 indicated that even that approach met resistance as, for example, Wisconsin, Minnesota, North Dakota, and South Dakota did not want to share organs with Illinois out of concern that Chicago-area hospitals, having so many sick patients, would get the largest share.

Congress, heavily lobbied by UNOS and by constituents energized by local transplantation programs, delayed the implementation of the new DHHS policy. Following recommendations in a 1999 report by the Institute of Medicine, the proposed policy would also create an advisory committee to help direct DHHS policy, would no longer require consideration of the amount of time a patient has been waiting for a transplant as an allocation priority criterion, and would seek to limit the "gaming" of the allocation system by programs.

The States Versus the Federal Government

The proposed DHHS rule has divided large transplantation programs from smaller ones. Smaller programs fear that without geographic protection, they will not obtain sufficient organs and will not survive economically. The institutions that sponsor these programs see them as important for reasons of money and prestige (e.g., a way to differentiate for marketing purposes the "cutting-edge" technology of one hospital from another). Large programs have, in turn, lost organs and business to smaller programs.

All of the programs have sought support from their state legislators, the smaller ones arguing that local control and priorities should prevail over federal regulation. Some states (including Louisiana, Wisconsin, Oklahoma, South Carolina, Florida, and Texas) have passed laws forbidding the out-of-state transfer of organs donated in their states if any of their state residents are prospective recipients. Such legislation has been rationalized on the premise that more organs will be donated if donors or families know that the organs will stay in their particular state, a hypothesis judged to be unfounded by research conducted in the Institute of Medicine 1999 report. Pennsylvania was scheduled in 2000 to launch a pilot program to pay $300 in funeral expenses for organ donors as another incentive for organ donations despite criticism that this was an indirect way of violating the previously mentioned U.S. legal prohibition on payments for organ donation.

Required Request Laws

In the mid-1980s, many U.S. state legislatures began adopting laws requiring hospitals to develop policies that facilitated the possibility of organ donation. These policies required the identification as possible donors all patients determined to be, or anticipated to soon become, brain dead, and the offering to the legal next of kin or other person authorized to make decisions for such patients an opportunity to donate the patient's organs.

Almost all U.S. states have now adopted varying forms of such "routine inquiry, required request" laws; federal law now mandates that all hospitals receiving Medicare or Medicaid funds make such donor inquiries. The theory behind this legal approach was that it would generate more kidneys and other organs available for transplantation, but that theory remains to be proved. Although organ donations have increased in some states and referrals to organ procurement agencies of potential donors have increased in all states, the actual number of available kidneys has remained the same nationally for 4 years.

This result has prompted some commentators to suggest that the problem is not a legal one but a psychological one on the part of attending physicians and nurses who do not wish either to be involved in or to see families "stressed" by organ donation requests at the time a loved one has died. Others, perhaps more pragmatic, have suggested that the better approach is to adopt "presumed-consent" laws similar to those adopted in a number of U.S. states that permit the removal of pituitary glands and corneas from eligible cadavers unless the patient objected in writing before death or the family objected at the time of death. This approach assumes, of course, that public and judicial reaction will be equally tolerant to the removal of kidneys without explicit consent.

There appears to be a deeply felt preference among physicians for the organ procurement process to be a voluntary one. In France, which has presumed-consent laws, physicians, for public relations reasons, seek family consent despite the laws and refuse to take organs when families object. It has been suggested that routine inquiry about organ donation in the event of sudden death should become part of the standard medical history. Congress in 1998 passed a law giving organ procurement organizations much more control over the organ and tissue donation process by requiring hospitals to work with them and threatening loss of Medicare eligibility for failure to do so.

SELECTION OF PATIENTS FOR TRANSPLANTATION

Equitable Selection and Access

The system of distribution of cadaveric kidneys is theoretically blind to the possibility of discrimination based on age, race, gender, and socioeconomic status. In practice, this equity has not always proved to be the case, and unanticipated distortions in the allocation of donor organs may occur. There is evidence to suggest that women, blacks, and low-income patients do not receive transplants at the same rate as white men with high incomes and that for-profit dialysis programs are less likely to refer their patients for transplantation than not-for-profit centers.

A patient must pass through several stages before actually receiving a transplant. First, he or she must be appropriately informed about available treatment options (see Chapter 1). The patient is then referred for transplantation evaluation (see Chapter 6). The transplant team, following a favorable consideration of objective medical factors, then offers the transplantation option to the patients they have helped educate. If the patient accepts, he or she is placed on the cadaveric waiting list both locally and nationally. When a suitable kidney eventually becomes available, the patient must have priority over other patients based on the scoring system described previously (see Chapter 3).

Such a complex system is inevitably prone to distortion. Are all patients with ESRD equivalently educated about their options? Do all dialysis units refer patients for evaluation expeditiously? Do all transplantation programs distribute kidneys fairly? Similarly, we must quantitate the medical and biologic factors (e.g., high levels of antibodies in multiparous women, excess of blood group O in blacks) that may have an effect on organ distribution.

Role of Perceived Noncompliance in Selection

One exclusionary factor that is not widely understood is the role of perceived or past noncompliance with medical regimens. This psychosocial issue affords great opportunity for discrimination because it can be used to deny access if used too loosely. Noncompliance is perhaps best measured by looking to objective criteria, such as the patient's past record of keeping medical appointments, taking prescribed drugs in the proper regimen, stopping substance abuse (smoking, alcohol, and drugs) with professional assistance and maintaining abstinence, and obtaining psychological or psychiatric therapy for diagnosed mental health problems (see Chapter 16).

A social support system in the form of friends or family is obviously crucial and can help a patient overcome physical and learning disabilities. On the contrary, the absence of a support network and the inability of the patient to understand or comply with the demands of a lifelong treatment regimen and to make medical appointments can be a legitimate reason for denying a transplant to a patient.

Foreign Nationals as Potential Recipients

Press reports during the 1980s of foreign nationals "buying their way to the front of the line" for kidney transplants raised the issue of whether organs donated by U.S. citizens and residents ought to be restricted to U.S. recipients. In 1985, some 300 of the about 6,000 cadaveric kidneys transplanted in the United States went to nonresident patients who came to the United States for the procedures. There was a suggestion that in communities with extensive publicity about foreign patients receiving transplanted kidneys, cadaveric donations fell below previous levels.

Although some argued that humanitarian considerations precluded the use of national citizenship as a criterion for acceptance as a recipient, others suggested that the donated organs are a national resource and that U.S. citizens and residents should at least have priority over foreign nationals. Others proposed a ceiling, or cap, on the number of nonresident aliens on any one program's waiting list, but then treating all on the list equally.

In response to this concern, the American Society of Transplant Surgeons adopted guidelines in 1986 limiting the transplantation of kidneys into foreign nationals to an average of "5% per year of the organs transplanted at any single center" and mandating that the charges for such transplantations be on the same basis as the charges to U.S. citizens. The UNOS board in 1988 adopted a somewhat similar policy that provided for the potential review by a UNOS committee of any program's transplantations involving foreign nationals and the automatic review of any UNOS member center that has foreign nationals constituting more than 10% of its recipients. In 1994, the UNOS board changed the percentage figure to 5%. The UNOS policy also requires that all patients accepted for kidney transplants be treated equally under UNOS guidelines for the distribution of organs.

RESOURCE ALLOCATION ISSUES

Future of End-Stage Renal Disease Program

There are congressional concerns about the dollar costs of the End-Stage Renal Disease Program under Medicare as part of the federal health care budget, and there are ongoing controversies within medicine regarding which activities should take funding and programmatic priority.

Kidney transplantation is unlike any other solid organ transplantation effort in that it usually has hemodialysis as a long-term fall-back modality. Heart, liver, and lung transplant recipients have no similar treatment mechanism. Thus, although kidney transplantation led the way and remains the volume leader in the transplantation community, there is a potential source of tension among the various organ transplantation teams.

This competitiveness was observed vividly when organ procurement teams jockeyed for position in terms of which organs were to be removed first. Collegial collaboration was mixed with a sense of a "pecking order" in which heart and liver teams were placed before kidney teams, partly because of their claim of a life-and-death time struggle and partly because of their greater media publicity. Fortunately, the technical aspects of multiorgan donation have been resolved, and the capacity to store organs for longer periods has helped defuse a potential source of tension. There may remain a sense of inequity over the full Medicare funding of kidney transplantations in contrast to the more limited federal funding of liver and heart transplantations.

We stand on the verge of significant technologic breakthroughs in clinical medicine that may radically alter the distribution of our resources. Human gene therapy has begun in closely monitored research trials at the National Institutes of Health and elsewhere. Those involved in the exploration of the human genome predict not only the identification of most of the genes but also the development of techniques to engineer proteins that can optimize gene functioning or even create new gene functions for particular kinds of organs. Cellular transplantation may replace surgical transplantations.

Thus, it may be possible to address ESRD as a disease process by totally different medical treatment approaches in the next century without the use of either hemodialysis or kidney transplantation, at least for some patients. Will we then, as a society, be willing to invest the large sums of money required to produce and clinically apply such treatment modalities? If the funding mechanism for health care is correctly perceived as a national combination of public and private funds, who will determine these priorities? Which diseases will get the greatest attention and funding? Will transplantation be as exciting as the new gene therapy approaches in the next several decades?

There remains the possibility that those in a position to influence these decisions (as much political and business decisions as they are medical and scientific) may decide that primary or preventive care treatment should take precedence over acute care programs, such as organ transplantation, and thus receive funding priority and greater patient access. These resource allocation or *rationing decisions,* as they are sometimes labeled, are going to become particularly difficult when those arguing for funding pit diseases with larger patient populations against those that are rarer, those with greater mortality against those with lesser morbidity, those that affect majority populations against those that affect only specific races or ethnic groups, and the like. Hospitals threatened with financial ruin may find in the future that transplantation programs, currently a significant "revenue enhancer," are less attractive if funding patterns change or if patient populations shift.

With health care spending spiraling ever higher and many patients and providers fighting for their share of that health care funding "pie," these issues will have to be faced, and they have enormous ethical implications. This all assumes, however, that the health care portion of the societal budget maintains its present significant percentage and growth pattern.

Future of Health Care Expenditures

In the United States, the seeming primacy of health care costs over other governmental expenses is being increasingly questioned. The relevant statistics offer some insight. Recently published data show that in 1997, overall health care costs in the United States passed the $1.1 trillion figure, 13 times higher than the 1970 cost, and represented almost 13.5% of the gross national product, or a per capita cost of almost $4,000.

Public Law 92-603, the law passed by Congress in 1972 to fund all ESRD care, through Medicare, has been the basis for federal expenditures for ESRD costs that amounted to $242 million in 1974 and that now exceed tens of billion dollars annually. No other potentially lethal chronic disease involving high treatment costs, including hemophilia, has been granted this across-the-board, categorical coverage under Medicare. Recent reports highlight concern in Congress about the increasing costs of the ESRD Program. Moreover, the costs per beneficiary of the ESRD Program to

Medicare, when compared with the other types of Medicare beneficiaries, is dramatic. In fiscal year 1996, Medicare paid an average of $5,012 in benefits for all types of its 38.1 million beneficiaries, but an average of $24,835 for the about 200,000 ESRD beneficiaries.

As talk of rationing and cost-containment becomes more fashionable, particularly in a context of national economic budgetary constraints, it will be interesting to see whether the U.S. public will continue to support such priorities for health care over potentially competing claims for law enforcement and prisons, education, and social welfare (to mention only three). Medicare budget cuts, even without a public debate about health care priorities, may reduce the ESRD Program under Medicare or, at the very least, prevent its expansion to treat new patients. The ESRD Program has had an average annual growth in recent years of 15%.

Some commentators suggest that, although Congress may have passed Medicare funding for ESRD in 1972 because it believed that saving life should take priority over other values, including cost and cost-effectiveness, the federal government's values may have shifted to place cost-containment higher than individual survival. If that is a correct assessment, future kidney transplantation programs in the United States will have to cope with the same issues of funding and insurance coverage that all other solid organ and bone marrow transplantation programs have been facing.

SELECTED READINGS

American Society of Transplantation. *The AST statement on ethics in organ transplantation.* 1999.

Cameron JS, Hoffenberg R. The ethics of organ transplantation reconsidered: paid organ donation and the use of executed prisoners as donors. *Kidney Int* 1999;55:724.

Childress JF. Ethical criteria for procuring and distributing organs for transplantation. *J Health Polit Policy Law* 1989;14:87.

Chugh KS, Jha V. Commerce in transplantation in third world countries. *Kidney Int* 1996;49:1181.

Gokol R. Cadaveric transplantation. *J Postgrad Med* 1993;39:105.

Institute of Medicine. *Non-heart-beating organ transplantation: medical and ethical issues in procurement.* Washington, DC: National Academy Press, 1997.

Institute of Medicine. *Organ procurement and transplantation: assessing current policies and the potential impact of the DHHS final rule.* Washington, DC: National Academy Press, 1999.

Kilner JF. *Who lives? Who dies? Ethical criteria in patient selection.* New Haven, CT: Yale University Press, 1990.

Kjellstrand CM, Dosseter JB, eds. *Ethical problems in dialysis and transplantation.* Dordrecht, The Netherlands: Kluwer Academic, 1992.

Moskop JC. Organ transplantation in children: ethical issues. *J Pediatr* 1987;110:175.

Qunibi W, Abulrub D, Shaheen F, et al. Attitudes of commercial renal transplant recipients toward renal transplantation in India. *Clin Transplant* 1995;9:317.

Ramos EL, Kasiske BL, Alexander SR, et al. The evaluation of candidates for renal transplantation: the current practices of U.S. transplant centres. *Transplantation* 1994;57:490.

Sade RM. Cadaveric organ donation: rethinking donor motivation. *Arch Intern Med* 1999;159:438.

Salahudeen AK, Woods HF, Pingle A, et al. High mortality among recipients of bought living-unrelated donor kidney. *Lancet* 1990; 336:725.

Simmons RG, Abess L. Ethics in organ transplantation. In Cerilli CG, ed. *Organ transplantation and replacement*. Philadelphia: JB Lippincott, 1988:691–702.

Spital A. When a stranger offers a kidney: ethical issues in living organ donation. *Am J Kidney Dis* 1998;32:676.

Takemoto S, Terasaki PI, Gjertson DW, et al. Equitable allocation of HLA-compatible kidneys for local pools and minorities. *N Engl J Med* 1994;331:760.

Nutrition in the Kidney Transplant Recipient

Susan Weil Guichard

The nutritional management of the renal transplant recipient is an important determinant of outcome in terms of both morbidity and mortality. Diet can be used to prevent and ameliorate many transplant-related complications, although the precise nutrient requirements of kidney transplant recipients continue to be incompletely defined. The following recommendations, which are based on available studies in the transplantation population and extrapolated data in comparable settings, provide a guide to nutrition care management in the pretransplantation, acute posttransplantation, and long-term posttransplantation periods.

PRETRANSPLANTATION NUTRITION MANAGEMENT

Major Concerns

In the pretransplantation period, a multidisciplinary approach should incorporate diet, lifestyle changes, and use of medications to aid in the correction or improvement of malnutrition, dyslipidemia, obesity, renal osteodystrophy, and hypertension. To varying degrees, the presence of these comorbidities in the pretransplantation patient is a predictor of related complications in the posttransplantation period. Although the etiology of these problems is multifactorial, it is reasonable to presume that aggressive nutritional management in the pretransplantation period may help minimize posttransplantation morbid events.

Malnutrition

The primary nutritional focus of the pretransplantation period is the prevention and treatment of malnutrition, which is clearly related to dialysis morbidity and mortality. At times, optimization of protein and calorie nutrition may seem to be at cross-purposes with other nutrition goals, such as phosphate restriction. Some element of malnutrition has been identified in up to 70% of the dialysis population, in whom a low serum albumin level is a powerful predictor of mortality risk. Inadequate dialysis may compound the effect of malnutrition on dialysis mortality.

It is unclear how these findings before transplantation specifically affect transplant outcome. Low serum albumin levels and other nutritional assessment parameters are predictors of surgical risk, and severely malnourished patients may be deemed inappropriate transplant candidates. Aggressive treatment of malnutrition with various forms of nutritional supplementation, as well as careful attention to adequacy of dialysis and a thorough evaluation of intervening causes of poor intake (e.g., medications, intercurrent illness, psychosocial issues), may improve transplant outcome and allow transplantation to be an option for patients who may otherwise have been excluded.

Obesity

Operative risk and wound healing can be negatively influenced by the presence of obesity, defined as a body mass index (BMI) of more than 30 kg/m^2 or more than 130% ideal body weight. An increased incidence of posttransplantation wound infections, delayed graft function, diabetes, dyslipidemia, and higher weight gains after transplantation has been observed in obese patients. A consistent correlation between obesity and graft survival has not been found, although patient survival may be reduced, largely as a result of cardiac death. It has been suggested that obese patients with a cardiac history should not undergo transplantation until weight loss to a BMI of less than 30 kg/m^2 has been achieved.

Dyslipidemia and Cardiovascular Disease

End-stage renal disease (ESRD) is associated with dyslipidemia, as evidenced by moderate hypertriglyceridemia with a normal total cholesterol; normal or increased triglyceride-rich low-density lipoprotein (LDL); decreased high-density lipoprotein (HDL); increased cholesterol-rich very-low-density lipoprotein (VLDL); and increased susceptibility of LDL to oxidation. In addition, decreased levels of apoprotein A-I and increased apoprotein B and C-III and lipoprotein (a) have been described. Atherosclerotic cardiovascular disease remains the major cause of death in the ESRD population, and these abnormalities may contribute to the increased incidence of cardiovascular disease in this population, although the correlation between these abnormalities and incidence of cardiac disease is less well established than in the general population. Dyslipidemia should be treated in the transplant candidate by a combination of diet, exercise, and lipid-lowering agents.

Assessment of Nutritional Status

Assessment of nutritional status by a renal dietitian should be incorporated into the transplant candidate selection process with a view to identifying those candidates in need of more intensive nutritional support and monitoring. Typical parameters of assessment may be unreliable or of limited value in patients with renal disease. For a thorough discussion of assessment of nutritional status, see Goldstein (1998) in the Selected Readings.

ACUTE POSTTRANSPLANTATION NUTRITION MANAGEMENT

Major Concerns

Protein Catabolism

The acute posttransplantation period generally refers to the 4- to 6-week period after surgery when the stress of surgery combined with the use of high-dose corticosteroids can lead to severe protein catabolism, particularly in patients with underlying malnutrition. Severe protein catabolism contributes to poor wound healing and an increased susceptibility to infection. The degree of protein catabolism can be assessed by the measurement of urea nitrogen appearance, although in patients without complications, this assessment is not warranted.

Fluid and Electrolyte Balance

During the postoperative period, fluid and electrolyte requirements vary depending on the level of renal function, volume status, and drug–nutrient interactions. Needs are reassessed daily, and routine ordering of a standard diet in the acute period should be avoided. Specific guidelines are discussed in the section on acute posttransplantation nutrient requirements.

Drug–Nutrient Interactions

Drug–nutrient interactions, important in the long-term management of the transplant recipient, should also be considered in the acute period. Table 18.1 lists both short- and long-term interactions with immunosuppressive agents.

Capsules are the most common form of cyclosporine administration, although liquid cyclosporine continues to be available and has specific administration recommendations. It can be effectively taken with a variety of beverages (juices or milk), provided the beverages are not heated, excessively chilled, or carbonated.

Table 18.1. Drug–nutrient interactions of immunosuppressive agents

Immunosuppressive Agent	Interaction
Corticosteroids	Polyphagia, glucose intolerance, hyperlipidemia, osteoporosis, gastritis and peptic ulcer disease, fluid retention, hypertension
Cyclosporine	Hypertension, glucose intolerance, hyperlipidemia, hyperkalemia, hypomagnesemia, hyperuricemia
Azathioprine	Leukopenia, thrombocytopenia, megaloblastic anemia, nausea and vomiting, pancreatitis
Antithymocyte globulin	Leukopenia, thrombocytopenia, hypotension, hyperglycemia (rare), diarrhea, nausea, vomiting
OKT3	Hypertension, pulmonary edema, nausea, vomiting, diarrhea
Tacrolimus	Anemia, leukocytosis, hypertension, hyperglycemia, hyperkalemia or hypokalemia, hyperuricemia, hypomagnesemia, nausea, abdominal pain, gas, vomiting, anorexia, constipation, diarrhea, leukopenia
Mycophenolate mofetil	Anorexia, nausea, epigastric pain, gas, diarrhea, abdominal pain
Sirolimus	Hypertriglyceridemia, hypercholesterolemia, leukopenia, hypokalemia

Liquid cyclosporine should be mixed and taken in a glass container rather than in a container made of foam, paper, or plastic, which adsorbs the medication. Patients are advised to be consistent in choice of beverage, proximity to eating, and timing of taking cyclosporine so that fluctuations in absorption can be avoided. The Neoral formulation of cyclosporine improves absorption characteristics and pharmacokinetic consistency, although both high-fat and low-fat diets may result in considerable interpatient and intrapatient variability.

Grapefruit juice contains a substance that inhibits the metabolism of cyclosporine and other substances in the liver by the P450 enzyme system (see Chapter 4) and causes a significant increase in cyclosporine area under the curve and an increase in the 24-hour trough cyclosporine concentration.

Acute Posttransplantation Nutrient Requirements

For many patients, a successful kidney transplantation represents a long-awaited opportunity to be liberated from the stringent dietary restrictions required while on dialysis. When providing dietary instruction, this need for "liberation" should be recognized and directed in a manner that will permit the patient a well-deserved sense of dietary freedom without potentially morbid dietary indiscretion. For some patients, it is hard to "loosen up" from years of compulsive dietary control, but dietary instruction serves to provide the confidence needed to allow these patients to enjoy their newly won freedom.

In the following sections, the recommendations listed as "per kilogram of body weight" should be based on actual body weight or body weight adjusted for obesity.

Protein

In the acute postoperative period, protein requirements are generally accepted to be 1.3 to 1.5 g/kg body weight. These levels are compatible with neutral or positive nitrogen balance, provided caloric intake is adequate. For patients who continue to require dialysis, these levels of protein intake do not result in an increased dialysis requirement and therefore are used in both the functioning and nonfunctioning graft. In the postoperative patient on dialysis or with evidence of protein depletion, protein is provided at the upper end of the recommended range.

Calories

For the uncomplicated patient, caloric requirements are 30 to 35 kcal/kg. This level appears to be compatible with maintaining or achieving neutral or positive nitrogen balance. Calorie needs may increase in the presence of fever, infection, or increased surgical or traumatic stress. In the stressed patient requiring nutritional support, caloric requirements can also be calculated using the Harris-Benedict equation to determine basal energy requirements with a stress factor of 1.5. The usefulness of this equation has not been systematically studied in transplant recipients.

Carbohydrates

Limitation of simple sugars and overall restriction of carbohydrates in combination with a high-protein diet may lessen cosmetic steroid side effects in the 3- to 4-week period after transplantation. The level of carbohydrate restriction used in one early study was 1 g/kg. It is unclear whether less severe levels of restriction combined with a high-protein intake have similar benefit. The side effects reported to improve are cushingoid facies and development of fat deposition patterns commonly seen with use of high-dose corticosteroids. Other effects, such as the development of steroid diabetes, do not correlate with dietary manipulation. Very-low-carbohydrate diets are not recommended because they necessitate high-fat intake for caloric adequacy.

Fat

Treatment of hyperlipidemia is a critically important issue in the long-term management of the transplant recipients. In the short-term period after surgery, however, manipulations in fat content or composition are unlikely to affect patient outcome. For the purpose of patient education, it is reasonable at this time to begin dietary fat and cholesterol modifications as discussed in the section on nutrition requirements for the stable posttransplantation patient.

Sodium

Posttransplantation hypertension and volume overload are common. Cyclosporine-related hypertension is, in part, salt dependent (see Chapter 9). In these circumstances, control of sodium intake to 2 g/day is appropriate. Normotensive patients who are edema free do not require strict sodium restriction.

Potassium

Hyperkalemia is often seen in the posttransplantation period and may be exaggerated by graft dysfunction and the use of cyclosporine, tacrolimus, beta-adrenergic blocking agents, angiotensin-converting enzyme inhibitors, and potassium-containing phosphorus supplements. Treatment of hyperkalemia may demand dietary potassium restriction and more aggressive measures. Adequate protein intake should not be compromised.

Phosphorus

Hypophosphatemia is a common finding after transplantation, primarily as a result of increased urinary excretion of phosphate both mediated by and independent of residual secondary hyperparathyroidism. In addition, glucocorticoid-induced gluconeogenesis in the renal proximal tubule contributes to phosphaturia. Increased intake of high-phosphorus foods may not be sufficient for repletion, and oral replacement is often necessary. Table 18.2 lists some available phosphate supplements, all of which contain potassium, sodium, or a combination of both.

In the presence of delayed graft function, the use of phosphate-binding antacids and modification of phosphorus intake to less than 1,000 mg/day may be temporarily warranted but should be discontinued as renal function improves to avoid severe hypophosphatemia.

Magnesium

Hypomagnesemia is a common postoperative finding secondary to cyclosporine- and tacrolimus-induced hypermagnesuria. Dietary

Table 18.2. Selected phosphorus and magnesium supplements

Product	Form	Mineral Content
K-Phos Neutral	Tablet	250 mg phosphorus, 45 mg (1.1 mEq) potassium, 298 mg (13 mEq) sodium
K-Phos Original	Tablet	114 mg phosphorus, 144 mg (3.7 mEq) potassium
K-Phos M.F.	Tablet	125.6 mg phosphorus, 44.5 mg (1.1 mEq) potassium, 67 mg (2.9 mEq) sodium
K-Phos No. 2	Tablet	250 mg phosphorus, 88 mg (2.3 mEq) potassium, 134 mg (5.8 mEq) sodium
Neutra-Phos	Powder	250 mg phosphorus, 278 mg (7.13 mEq) potassium, 164 mg (7.13 mEq) sodium
Uro-Mag	Capsule	140 mg magnesium oxide, 84.5 mg (6.93 mEq) elemental magnesium
Mag-Ox 400	Tablet	400 mg magnesium oxide, 241.3 mg (19.86 mEq) elemental magnesium
Mag-Tab SR	Caplet	84 mg (7 mEq) elemental magnesium as magnesium lactate

replacement of magnesium is likely to be inadequate, necessitating the use of magnesium supplements (Table 18.2).

Fluid Intake
Early posttransplantation fluid management is discussed in Chapter 8. For a normovolemic patient with a well-functioning graft, a reasonable minimum fluid intake is 2,000 mL/day. For an oliguric patient, a volume of fluid should be provided to equal urine output plus a minimum of 500 to 750 mL to cover insensible losses. Variations should be determined by volume status and blood pressure, typically erring on the positive side, as urine output increases.

Vitamins
Replacement of water-soluble vitamins containing B complex and up to 100 mg of vitamin C should be continued as long as posttransplantation dialysis is required. The efficacy of routine supplementation of water-soluble vitamins after the patient no longer requires dialysis has not been well studied. 1,25-Dihydroxyvitamin D$_3$ replacement may be warranted in the immediate postoperative period if the patient is hypocalcemic.

Trace Minerals
IRON. A transferrin saturation (iron/total iron-binding capacity) of less than 20% or a serum ferritin level of less than 100 ng/mL is indicative of iron deficiency. A baseline evaluation of iron status should be performed preoperatively because iron deficiency is commonly found in the dialysis population in conjunction with

erythropoietin therapy. If oral iron replacement is warranted, intake should be scheduled so that it does not coincide with antacid therapy to avoid interference with iron absorption.

OTHER TRACE MINERALS.   Posttransplantation trace mineral requirements have not been well investigated. Zincuria has been associated with steroid therapy, although its clinical significance is not well substantiated. Routine supplementation of trace minerals is not indicated in patients on an oral diet who do not have postoperative complications.

NUTRITIONAL SUPPORT IN THE POSTTRANSPLANTATION PERIOD

In nutritionally high-risk patients, early nutritional support is indicated. Use of aggressive nutritional support in patients with ESRD and septic complications, including posttransplantation patients, has been shown to reduce mortality rates.

In the typical posttransplantation course, progression to oral intake and solid foods usually occurs within 2 to 3 postoperative days. The length of hospitalization may be less than 1 week, and aggressive nutritional support is rarely necessary. The following guidelines, however, can be used for either recent or long-term transplant recipients who may be at high nutritional risk or may be undergoing additional major surgical procedures. The guidelines may be particularly pertinent for recipients of combined pancreas–kidney transplants, who may not be able to tolerate oral nutrition for prolonged periods (see Chapter 14).

Indications for Aggressive Nutritional Intervention

Delayed Oral Intake

Nutritional support in the form of parenteral nutrition may be warranted if postoperative oral intake is delayed for more than 5 days because of complications such as protracted ileus or intractable nausea and vomiting. The decision to begin nutritional support requires consideration of the overall nutritional status of the patient, as evidenced by anthropometric and laboratory data. Nutritional support may be necessary even in patients who are adequately nourished before transplantation, who will become catabolic with the combination of high-dose corticosteroids and surgery.

Inadequate Intake

Any patient unable to sustain adequate intake to meet protein and calorie needs after the fourth or fifth postoperative day is considered a potential candidate for some type of nutritional intervention. The decision to intervene will again depend on the nutritional status of the patient, degree of catabolism (either measured by urea generation rate or estimated by type and degree of surgical or medical complication), amount of intake deficit, and assessment of the cost–benefit risks of initiating support.

Choice of Feeding Modality

Oral Supplements

Supplements are considered 4 to 5 days after surgery in any patient in whom protein and calorie needs are not being met on a standard diet. Correctable reasons for inadequate oral intake should be assessed, such as overly restrictive diet, unnecessarily slow progression to a full diet, and interference with meals by dialysis, scheduled tests, and procedures.

Tube Feeding

Tube feeding is considered in the postoperative period in any patient with a functional gastrointestinal tract who, by 7 days after surgery, is unable to maintain adequate protein and calorie nutrition with the use of diet or oral supplements. Tube feeding is rarely required after kidney transplantation. Small bowel access and use of continuous feeding are preferred when tube feeding is indicated. Tube feeding is preferred over parenteral nutrition because of a decreased risk for infection related to the avoidance of central line use and because of the production of secretory immunoglobulins, which help to prevent adverse bacterial growth in the intestinal mucosal lining. The maintenance of normal intestinal function and integrity, a decreased potential for electrolyte imbalance, and cost savings are other benefits of enteral feeding.

A wide variety of oral and enteral products are commercially available to meet the needs of the transplant recipient (see Selected Readings).

Total Parenteral Nutrition

A mixture of both essential and nonessential amino acids, fat, and dextrose should provide a daily intake of 1.5 g protein/kg and 30 to 35 kcal/kg. Ideally, calorie requirements are assessed by indirect calorimetry.

Dietary Considerations During Acute Rejection Episodes

During acute rejection episodes, provision of optimal protein and calorie intake is the primary nutritional concern. High-dose steroids produce a dose-related increase in protein catabolic rate, and with rising creatinine and blood urea nitrogen levels, there may be an inclination to restrict protein intake. Protein restriction in this setting leads to severe catabolism, and a daily protein intake in the range of 1.3 to 1.5 g/kg is appropriate. Minimum daily calorie requirements during rejection therapy are 33 to 35 kcal/kg.

Special Considerations for the Simultaneous Pancreas–Kidney Recipient

For the well-functioning combined pancreas–kidney transplant, nutritional guidelines are essentially the same as for solitary kidney transplants, except with regard to fluid and electrolyte intake. In the bladder-drained pancreas transplant, persistent exocrine pancreatic drainage into the bladder results in sizable urinary losses of sodium chloride and sodium bicarbonate (see Chapter 14). Extracellular fluid volume contraction and metabolic acidosis may ensue. Sodium and bicarbonate intake often need to be supplemented. Enteric drainage of the exocrine pancreas secretions is being increasingly employed and averts these metabolic complications.

LONG-TERM NUTRITION MANAGEMENT

Major Concerns

Hyperlipidemia

Accelerated atherosclerosis is commonly seen in transplant recipients and remains the main cause of long-term mortality in the transplantation population. Hyperlipidemia, a known risk factor for atherosclerotic disease, is associated with numerous factors in the posttransplantation patient, including diabetes and glucose intolerance, use of glucocorticoids and cyclosporine, obesity, genetic predisposition, use of certain diuretics and beta-adrenergic blocking agents, nephrotic syndrome, hypothyroidism, ovarian failure of menopause, and inappropriate diet. There is evidence to suggest that chronic allograft failure may be enhanced by the presence of hyperlipidemia.

Transplant recipients typically present with elevated VLDL cholesterol levels and elevated LDL levels. HDL levels are typically normal or elevated; however, the cardioprotective HDL2 fraction may remain low. The effect of transplantation and immunosuppressive agents on atherogenic lipoprotein (a) levels is unclear. The hyperlipidemic effect of corticosteroids is well established and is thought to result from increased hepatic VLDL synthesis and a resultant increase in cholesterol and triglycerides. Cyclosporine and sirolimus adversely affect lipid levels independent of steroid use, although the mechanism is not fully understood.

Diet therapy and exercise may be at least partially effective in lipid reduction after transplantation, although the "statin" drugs are usually required, and their introduction should not be delayed.

Homocysteine

Homocysteine is a sulfur-containing amino acid, which is formed from the essential amino acid methionine. It has been identified as a risk factor for the development of cardiovascular disease in the general population. A high prevalence of hyperhomocysteinemia has also been identified in the renal transplantation population and is associated with increased cardiovascular risk. Several B complex vitamins play a role in the metabolic pathway of methionine. Pyridoxine (vitamin B_6) is a cofactor for cystathionine-beta-synthase, by which homocysteine is transformed to cystathionine—the initial step in the transsulfuration pathway and renal excretion of sulfur. Roughly half of the homocysteine formed from a normal diet is remethylated to methionine by a pathway requiring folic acid and vitamin B_{12}. A deficiency of these vitamins or decrease in renal function can result in elevated homocysteine levels. High-dose B complex supplementation (folic acid, 5 mg/day; vitamin B_6, 50 mg/day; vitamin B_{12}, 0.4 mg/day) can reduce homocysteine levels in transplant recipients. There is currently no evidence of reduction of cardiovascular risk as a result of B vitamin therapy; thus, it is premature to make firm recommendations for administration.

Obesity and Weight Gain

Hyperphagia associated with steroid therapy, together with a sense of liberation from the dietary constraints of dialysis and an increased sense of well-being, contributes to the propensity for weight gain after transplantation. If obesity ensues, it may contribute to the development or exacerbation of hypertension, hyperlipidemia, cardiovascular disease, and steroid-induced diabetes.

The reported prevalence of posttransplantation obesity varies considerably. The degree of weight gain does not appear to correlate with corticosteroid dose, donor source, rejection history, length of time on dialysis before transplantation, or posttransplantation renal function. Demographic factors such as female sex and black race have been associated with the most weight gain in the first posttransplantation year. Not surprisingly, pretransplantation obesity may be predictive of a posttransplantation propensity for weight gain.

MANAGEMENT OF OBESITY.   In addition to limitation of caloric intake, management of posttransplantation obesity includes behavior modification, an exercise program, and early intensive nutritional counseling. Frequent follow-up by members of the health care team, including a physician, dietitian, and nurse, along with group support techniques, may optimize adherence to weight management programs.

Bone Disease

Diet plays both a palliative and a preventive role in certain posttransplantation bone abnormalities. Osteoporosis has been associated with long-term glucocorticoid use as a result of decreased intestinal absorption of calcium, increased urinary calcium excretion, decreased production of skeletal growth factors, and decreased bone formation by osteoclasts. Along with calcineurin-phosphatase inhibitors (cyclosporine and tacrolimus), glucocorticoids also increase bone resorption and decrease gonadal hormone synthesis. Hyperparathyroidism may persist long after transplantation and may influence the severity of bone loss. Provision of adequate calcium and phosphorus intake may attenuate these problems. Weight-bearing exercise is also beneficial. A low-purine diet may be useful for patients with gout or severe hyperuricemia. Additional manifestations of transplant-related bone disease are reviewed in Chapter 9.

Hypertension

The prevalence of hypertension is reported in most series to be about 50% in transplant recipients. Hypertension is an important risk factor for cardiovascular disease as well as for graft survival. Although posttransplantation hypertension is multifactorial in origin, cyclosporine-related hypertension is a common contributing component (see Chapter 9). Sodium sensitivity is a hallmark of cyclosporine-related hypertension, and patients treated with either cyclosporine or tacrolimus who are hypertensive should probably be on a sodium-controlled diet. Routine sodium restriction of all transplant recipients is not justified, and possible adverse consequences of dietary sodium restriction in the nontransplantation population should also be considered in deciding whether sodium restriction is appropriate. Calcium-channel blocking agents have improved efficacy in the salt-replete hypertensive person. In animal models, sodium depletion enhances the nephrotoxicity of cyclosporine and tacrolimus as well as enhancing the growth of cysts in cystic renal disease.

Weight loss in the obese hypertensive patient may also play an important role in its treatment. Exercise provides a beneficial adjuvant. The beneficial effect of other nonpharmacologic influences, such as calcium, potassium, and magnesium intake, and avoidance of alcohol use have not been well defined.

Posttransplantation Diabetes Mellitus

Posttransplantation diabetes mellitus develops in about 20% of transplant recipients, with risk factors including advanced age, obesity, glucocorticoid and cyclosporine or tacrolimus use, certain human leukocyte antigen types (A30 and Bw42 antigens), and cadaveric donor source.

Corticosteroids have been shown to produce peripheral insulin resistance and to cause an alteration in pancreatic beta-cell insulin secretion. Cyclosporine also appears to alter peripheral insulin sensitivity and to diminish islet cell function. The percentage of weight gain is not clearly associated with the development of glucose intolerance. The presence of posttransplantation diabetes appears to be associated with decreased graft survival rate and increased risk for infection and is a risk factor for the development of cardiovascular disease.

Diet, weight loss if appropriate, and exercise, along with decreased dosing of corticosteroids and cyclosporine when possible, provide the basis for initial management. Oral hypoglycemic agents or insulin may be warranted in diagnosed cases.

Progression of Renal Disease in Kidney Transplants

The role of diet in the progression of renal disease in the transplanted kidney requires further study. The potential deleterious effect of excess protein on the kidney versus the known effect of protein wasting from chronic corticosteroid therapy implies conflicting recommendations. Several short-term studies indicate that a low protein intake of 0.55 g/kg may be helpful in the presence of chronic graft loss and may help decrease the proteinuria associated with the chronic rejection. Protein status must be closely monitored to avoid exacerbation of hypoalbuminemia, a predictor of mortality in the transplant recipient. The long-term efficacy of low protein intake and the optimal dose of protein remain to be determined in long-term studies. Evidence of continued protein wasting has been described even with low doses of corticosteroids, necessitating ongoing assessment of nutritional status. Hamar and colleagues described predictors of graft failure in a retrospective study of 184 transplant recipients. Predictors of early graft failure included elevated serum triglycerides (more than 300 mg/dL) and elevated cholesterol (more than 250 mg/dL). Low levels of cholesterol, triglycerides, and glucose both before and after transplantation predicted prolonged graft survival. A retrospective, multivariate analysis of 675 transplant recipients by Massy's group (see Selected Readings) defined chronic rejection risk factors that were independent of acute rejection and proteinuria and not attributable to immune mechanisms. These risk factors included low serum albumin levels (less than 3.5 g/dL) and high triglyceride levels (more than 200 mg/dL).

Hypoalbuminemia

In addition to its possible role as a risk factor for decreased renal graft survival, a retrospective analysis of 232 simultaneous pancreas–kidney transplant recipients by Becker and coworkers (see Selected Readings) indicated that hypoalbuminemia was associated with increased risk for cytomegalovirus infection, graft loss, and decreased survival rate. Low albumin levels have also been described as a strong independent risk factor for all causes of mortality after renal transplantation.

Foodborne Infectious Complications

Even the nonnutritionally compromised transplant patient may be susceptible to an increased incidence of infection (see Chapter 10). Infectious complications in the renal transplant recipient have been reported to occur at a level 10 times higher than anticipated in the presence of malnutrition, defined as a serum albumin of less than 2.8 g/dL. An awareness of potentially pathogenic organisms commonly found in food may provide an often-ignored, relatively simple, preventive measure. Providing education on safe and sensible food habits may help minimize the morbidity associated with certain posttransplantation infectious disease complications.

Food vehicles for *Listeria monocytogenes* include raw milk, soft cheeses, and hot dogs. Pasteurization and proper food handling technique may help minimize the risk for contamination. *Nocardia asteroides,* although ubiquitous in the environment and not uncommonly nosocomially acquired, can be present in decaying vegetables. *Salmonella* species infections are associated with undercooked, contaminated meat, poultry, and eggs as well as raw milk. Raw seafood and raw fruits and vegetables also present an increased risk. Prevention includes proper food handling, preparation, and pasteurization. The potential for *Legionella* species infection exists in areas with a contaminated or unsafe water supply.

Use of Herbal Supplements

The use of herbal medicines and inclusion of herbal medicines in food items, such as juices, is increasingly common. In the United States, herbal medicines are regulated as food products and dietary supplements and therefore are not tested for safety or efficacy by the Food and Drug Administration. These products pose a special potential risk for transplant recipients for several reasons. One concern is the lack of information about drug–nutrient interactions and whether these substances increase or decrease the effectiveness of immunosuppressants or other prescribed medications. A second related concern is that certain herbs, such as echinacea and astralagus, appear to contain immune-enhancing properties and may enhance elements of the immune system that are intentionally being suppressed. Some herbal preparations have been found to contain heavy metals and toxic botanicals. Because there are no sanitation standards for herbal medicines, the potential for microbial contamination poses a particular risk for the immune-suppressed patient. Until and unless adequate research and appropriate regulations exist, herbal product use should be discouraged in transplant recipients.

Nutrient Recommendations for the Stable Posttransplantation Patient

Protein and Calories

Protein requirements for stable posttransplantation patients are not well defined, with muscle wasting identified even at corticosteroid doses of 0.20 mg/kg/day. A daily protein intake ranging from 0.55 to 1.0 g/kg has been recommended for stable posttransplantation patients. Negative nitrogen balance has been reported in short-term studies of protein intake levels of 0.6 g/kg/ day unless calorie intake is maintained above 25 kcal/kg/day. These levels may be difficult to achieve even in patients who are not experiencing complications. A daily protein intake approaching 1 g/kg, combined with an adequate calorie intake, appears to be compatible with neutral or positive nitrogen balance.

For stable transplant recipients who require weight reduction, a daily calorie intake of 25 kcal/kg ideal body weight is a reasonable starting point. Caloric restriction should be combined with exercise, behavior modification techniques, and regular team follow-up.

Fat

Given the incidence of posttransplantation hypercholesterolemia, the propensity toward weight gain, and the potential contribution of lipids to decreased graft survival, a reduced fat and reduced cholesterol diet is appropriate for most long-term patients.

The recommendations of the National Cholesterol Education Program (NCEP) appear to be of some benefit for lipid control in this group. For patients who ultimately require pharmacologic management for control of hypercholesterolemia, diet guidelines should continue to be encouraged as adjunctive therapy. NCEP guidelines are listed in Table 18.3.

Table 18.3. Nutrient recommendations for cholesterol control

Nutrient	Recommended Intake
Total fat	≤30% total kcal[a]
Saturated fatty acids	8–10% total kcal[b]
	<7% total kcal if not responsive to initial diet
Polyunsaturated fatty acids	Up to 10% kcal[b]
Monounsaturated fatty acids	Up to 15% kcal[c]
Cholesterol	<300 mg
	<200 mg if not responsive to initial diet
Total calories	Individualized level to achieve or maintain ideal body weight

[a] 60 g/day on an 1,800-kcal diet.
[b] 20 g/day on an 1,800-kcal diet.
[c] 20–30 g/day on an 1,800-kcal diet.

Fish Oil

Further studies are needed to clarify and evaluate the effect of n-3 fatty acids, in the form of fish oil or flaxseed oil, as an adjunct to immunosuppressive therapy. Supplemental fish oil in the amounts of 3 to 6 g/day may have a positive effect on glomerular filtration rate, effective renal plasma flow, and blood pressure in cyclosporine-treated patients. The potential beneficial effects of n-3 fatty acids are in decreasing the production of compounds that contribute to inflammation, vasoconstriction, platelet activation, and chemotaxis. Diminished renal thromboxane A_2 production by fish oil also appears to improve proteinuria and cyclosporine-induced vasoconstriction. Castro and colleagues (see Selected Readings) demonstrated, in a randomized 3-month study of 43 transplant recipients, that fish oil was as effective and safe as low-dose simvastatin in correcting posttransplantation hyperlipidemia. The precise role of fish oil in this setting remains controversial.

Sodium

Sodium restriction to 2 to 3 g/day is warranted in cyclosporine-treated patients with hypertension. In normotensive, nonedematous patients, strict sodium restriction is not warranted. Sodium restriction may be of little benefit in hypertensive transplant patients not receiving cyclosporine.

Potassium

Hyperkalemia, associated with the use of cyclosporine and tacrolimus, may continue to be observed in otherwise stable transplant recipients. Guidelines as discussed in the section on acute posttransplantation management continue to apply in this setting. Potassium levels up to 5.5 mEq/L are common and are rarely a source of concern in stable patients.

Calcium, Phosphorus, and Vitamin D

In the absence of hypercalcemia, calcium should be provided at the level of 1,000 to 1,500 mg/day by diet, supplements, or both. If hypocalcemia or evidence of secondary hyperparathyroidism persists, vitamin D therapy in the form of active 1,25-dihydroxyvitamin D_3 is instituted. Hypophosphatemia may persist into this period, necessitating phosphate supplementation. Hypercalcemia may persist in as many as one third of patients in the first year and subsequently in as many as 10% after 1 year as a result of secondary hyperparathyroidism. When related to secondary hyperparathyroidism, hypercalcemia may respond to judiciously monitored 1,25-dihydroxyvitamin D_3 therapy.

Magnesium

Hypomagnesemia may persist into the long-term posttransplantation period, and magnesium supplements are often prescribed (Table 18.3). Magnesium supplementation may favorably influence the blood lipid profile, primarily by increasing HDL cholesterol levels. The role of magnesium in controlling blood pressure in this population remains equivocal.

Vitamins and Trace Minerals

To ensure adequate intake of vitamins and trace minerals, water-soluble vitamin supplementation is warranted for patients on diets restricting protein (to less than 60 g/day), potassium, or calories (to less than 1,200 kcal/day). Supplementation is not otherwise routinely warranted. Vitamin A levels are typically elevated in kidney transplant recipients; thus, vitamin A should not be supplemented. High doses of vitamin C should probably be avoided based on extrapolated information about oxalate in patients with renal dysfunction. Impaired urinary oxalate clearance in renal insufficiency may be the cause of increased tissue and plasma oxalate load. High concentrations of plasma oxalate may cause calcium oxalate deposition and urinary calcium oxalate calculi. Ascorbic acid provides a primary metabolic pathway for oxalate synthesis, and plasma levels correlate to vitamin C intake. The appropriate dose in transplant recipients is yet to be determined. Iron supplementation may be appropriate. Zinc supplementation may be warranted with the long-term use of corticosteroids, although specific needs have not been determined. A study by Vela and colleagues (see Selected Readings) suggests that Vitamin E supplementation may have a protective effect by reducing oxidative stress associated with the development or progression of vascular lesions seen in chronic rejection. The optimal intake of folic acid, pyridoxine, and vitamin B_{12} is also not known.

Alcohol

Conflicting studies are available regarding the effect of alcohol consumption on cyclosporine metabolism. Data suggest that excessive alcohol intake increases the absorption and therefore potential toxicity of cyclosporine, although moderate amounts may be tolerated without a marked effect on absorption. Heavy alcohol use has also been associated with increased risk for avascular necrosis. Other nonroutine medications should be screened for drug and alcohol interactions. Alcohol intake should be discouraged in patients with poorly controlled hypertension and used with caution in diabetic patients to avoid severe hypoglycemia.

Exercise

Physical training is a vital part of posttransplantation management of the transplant recipient. It attenuates some of the side effects of immunosuppressive therapy, such as protein catabolism and muscle wasting, hyperlipidemia, obesity, hypertension, and osteoporosis. Glucose control in diabetic patients can also be improved with a regular exercise program. Quality of life may also improve as a result of a regular exercise program. Although the optimal exercise program is not defined in the transplantation population, recommendations for the general population, which include cardiovascular conditioning and muscle strengthening, are appropriate for most patients.

Nutrient Recommendations for the Pregnant Transplant Recipient

The protein needs of stable pregnant transplant recipients are 0.8 g/kg pre-gravida ideal or adjusted body weight plus 10 g/day. Caloric requirements can be calculated using basal energy expenditure times an activity factor of 1.2 to 1.4; an additional 300 kcal/ day should be consumed in the second and third trimesters. Other nutrient requirements are the same as for nontransplanted pregnant women, although close monitoring is appropriate in terms of weight gain and glucose control because of the risk for glucose intolerance. Residual secondary hyperparathyroidism may also require adjustments in phosphorus, calcium, and vitamin D intake.

SELECTED READINGS

Arnadottir M, Berg A. Treatment of hyperlipidemia in renal transplant recipients. *Transplantation* 1997;63:339.

Becker BN, Becker YT, Heisey DM, et al. The impact of hypoalbuminemia in kidney-pancreas transplant recipients. *Transplantation* 1999;68:72.

Bennett WM. Drug interactions and consequences of sodium restriction. *Am J Clin Nutr* 1997;65:678.

Bertolas JA, Hunsicker LG. Nutritional requirements of renal transplant patients. In: Mitch WE, Klahr S, eds. *Handbook of Nutrition and the Kidney*, 3rd ed. Philadelphia: Lippincott-Raven, 1998.

Bostrom AG, Culleton BF. Hyperhomocysteinemia in chronic renal disease. *J Am Soc Nephrol* 1999;10:891.

Brookhyser J, Wiggins K. Medical nutrition therapy in pregnancy and kidney disease. *Adv Ren Replace Ther* 1998;5:53.

Castro R, Quieros J, Fonseca I, et al. Therapy of post-renal transplantation hyperlipidemia: comparative study with simvastatin and fish oil. *Nephrol Dial Transplant* 1997;12:2140.

Clinical practice guidelines for nutrition in chronic renal failure. *Am J Kidney Dis* 2000;35(6 suppl 2).

Dimeny E, Fellstrom B. Metabolic abnormalities in renal transplant recipients: risk factors and predictors of chronic graft dysfunction. *Nephrol Dial Transplant* 1997;12:21.

Drafts HH, Anjun MR, Mulloy LL, et al. The impact of pre-transplant obesity on renal transplant outcomes. *Clin Transplant* 1997;11:493.

Foote J, Cohen B. Medicinal herb use and the renal patient. *J Ren Nutr* 1998;8:40.

Goldstein DJ. Assessment of nutritional status in renal diseases. In: Mitch WE, Klahr S, eds. *Handbook of Nutrition and the Kidney*, 3rd ed. Philadelphia: Lippincott-Raven, 1998.

Guijarro C, Massy ZA, Weiderker MR, et al. Serum albumin and mortality after renal transplantation. *Am J Kidney Dis* 1996;27:117.

Gupta BK, Glicklich D, Tellis VA. Magnesium repletion therapy improves lipid metabolism in hypomagnesemic renal transplant recipients. *Transplantation* 1999;67:1485.

Klauser RM, Irschik H, Kletzmayr J, et al. Pharmacokinetic cyclosporine A profiles under long-term Neoral treatment in renal transplant recipient: does fat intake matter? *Transplant Proc* 1997; 29:3137.

Markell MS, Armenti V, Danovitch G, et al. Hyperlipidemia and glucose intolerance in the post-renal transplant patient. *J Am Soc Nephrol* 1994;4(Suppl 1):37S.

Massy ZA, Guijarro C, Wiederkehr MR, et al. Chronic renal allograft rejection: immunologic and non-immunologic risk factors. *Kidney Int* 1996;49:518.

Modlin CS, Flechner SM, Goormastic M, et al. Should obese patients lose weight before receiving a kidney transplant? *Transplantation* 1997;64:599.

Painter P. Exercise after renal transplantation. *Adv Ren Replace Ther* 1999;6:159.

Patel MG. The effect of dietary intervention on weight gains after renal transplantation. *J Ren Nutr* 1998;8:137.

Rodino MA, Shane E. Osteoporosis after organ transplantation. *Am J Med* 1998;104:459.

Vela JP, Cristol JP, Maggi MF, et al. Oxidative stress in renal transplant recipients with chronic rejection: rationale for antioxidant supplementation. *Transplant Proc* 1999;31:1310.

Windus DW, Lacson S, Delmez JA. The short-term effects of a low-protein diet in stable renal transplant recipients. *Am J Kidney Dis* 1991;17:693.

19

Psychosocial and Financial Issues in Kidney Transplantation

Marcy H. Gitlin, Terri H. Sayama, and Robert S. Gaston

The diagnosis of advancing kidney disease is life changing not only for the patient but also for family members. Many questions and concerns may arise that can be addressed by the social worker who is highly invested in patient care and treatment and who should be an intrinsic part of the transplant team. Questions may include the following:

What treatment choice is best for me? How will my life change because of my illness?
How will my illness affect my family?
How will I pay for my treatments?
Will I be able to continue working and return to my daily activities?

The nephrology or transplantation social worker can help patients understand and cope with their feelings and adjust to a new lifestyle with dialysis or a transplant. The social worker can assist patients with their concerns about employment, insurance, changing roles in marriage and family life, problems with sex and intimacy, and concerns about death and dying.

The social work team member is expert on community resources and may refer patients and family members to the appropriate programs that they need, including vocational rehabilitation, Social Security disability, home health care services, medical equipment, support groups, and financial assistance.

When a patient begins their assessment for transplant candidacy, it is recommended that a comprehensive psychosocial assessment be completed by the transplant team social worker. It is during this process that compliance, family system dynamics, financial resources, and mental health are examined. The areas to be covered in a social work assessment are listed in Table 19.1.

This chapter discusses the psychosocial benefits and potential risks of transplantation; concerns with patient nonadherence; and information regarding Social Security disability, vocational rehabilitation, financial concerns, and psychosocial assessment.

PSYCHOSOCIAL BENEFITS OF TRANSPLANTATION

The quality of life for transplant recipients is generally better than the quality of life for dialysis patients. About 80% of transplant recipients have been shown to function psychosocially at nearly normal levels, compared with about 50% of dialysis patients. Dialysis patients show more morbidity on the General Health Questionnaire (GHQ), which evaluates loss of emotional control and

Table 19.1.   Major areas covered in psychosocial assessment

Illness Assessment

1. Illness history and effect on patient's functioning, understanding, reaction, and adjustment
2. Patient's knowledge of transplantation, process of being referred to transplantation center, understanding of the assessment process for candidacy, feelings about transplantation

Patient Assessment

1. Personal
   Age, life-cycle stage
   Physical functioning
   Intellectual functioning
   Emotional functioning
   Sexual functioning
   Major life stressful events
   Coping style and approaches
   Religious beliefs and faith
   History of substance abuse
   Ability to comply with medical regime
2. Educational
   Level of education attained
3. Vocational
   Type of occupation
   Length of employment
   Stability of present or recent job
4. Financial
   Sources of income and other resources, their adequacy for current lifestyle, their adequacy for transplantation and for future medical needs

Support System Assessment

1. Family
   Composition—spouse and children; age, education, occupation, needs, availability
   Role structure—effect of illness on roles
   Interactions—patterns and quality of communication
   Functioning—quality of family life
   Problem solving approach and skills
2. Social
   Extended family—quality of contacts
   Friends, neighbors, colleagues—quality of relationships
   Others—religious, cultural, and social affiliations
3. Environmental
   Housing and transportation
   Need for relocation
   Need for travel alternatives

depression, compared with transplant recipients and healthy control subjects. It is important to note, however, that these studies do not address the effects of transplant failure, which may result in significant decrease in quality of life.

The obvious benefit of kidney transplantation is freedom from the constraints of dialysis. Successful transplantation permits much more personal time and independence for an individual who is freed of the necessity of being connected to a machine several times a day or at night or of going to an outside facility two to three times a week for several hours each visit. On average, patients spend 40 to 50 hours a month receiving hemodialysis, 60 to 70 hours receiving chronic ambulatory peritoneal dialysis (CAPD), or 280 hours receiving chronic cycling peritoneal dialysis (CCPD).

Significant psychosocial stress is associated with dialysis. Patients are faced with the conflict of maintaining independence despite being forced to depend on a machine, with difficulties in remaining financially solvent, with reduced activity in the family household, and with loss of spontaneity.

Transplantation permits greater flexibility and more convenience when traveling. Patients need not worry about having to make arrangements ahead of time or about having to travel only to those cities that have dialysis centers. For many patients who have been treated with dialysis, transplantation offers the freedom to plan a vacation (more than a weekend getaway). Many patients report they have not taken an extended trip since commencing dialysis because of the inconvenience and concerns about being too far away from their dialysis center or going to an unfamiliar dialysis unit.

Transplant recipients also have greater dietary flexibility (see Chapter 18). Specifically, the fluid restrictions of patients receiving dialysis are often difficult to adhere to in warmer climates or during the summer seasons. Many patients complain of having a difficult time finding enough protein in their diet without having to eat foods previously considered unhealthy (e.g., red meat, starchy carbohydrates).

Transplant recipients generally have more energy and stamina and can spend more time dealing with issues outside their own health problems. The time saved by no longer needing dialysis is about 50 hours a month—2600 hours a year! This results in an increased earning potential and increased family and personal time. The long-term complications of dialysis may be avoided by transplantation (see Chapter 1), and many patients view transplantation as a symbol of freedom and restored health.

Ideally, after receiving a kidney transplant, patients are able to return to work or school. Patients are encouraged to engage in vocational rehabilitation while they are receiving dialysis because the waiting time for a cadaveric transplant may be years, during which time they may complete training courses or school programs. Social Security offers vocational training for patients while they are receiving disability benefits and assists with job placement to help individuals get back into the work force when they are medically able.

Successful kidney transplantation is more cost-effective than hemodialysis and provides a relative net saving after a period of about 3 years. Although cost data vary from center to center, transplantation costs average $61,000 by the end of the first year, with cumulative costs decreasing each successive year, because of reduction in dosage of immunosuppressive drugs. The reduction continues, so that the total cost is about $70,000 by the end of the second year and $77,000 by the end of the third year. These figures do not reflect the costs associated with rehospitalization. The cost of providing dialysis is about $35,000 per year. Therefore, kidney transplantation is a more cost-effective alternative than dialysis if the graft remains viable for more than 2 years and if there are no hospital readmissions after initial surgery, in which case the cost advantage will be delayed. Failed transplantations are clearly expensive, although the financial effects of transplant failure have not been systematically studied.

PSYCHOSOCIAL RISKS OF TRANSPLANTATION

The social worker can offer support for the patient, family, and friends with issues that can have a negative effect on transplant results. These include the hesitancy to leave the dependent sick role, concerns about reentering the workforce, importance of being needed rather than needing, maintenance of hope during periods of rejection, and the need to escape feelings of distinctiveness both in terms of psychological and physical symptoms.

Although patients are educated about medication side effects, until they are faced with them, it is uncertain how they will cope. Patients who have a prior psychiatric history of anxiety or depression are particularly susceptible to an exacerbation of their symptoms after immunosuppressive therapy begins, although patients with no prior history are also at risk (see Chapter 16). Family members should be comforted by the assurance that such symptoms are generally temporary and treatable. The physical side effects of transplant medications, such as hirsutism, gum overgrowth, and weight gain, may affect body image in a manner that is not always easy to detect, and sensitive probing may be required. Side effects are almost inevitable after transplantation and can cause patients to stop or skip doses of their medication. Patients should be systematically questioned about how they feel about these side effects.

Multiple lifestyle changes occur for the transplant recipient. The patient's roles within their family system and work environment may change. Their capacity to reenter the workforce after many years may be changed. There may risk losing financial support, such as disability income and health insurance. Personal relationships may be at risk, and posttransplantation stress may lead to divorce and separation. Sexual functioning may change after transplantation (see Chapter 9) and engender new hopes and fears. The newly found posttransplantation freedom may be a threat to patients whose identity has been associated with their sick-role as a dialysis patient. The shift to health may be difficult, and an identity crisis may occur. Counseling and support groups can aid in this transition. Employment is a topic that weighs heavily on many patients who have been receiving disability payment from various sources and is often tied to their health insurance coverage. Patients may be concerned about losing the benefits that they have come to rely on. They may struggle with striving to become independent versus remaining dependent.

Many patients live in fear of suffering rejection episodes and losing their transplants or of suffering other catastrophic complications. These fears are not irrational, although they may be exaggerated; they can best be addressed by an open and factual discussion of the extent of the risk at all phases of treatment. Patients may also suffer feelings of guilt about having received a kidney at someone else's expense. They should be assured that these are common feelings and reminded that they are deserving beneficiaries of the wishes of the donor and the donor's loved ones.

NONADHERENCE (NONCOMPLIANCE)

Graft survival is dependent on providing adequate long-term pharmacologic immunosuppression. As a consequence, transplant recipients who do not adhere to the often complex medical regimens are at substantial risk for graft loss. The term *noncompliance* is used to indicate failure of transplant recipients to ingest medications as prescribed, for whatever reason. Few patients consciously decide to discontinue immunosuppression. For most, noncompliant behavior evolves gradually as a consequence of many interacting variables. The term *nonadherence* is sometimes preferred because it is less pejorative.

Noncompliance with medical therapies has been shown to affect treatment outcomes in many chronic diseases, and it has been estimated that only about half of the 1.6 billion prescriptions written in the United States each year are taken properly. To quote the former Surgeon General, Dr. C. Everett Koop, "Drugs don't work in patients who don't take them"! A series of variables has been linked to medication noncompliance (Table 19.2), each of which is evident in transplant immunosuppressant regimens. In renal transplantation, clinically important noncompliance occurs in 15% to 20% of recipients, substantially increasing the risk for adverse immunologic events and even death. Occasional noncompliance is widespread, although its clinical significance is difficult to assess. Both multiple and late episodes of acute rejection predict subsequent graft loss to chronic rejection (see Chapter 9), and medication noncompliance significantly enhances the risk for both. Noncompliance increases the risk for graft loss three- to five-fold and has been

Table 19.2.   Attributes of pharmacologic therapies that enhance the risk for noncompliance

Multiple medications
Prolonged duration of therapy
Short dosing intervals
Palatability of medication
Definable adverse effects
Financial expense
Beliefs about severity of illness
Failure to understand treatment regimen
Increasing intervals between contacts with providers

Adapted from Cramer, J.A.: Practical issues in medication compliance. Transplant. Proc. *31* (Suppl 4A):7S, 1999, with permission.

found to be the most common cause of graft loss beyond 6 months of transplantation.

Several demographic variables appear to affect the likelihood of noncompliance. Diabetic patients, accustomed to the demands of living with chronic illness, are less likely to have problems with compliance. Younger patients and those with limited educational backgrounds are more likely to be noncompliant. Psychiatric illness and a history of substance abuse also increases risk. At least some noncompliant behavior is attributable to either financial hardship or the relative inability to procure appropriate medication when no funds are available. Low socioeconomic status is a strong predictor of noncompliance and poorer long-term outcomes in renal transplantation. Knowledge of these demographic risk factors, however, is of only limited benefit in dealing with individual patients. It does little to facilitate identification of noncompliant behavior early enough to allow remedy, nor does it provide insight into what that remedy should be.

The interventions required to alter noncompliant behavior vary from patient to patient. At the least, transplant recipients must have access to immunosuppressants, the annual cost of which may exceed that of housing for many patients (Table 19.3). For patients with private insurance or Medicaid coverage, finances may not pose a significant problem. A substantial number of renal allograft recipients, however, have only Medicare to assist with payment for medications, coverage that currently expires at 44 months. Beyond that time limit, patients must navigate (usually with the assistance of social workers) a complex network of indigent care programs and state kidney networks. There is a significant risk for late rejection and graft loss in patients forced to discontinue cyclosporine because of financial hardship; when patients are provided with this drug, outcomes improve dramatically. Extension of Medicare coverage for immunosuppressants from 1 to 3 years has been shown to attenuate income-related differences in long-term graft survival. The Institute of Medicine has recommended elimi-

Table 19.3.   Financial costs of commonly used immunosuppressive regimens in the United States

Immunosuppressive Regimen	Cost Per Annum[a]
Neoral, MMF, prednisone	$13,000
Neoral, sirolimus, prednisone	$12,900
Tacrolimus, MMF, prednisone	$12,800
SangCyA, MMF, prednisone	$11,400
Tacrolimus, azathioprine, prednisone	$7,480
Neoral, prednisone	$6,500
SangCyA, azathioprine, prednisone	$5,500

[a] Annual charges (for an average patient weighing 70 kg, at a retail pharmacy in Birmingham, Alabama, 12/99), assuming the following medication doses:
   Cyclosporine (Neoral or SangCyA): 4 mg/kg/day
   Mycophenolate mofetil (MMF): 2000 mg/day
   Tacrolimus: 0.1 mg/kg/day
   Sirolimus: 2 mg/day

nating of all time limits on Medicare immunosuppressant coverage, and the issue is currently under advisement by Congress.

In addition to ensuring financial access to proper medications, other interventions may improve patient compliance. Electronic monitoring of drug dosing can allow earlier detection of noncompliance, although such devices have not become widely accepted. Drug regimens should be simplified, with optimal compliance a more compelling goal than optimal pharmacokinetics. Patients should be helped to develop daily routines that foster compliance. The facilitation of adherence of transplant recipients to their medical regimen requires both recognition of its importance in ensuring long-term graft survival and ongoing trust between patient and provider.

DISABILITY INSURANCE FOR TRANSPLANT RECIPIENTS

Many transplant recipients have legitimate financial concerns. How can I afford this? The medical expenses, including prescriptions, at least initially, are covered by insurance. The financial counselor, who should be an integral part of the transplant team, is the person who has detailed knowledge of these financial matters. There are other expenses, non-medical that also need consideration.

For transplant recipients, the estimated time off work is approximately 3 months, although some patients return sooner. The close medical supervision required after transplant makes it difficult for most people to resume work during this time. One main reason patients might return to work sooner than medically recommended is a financial one. Most disability plans do not compensate recipients for their total lost wages. This financial hardship is what makes people feel the pressure to return to work. Recipients who are on Social Security Disability Insurance (SSDI), or Supplemental Security Income (SSI), at the time transplant will continue to receive the same benefits after transplant, so they do not feel the same time pressure as those who are not. The various programs explained are available to recipients.

State Disability Insurance

State Disability Insurance (SDI) varies from state to state. It is available for recipients who are employed and paying state income taxes. SDI eligibility begins 1 week after the patient stops working (usually at time of transplant) and can possibly continue for up to one year. Most recipients are able to return to work in the 3-month period described above. Some states do not have SDI. They often have company sponsored programs. Recipients, in the pretransplant phase, need to be advised to speak to their employment human resources department to find out what disability programs will be available to them.

Social Security Disability Income

Social Security Disability Income (SSDI) is long-term disability for patients who are considered "permanently" disabled for at least 1 year. Patients who run out of temporary disability and yet are still unable to return to work often apply for SSDI, even before 1 year of being disabled, because the eligibility process can take several months.

Social Security payments are monthly and are based on a patient's individual earnings in the highest quarter. Patients with ESRD who are receiving dialysis or who have undergone transplantation are eligible for SSDI if they have paid into Federal Insurance Contribution Act (FICA) taxes. Patients are encouraged to continue working even after beginning dialysis treatment because they may "flex" their work hours or cut down to part-time work. Patients may choose CAPD or CCPD so that they do not interrupt their work schedules by having to go to a hemodialysis center several times a week. Patients receiving SSDI may return to work on a limited basis without having their Social Security benefits stopped. They may still collect SSDI as long as they do not earn more than $500 per month for more than 8 months.

Patients should be encouraged to return to work after transplantation because many of them lose their benefits and insurance. Some patients continue on SSDI if they have additional disabling conditions besides ESRD (e.g., diabetes, retinopathy, blindness, or other physical disabilities).

Supplemental Security Income

SSI is a federally funded program administered by the Social Security Administration (SSA). This benefit provides monthly cash benefit to persons who have disabilities, and limited income and resources. To be eligible both financial and disability criteria must be met. This disability must be medically-determined mental and/or physical condition that is expected to last a year or longer. Often patients receive this in addition to their SSDI. The SSI amount varies from state to state, depending on each state's cost of living. And similar to SSDI recipients, SSI recipients should be encouraged to return to work after transplant, because they may no longer have a qualifying disability and may lose this benefit within a few years after the transplant.

Consolidated Budget Reconciliation Act

The Consolidated Budget Reconciliation Act (COBRA) of 1985 provides additional help to employees and their dependents who would normally lose their health insurance coverage because of job loss, divorce, or the death or retirement of a spouse. This is a federal law that requires companies with 20 or more employees to extend their insurance coverage to employees and their dependents for 18 months (up to 36 months) when benefits would otherwise end. Although a person may receive extended coverage through COBRA, they are still fully responsible for premium payments to the group health plan.

An employee covered by a group health plan may continue coverage for up to 18 months if the employee left work voluntarily or involuntarily (for reasons other than misconduct) or the working hours are reduced beyond the minimum amount to qualify for health benefits. Patients considered disabled under Social Security guidelines at the time work is discontinued may choose to continue their health coverage for up to 29 months, after which time they becomes eligible for Medicare. They must show that they are insurable to continue coverage. People who leave work because of disability may be able to keep their life insurance policy if there is a disability waiver. The insurer must be notified and proof of disability provided.

Family Medical Leave Act

The Family Medical Leave Act (FMLA) requires employers to provide up to 12 weeks of unpaid job-protected leave to "eligible" employees for certain family and medical reasons that make the employees unable to perform their work. Employees are eligible if they have worked for an employer for at least 1 year (minimum of 1,250 hours over the previous 12 months) and if there are at least 50 employees within 75 miles.

The employee may be required to provide advance leave notice and medical certification. Leave may be denied if requirements are not met. The employee ordinarily must provide 30 days' advance notice when leave is foreseeable. An employer may require a medical certificate (and may require a second opinion at the employer's expense) to support a request for leave because of a serious health condition.

For the duration of FMLA leave, the employer must maintain the employee's health coverage under any group health plan. Upon return from FMLA leave, most employees must be restored to their original or equivalent positions with equivalent pay, benefits, and other employment terms.

The use of FMLA leave cannot result in the loss of any employment benefit that accrued before the start of an employee's leave. The U.S. Department of Labor is authorized to investigate and resolve complaints of violations. An eligible employee may bring a civil action against an employer for violations.

Vocational Rehabilitation

Many transplant recipients are not working at the time of the transplantation for various health reasons. They may be eligible for vocational rehabilitation together with patients who are unable to return to their prior employment because their job responsibilities are in conflict with transplant-related restrictions.

Vocational rehabilitation is a service that provides people with disabilities the tools they need to be able to return to work, enter a new line of work, maintain work, or start work for the first time. After transplantation, it is important that patients enter a rehabilitation program as soon as they are well enough, to protect their disability coverage.

The Social Security Administration (SSA) can help people with disabilities get the vocational rehabilitation services they need. Patients need to inquire at their local SSA office about these services; they may also contact their state rehabilitation agency. Vocational rehabilitation providers furnish a variety of services designed to provide the training or other services that are needed to help patients acquire gainful employment.

When a person is able to return to work, special rules, called *work incentives,* help them retain their current cash benefits (SSDI, SSI) and health insurance coverage (Medicare, Medicaid) during a trial work period. There are different work incentives for people who receive SSDI and SSI benefits. These incentives help people with disabilities to work by allowing them to test their ability to work for a specified period of time without losing any benefits.

SELECTED READINGS

Gaston RS, Hudson SL, Ward M, et al. Late allograft loss: noncompliance masquerading as chronic rejection. *Transplant Proc* 1999; 31:(Suppl 4A):21S.

Greenstein S, Siegal B. Compliance and noncompliance in patients with a functioning transplant: a multicultural study. *Transplantation* 1998;66:1718.

Kalil RSN, Heim-Dutoy KL, Kasiske BL. Patients with a low income have a reduced allograft survival. *Am J Kidney Dis* 1992;20:63.

Levenson J, Glochescki S. Psychological factors affecting end-stage renal disease. *Psychosomatics* 1991;32:4.

Markell SM, DiBenedetto A, Maursky V, et al. Unemployment in inner-city renal transplant recipients: predictive and sociodemographic factors. *Am J Kidney Dis* 1997;29:881.

Prieto LR, Miller DS, Gayowski T, et al. Multicultural issues in organ transplantation: the influence of patients' cultural perspectives on compliance with treatment. *Clin Transplant* 1997;11:529.

Rudman L, Gonzales MH, Borgida E. Mishandling the gift of life: noncompliance in renal transplant patients. *J Appl Soc Psychol* 1999; 29:4.

Sanders CE, Julian BA, Gaston RS, et al. Benefits of continued cyclosporine through an indigent drug program. *Am J Kidney Dis* 1996; 28:572.

Thamer M, Henderson SC, Fox Ray N, et al. Unequal access to cadaveric transplantation in California based on insurance status. *Health Services Res* 1999;34:879.

Subject Index

A

ABO blood group, distribution of kidney transplants, 53

Abscess
features and imaging, 279–280
pancreas transplantation complication, 326

Accelerated acute rejection, 32–33, 37, 173–174

Acquired cystic disease, dialysis complication, 12

Acute rejection. *See* Rejection, renal graft

Acute transplant glomerulopathy, 295–296

Acute tubular necrosis (ATN)
fine-needle aspiration cytology, 310
histopathology, 302
imaging, 283, 285
kidney donors, 124
posttransplantation patients course, 170–172
immunologic consequences, 172
oliguria etiology, 171
prevention and management, 173

Adenovirus, 260

Adherence. *See* Compliance

Age
donors for cadaveric renal transplantation, 121–123
effects on transplantation outcome
donor age, 59, 194
recipient age, 58–59, 141–142
pediatric kidney transplantation
donor age, 337
effects on growth, 359
recipient age, 336–337

Alcohol, posttransplantation effects, 408

Allogeneic graft, definition, 17

Allograft failure. *See* Late renal allograft failure

Allorecognition
accessory molecules, 25–26
cytokine functions, 31
pathways, 22–23
T cell receptor–CD3 antigen complex, 23–25

Alport's syndrome
effects on pediatric kidney transplantation outcome, 340
primary disease effects on transplantation outcome, 136–137

Amphotericin B
calcineurin inhibitor interactions, 71
formulations and toxicity, 252–253

Amyloidosis
dialysis complication, 11–12
primary disease effects on transplantation outcome, 137

Anemia, posttransplantation, 180–181, 214

Angiotensin-converting enzyme inhibitors
calcineurin inhibitor interactions, 71
late posttransplantation period
hypertension control, 208
reduction of proteinuria, 204–205

Anti-glomerular basement membrane disease, recurrence effects on pediatric kidney transplantation outcome, 341

Anti-HLA antibodies
classification of patient groups, 49
enzyme-linked immunosorbent assay, 49
flow cytometry crossmatch, 51–52
panel-reactive antibody, 49, 51
microcytotoxicity test, 44, 46, 48–49
panel-reactive antibody, 48–49
pretransplantation crossmatch, 51

Anti-HLA antibodies (*contd.*)
  T warm antibody, 48
  tissue typing, 44
Anuria, postoperative evaluation
    and management,
    166–168
Anxiety, treatment of, in post-
    transplantation period,
    376
Apoptosis, promotion of graft
    acceptance, 97
Arteriovenous fistula, imaging,
    288
Aspergillosis
  diagnosis, 250–252
  postoperative syndromes, 250
  prophylaxis, 252
  treatment, 252–253, 255
Aspirin, late posttransplantation
    period use, 211
Atgam
  dose and administration, 90
  indications, 85
  mode of action, 89
  side effects, 90
ATN. *See* Acute tubular necrosis
Autologous graft, definition, 17
Azathioprine
  dose and administration, 82,
    104
  history of use, 62, 81
  mode of action, 81
  pregnancy, 218
  side effects, 81–82

B
Bacteremia, diagnosis, 231
Banff 97 classification, 304–305
Barbiturates, calcineurin
    inhibitor interactions, 69
Basiliximab
  dosage and administration, 91
  indications, 85
  mechanism of action, 90–91
  side effects, 91
Biopsy. *See also* Fine-needle
    aspiration cytology
  core needle biopsy
    complications, 291–292
    technique, 290–291
  diagnostic capability, 290–291
  histopathologic findings in
    major causes of allograft
    dysfunction, 293

indications, 290
  protocol biopsy, 178, 205, 290
  specimen handling, 292
BK virus, 260, 303
Bleeding, postoperative,
    154–155, 168
Blood transfusion
  with immunosuppression
    therapy, 99
  presensitization and graft
    survival in children, 338
Bone loss. *See* Osteopenia;
    Osteoporosis
Bone marrow transplantation,
    with immunosuppression
    therapy, 99
Brain-dead donor
  diagnosis of brain death,
    124–125, 380–381
  management, 125–126

C
Cadaveric renal transplantation
  age of donors, 121–123
  brain-dead donors
    diagnosis of brain death,
      124–125, 380–381
    management, 125–126
  characteristics of donors, 121
  children as recipients, 333,
    335
  contraindications, 121–124
  failure. *See* Late renal allo-
    graft failure
  family consent, 120–121
  immunosuppressive therapy
    protocols, 102–105
  infants as donors, 121–122
  ischemia times, 127
  non–heart-beating donors, 124
  organ harvesting
    kidneys alone, 126–127
    kidneys with other organs,
      127
    pharmacologic adjuncts, 127
  outcomes versus live donor
    grafts, 55–56, 182–183
  preoperative factors promot-
    ing ischemic injury,
    171–172
  preservation of kidneys
    cold storage, 127–128
    Collins solution, 128
    machine perfusion, 127–128

University of Wisconsin solution, 128
reevaluation of patients on waiting list, 144
sequence of events, 120–121
supply and demand, 3, 9, 52, 111, 333, 380
tissue typing, 47
UNOS point system for allocation, 54

Calcineurin inhibitors. *See* Cyclosporine; Tacrolimus

Calcium, supplementation in late posttransplantation period, 212, 407

Calcium channel blockers
calcineurin inhibitor interactions, 70
immunosuppression therapy inclusion, 104–105
late posttransplantation period hypertension control, 208

Cancer
contraindication for kidney transplant recipients, 130
late posttransplantation period, 188–191
screening
late posttransplantation period, 209–210
transplant recipients, 132–133
transmission by donor organs, 124

Candidiasis
diagnosis, 250–251
postoperative syndromes, 249–250
prophylaxis, 252
treatment, 252–253, 255

CAPD, 7–9, 13

Carbamazepine, calcineurin inhibitor interactions, 69

Cardiovascular disease (CVD)
diabetic transplant recipient screening, 314–316
dialysis complications of, 10
late posttransplantation period risk factors
coagulation abnormalities, 186
diabetes, 185
hematocrit elevation, 186
homocysteine elevation, 187

hyperlipidemia, 185
hypertension, 186
infection, 187
overview, 183–184
oxidative stress, 186–187
smoking, 185
pancreas transplantation outcomes in diabetics, 329
pediatric kidney recipient evaluation, 344–345
posttransplantation, 362
primary disease effects on transplantation outcome, 139–140, 184–185

Carrel patch, artery anastomosis, 148

CCPD, 7–9

CD3
anti-CD3 immunotoxin for immunosuppression therapy, 97
T cell receptor complex, 23–25

Child kidney transplantations
access to transplantation, 333, 335
acute rejection
diagnosis, 355
incidence, 354–355
refractory rejection, 356–357
treatment, 355–356
compliance
adolescent kidney recipients, 344, 357
improvement strategies for, 358
incidence, 357
measurement, 357
prediction, 357
psychological intervention, 358
donor evaluation, 343
en bloc transplantation, 151
end-stage renal disease
etiology, 333–335
incidence, 332–333
evaluation of recipient
cardiovascular disease, 344–345
infection, 345
nephrotic syndrome, 347
neuropsychiatric development, 343–344
peritoneal dialysis patients, 346–347

Child kidney transplantations, evaluation of recipient (*contd.*)
portal hypertension, 347
psychoemotional status, 344
renal osteodystrophy, 346
urologic problems, 345–346
Wilms' tumor, 347
growth
age of recipient, effects on, 359
allograft function effects, 360
corticosteroid dosing, 359
growth hormone therapy, 359–360
retardation assessment, 358
hypertension and cardio-vascular disease, post-transplantation, 362
immunosuppressive therapy
antibody induction, 354
corticosteroids, 351–353
cyclosporine, 351, 353
mycophenolate mofetil, 354
regimens, overview, 349–351
tacrolimus, 351, 353–354
tapering of dose, 352
infection, posttransplantation
antibiotic prophylaxis, 362
bacterial infection, 360–361
viral infection, 361–362
intraoperative management, 348–349
nutritional support, 348
postoperative management, 349
predialysis transplantation, 347–348
preoperative preparation, 348
prognostic factors influencing graft survival
age of donor, 337
age of recipient, 336–337
antibody induction, 339
cohort year, 339
donor source, 336
HLA matching, 338
immunological factors, 338
metabolic diseases, 342–343
presensitization, 338
race, 337–338
recurrence of original renal disease, 339–342

technical factors and delayed graft function, 338–339
transplantation center volume, 339
rehabilitation, 362–363
sexual maturation following transplantation, 360
surgical considerations, 150
survival of patients and grafts, 336
timing, 335
Chimerism, induction, 35–36, 99
Cholelithiasis, primary disease effects on transplantation outcome, 140
Chronic allograft nephropathy
clinical presentation, 192
differential diagnosis, 299
histopathology, 192, 194, 298–299
risk factors
alloantigen-dependent, 191–193
alloantigen-independent, 191, 193–196
Chronic rejection. *See* Rejection, renal graft
Clinical trials, immunosup-pressive drugs
acute rejection episodes as end points, 93–96
design, 93
overview of procedures, 92–93
Clostridium difficile, manage-ment of infection, 235, 240
CMV. *See* Cytomegalovirus
COBRA. *See* Consolidated Bud-get Reconciliation Act
Coccidioidomycosis, serologic testing, 225
Cold ischemia time, 127
Collins solution, kidney storage, 128
Compliance
chronic allograft nephrop-athy, noncompliance as risk factor, 193
ethics of perceived noncompli-ance in selection, 389
late allograft failure role of noncompliance, 198–199, 415–416

noncompliance as contraindication for kidney transplant recipients, 132
pediatric kidney recipient
  adolescent compliance, 344, 357
  improvement strategies, 358
  incidence, 357
  measurement, 357
  prediction, 357
  psychological intervention, 358
prevention of noncompliance in late posttransplantation period, 203–204
psychiatric evaluation of kidney recipients, 371–372
psychosocial issues of noncompliance, 415–417
reasons for noncompliance, 198–199
risk factors for noncompliance, 415
Computed tomographic angiography (CTA), donor evaluation, 273–274
Computed tomographic urography (CTU), donor evaluation, 273–275
Congenital nephrotic syndrome, recurrence effects on pediatric kidney transplantation outcome, 341–342
Consolidated Budget Reconciliation Act (COBRA), 418
Continuous ambulatory peritoneal dialysis (CAPD), 7–9, 13
Continuous cycling peritoneal dialysis (CCPD), 7–9
Contraindications, kidney transplant recipients
  chronic infection, 130–131
  malignancy, 130
  noncompliance history, 132
  psychiatric illness, 132
  severe extrarenal disease, 131–132
Core needle biopsy. See Biopsy
Corticosteroids
  cadaveric renal transplantation protocols, 104

calcineurin inhibitor interactions, 71
complications, 83
cytokine expression inhibition, 82–83
growth retardation and dosing, 359
history of use, 62, 82
immunosuppression mechanisms, 82, 83
osteopenia induction and prevention, 211–212
pediatric kidney transplantation, 351–353, 355, 359
prednisolone, 62, 84, 217, 353
pregnancy, prednisone use, 217
preparations, 83–84
pulse steroids in rejection management, 106–107
receptors, 82–83
withdrawal, 105–106, 202
Costs. See Health care costs
Creatinine
  late posttransplantation period monitoring, 204
  posttransplant elevation, 177–178
Cross-reacting group matching, 47–48
Cryptococcosis
  postoperative syndromes, 249–250
  treatment, 252–253, 255
CTA. See Computed tomographic angiography
CTU. See Computed tomographic urography
CVD. See Cardiovascular disease
Cyclosporine
  cadaveric renal transplantation protocols, 102–103
  chronic allograft nephropathy risk factor, 194
  comparison with tacrolimus, 64, 100
  concentration monitoring, 68–69, 178–179
  cosmetic complications, 76
  distribution, 67
  drug interactions
    lipid-lowering agents, 71
    nephrotoxicity enhancers, 71
    nutrient interactions, 396–397

Cyclosporine, drug interactions
(*contd.*)
  P450 inducers, 69–70
  P450 inhibitors, 70–71
  psychotropic drugs, 378
  sirolimus, 80
fine-needle aspiration cytol-
    ogy of nephrotoxicity, 311
formulations, 65–67, 103
gastrointestinal toxicity, 75
generic formulations, 66–67
glucose intolerance as a side
    effect, 76
gout and, 77
histopathology of nephro-
    toxicity
  acute toxicity, 299–300
  chronic toxicity, 301
  differential diagnosis,
    301–302
  vascular effects, 300–301
history of use, 62
hyperlipidemia as a side
    effect, 76
malignancy and, 77
mechanism of action, 28–29,
    63, 65
metabolism, 67–68
nephrotoxicity
  acute microvascular disease,
    74
  amelioration, 75
  chronic interstitial fibrosis,
    73–74
  electrolyte abnormalities,
    74–75
  hypertension, 74
  renal blood flow and filtra-
    tion rate decrease, 72–73
neurotoxicity, 76
pediatric kidney transplanta-
    tion, 351, 353
pregnancy and, 218
residual host defense, 65
structure, 63
therapeutic ranges, 103
thromboembolism association,
    77
withdrawal, 202
Cytokines
  calcineurin inhibition effects
    in immunosuppression,
    65
  expression inhibition by corti-
    costeroids, 82–83
  release in acute rejection, 33
  types and functions, 29–31
Cytomegalovirus (CMV)
  cardiovascular disease risk
    factor, 187
  classification of infection,
    255–256
  diagnosis, 256–258
  graft rejection role, 34–35
  pediatric kidney recipient
    evaluation, 345
  posttransplantation, 361
  prophylaxis, 258–259
  serologic testing, 225–226
  syndromes, 256
  treatment, 258

D
Daclizumab
  dosage and administration, 91
  indications, 85
  mechanism of action, 90–91
  side effects, 91
Delayed graft function (DGF)
  chronic allograft nephropathy
    risk factor, 193–194
  differential diagnosis,
    170–171
  effect on graft survival, 172
  pediatric kidney transplanta-
    tion, 338–339
  prevention and management,
    173
Delirium, treatment in post-
    transplantation period,
    375
Delusion, treatment in post-
    transplantation period,
    378
Demographics, end-stage renal
    disease
  United States, 2–3
  worldwide, 3
Department of Health and
    Human Services, 387
Depression, treatment in post-
    transplantation period,
    376–377
DGF. *See* Delayed graft function
Diabetes mellitus
  cardiovascular disease risk
    factor, 185
  effects on transplantation out-
    come, 135

end-stage renal disease association, 2–3, 313
impact on renal patient survival, 14
insulin requirements after
transplantation, 316–317
kidney–pancreas transplantation
indications, 329
nutrition, 401
outcomes, 321–322
pancreas transplantation
following kidney, 321
preuremic pancreas trans-
plantation, 321
simultaneous transplanta-
tions, 321
late posttransplantation
period, 197–198
nutritional management, 404
pancreas transplantation. *See*
Pancreas transplantation
posttransplantation complications
bone disease, 319
hyperlipidemia, 319
hypertension, 318–319
neuropathy, 318
peripheral vascular disease,
318
pseudorejection, 317
recurrent diabetic
nephropathy, 319
rejection, 317
retinopathy, 318
urinary tract infection, 317
predialysis transplantation
recommendations, 316
pregnancy following transplantation, 319
preoperative assessment for
kidney transplantation.
See also Recipient evaluation, kidney trans-
plantation
cerebrovascular disease, 316
coronary artery disease,
314–316
infection, 316
peripheral vascular disease,
316
preoperative preparation,
316–317
Diltiazem, calcineurin inhibitor
interactions, 70

Disability insurance
Social Security disability
income, 417–418
state programs, 417
DNA typing, human leukocyte
antigens, 46–47

E
EBV. *See* Epstein-Barr virus
ELISA. *See* Enzyme-linked
immunosorbent assay
End-stage renal disease (ESRD)
costs of therapy, 14
demographics. *See* Demo-
graphics, end-stage renal
disease
epidemiology in children,
332–335
initiation of therapy, 15–16
neuropsychiatric effects in
children, 343–344
survival. *See* Survival
Enzyme-linked immunosorbent
assay (ELISA), anti-HLA
antibodies, 49
Epstein-Barr virus (EBV)
pediatric kidney recipient
evaluation, 345
posttransplantation, 361
posttransplantation lymphoproliferative disease role,
213
serologic testing, 225
Erythrocytosis, posttransplantation, 214–215
Erythromycin, calcineurin
inhibitor interactions, 70
ESRD. *See* End-stage renal
disease
Ethical and legal issues in
kidney transplantation
allocation of organs, 385–386
anencephalic organ donors,
385
cadaveric organ donors
determination of death,
380–381
shortage, 380
financial inducement for
donation, 371, 383–384
gifting of kidneys, 384–385
living donor ethical dilemmas,
381–383

Ethical and legal issues in
kidney transplantation
(*contd.*)
organ donor card, family veto,
386
required request laws, 388
resource allocation issues,
390–392
selection of patients for transplantation
equitable selection and
access, 388–389
foreign nationals as potential recipients, 389–390
perceived noncompliance in
selection, 389
tensions within the U.S.
transplantation system
states versus federal
government, 387–388
United Network for Organ
Sharing versus Depart-
ment of Health and
Human Services, 387
xenografts, 385
Exercise, posttransplantation
benefits, 408

F

Fabry's disease, primary disease
effects on transplantation
outcome, 138
Family Medical Leave Act
(FMLA), 418–419
Fever
OKT3 side effect, 87
posttransplantation, 177, 233
Fine-needle aspiration cytology
acute cellular rejection
differential diagnosis, 309
immunochemical stains, 308
May-Grünwald-Giemsa
stain, 308
acute tubular necrosis, 310
calcineurin inhibitor nephrotoxicity, 311
diagnostic uses and limitations, 306
donor kidneys, 305
indications, 306
infection
bacterial infection, 309–310
differential diagnosis, 309

fungal infection, 309–310
viral infection, 309
interpretation of
leukocytes, 307
parenchymal cells, 307
processing, 306–307
technique, 306
Fish oil supplementation, 407
FK506. *See* Tacrolimus
Flow cytometry
crossmatch, 51–52
panel-reactive antibody, 49,
51
Fluconazole
calcineurin inhibitor interactions, 70
indications for use, 253, 255
FMLA. *See* Family Medical
Leave Act
Focal segmental glomerulosclerosis (FSGS)
histopathology, 303
late posttransplantation
period, 196–197
primary disease effects on
transplantation outcome,
136
recurrence effects on pediatric
kidney transplantation
outcome, 339–340
FSGS. *See* Focal segmental
glomerulosclerosis
FTY720, immunosuppression
therapy, 96
Fungemia, diagnosis, 231

G

Gastrointestinal complications,
kidney transplantation
surgery, 158–159
Glomerular filtration rate (GFR)
calcineurin inhibitor effects,
72–73
donor criteria, 115
initiation of renal replacement therapy, 15–16
isotopic techniques for measurement, 289
pediatric growth, allograft
function effects, 360
pregnancy, 217
Glucose intolerance, calcineurin
inhibitor side effect, 76

Goodpasture's syndrome, primary disease effects on transplantation outcome, 136

Gout, calcineurin inhibitor side effect, 77

Graft rejection. *See* Rejection, renal graft

Growth hormone, pediatric kidney recipient therapy, 359–360

H

Half-life, allografts, 182–183

Hallucinations, treatment in posttransplantation period, 387

Health care costs. *See also* Medicare
immunosuppressive therapy, 416–417
rationing, 391–392
transplantation versus dialysis, 413–414
United States, 391

Hematocrit
elevation as cardiovascular disease risk factor, 186
posttransplantation levels, 215

Hematoma, features and imaging, 276

Hematuria, pancreas transplantation complication, 326

Hemodialysis
adequacy, 5–6
comparison with peritoneal dialysis, 7–8
complications, 1, 4–6
acquired cystic disease, 12
amyloidosis, 11–12
cardiovascular disease, 10
renal osteodystrophy, 10–11
uremic neuropathy, 11
vascular access failure, 12
costs, 14
effects on transplantation outcome, 60
efficiency, 1, 5–6
facilities, 3
initiation of therapy, 15–16
posttransplantation dialysis, 168–169
principle, 4

psychosocial stress, 413
quality of life, 15
survival of patients, 13–14
technical advances, 9
vascular access, 6–7

Hemolytic-uremic syndrome (HUS)
calcineurin inhibitor nephrotoxicity, 74, 175, 300–301, 341
histopathology, 300–301
recurrence effects on pediatric kidney transplantation outcome, 341

Henoch-Schönlein purpura, recurrence effects on pediatric kidney transplantation outcome, 341

Hepatitis B
antiviral therapy, 266–267
donor disease effect on recipients, 270
effects on transplantation outcome, 263
natural history, 263–265
phases of chronic infection, 264
pretransplantation liver biopsy, 265–266
progression following renal transplantation, 265
serologic testing, 225, 263

Hepatitis C
antiviral therapy, 269
donor disease effect on recipients, 270
natural history, 268
pretransplantation liver biopsy, 269
progression following renal transplantation, 268
recommendations in transplantation, 269–270
serologic testing, 225, 267–268

Hereditary nephritis, patients as donors, 116

Herpes simplex virus (HSV)
management of infection, 259–260
pediatric recipient infection, 362

Histamine blockers, calcineurin inhibitor interactions, 70–71

Histoplasmosis, serologic testing, 225
HIV. *See* Human immunodeficiency virus
HLA. *See* Human leukocyte antigen
Homocysteine
  cardiovascular disease risk factor, 187
  effects on graft survival, 195
  nutritional management, 402
HSV. *See* Herpes simplex virus
Human herpesviruses, 260
Human immunodeficiency virus (HIV)
  contraindication for kidney transplant recipients, 131
  serologic testing, 224–225
  transmission in transplantation, 123, 225
Human leukocyte antigen (HLA)
  class I antigens, 19–20, 39
  class II antigens, 20, 39
  genotypes, 43
  heredity, 41–42
  linkage disequilibrium, 43
  matches and mismatches, 43–44
  nomenclature, 39, 41
  phenotypes, 42–43
  specificities, 40–41
  structure, 41
  tissue typing. *See* Anti-HLA antibodies; Tissue typing
  twins, 43
Humanized anti-Tac. *See* Basiliximab; Daclizumab
HUS. *See* Hemolytic-uremic syndrome
Hyperacute rejection, 32
Hypercalcemia, posttransplantation, 180
Hyperchloremic metabolic acidosis, posttransplantation, 180
Hyperkalemia
  calcineurin inhibitor association, 74–75
  posttransplantation, 180, 398, 407
Hyperlipidemia
  cardiovascular disease risk factor, 185, 395

chronic allograft nephropathy risk factor, 195
  in diabetic kidney transplant recipients, 319
  immunosuppressive therapy tailoring, 202–203
  late posttransplantation period management, 205–206
  nutritional management, 395, 402, 406
Hyperoxaluria
  primary disease effects on transplantation outcome, 138
  type I effects on pediatric kidney transplantation outcome, 342
Hypertension
  advantages and disadvantages of specific antihypertensive agents, 207–208
  calcineurin inhibitor association, 74
  cardiovascular disease risk factor, 186
  chronic allograft nephropathy risk factor, 195
  combination therapy, 208
  in diabetic kidney transplant recipients, 318–319
  late posttransplantation period management, 206–209
  nutritional management, 403–404
  in pediatric kidney recipients, 362
  renal artery stenosis association, 208–209
Hypoalbuminemia, effect on transplantation outcome, 405
Hypomagnesemia
  calcineurin inhibitor association, 75
  posttransplantation, 180, 212, 398–399, 407
Hypophosphatemia
  late posttransplantation period, 212
  posttransplantation, 180, 398

I

IL-2. *See* Interleukin-2
Immunizations
  late posttransplantation
    period, 210–211
  pediatric kidney recipient
    evaluation, 345
  pretransplantation period,
    225, 227
  varicella zoster virus, 262
Immunoglobulin A nephropathy, recurrence effects on
  pediatric kidney trans-
  plantation outcome, 341
Immunologic evaluation of
  transplantation candi-
  dates. *See* Anti-HLA antibodies; Tissue typing
Immunosuppressive therapy.
    See also specific drugs
  acute rejection management,
    106–108
  cadaveric transplants, 102–105
  cancer risks, 191
  children
    antibody induction, 354,
      416–417
    corticosteroids, 351–353
    cyclosporine, 351, 353
    mycophenolate mofetil, 354
    regimens, overview of,
      349–351
    tacrolimus, 351, 353–354
    tapering of dose, 352
  chronic allograft nephropathy
    risk reduction, 193
  clinical trials
    acute rejection episodes as
      end points, 93–96
    design, 93
    overview of procedures,
      92–93
  compliance. *See* Compliance
  historical perspective, 62–63
  interference with T cell acti-
    vation, 28–29
  live donor transplants, 105
  nutrient interactions,
    396–397
  pancreas transplantation, 327
  pregnancy
    azathioprine, 218
    cyclosporine, 218
    mycophenolate mofetil, 218
    prednisone, 217

protocol design
  adjunctive agent selection,
    100–101
  antibody induction therapy,
    101
  calcineurin inhibitor selec-
    tion, 100
  components, 99–100
  duration, 102
  overview, 99–100
  risk stratification of
    patients, 101–102
  psychotropic drug inter-
    actions, 378–379
  reduction in late posttrans-
    plantation period,
    200–203
  tailoring, 202–203
  withdrawal protocols, 105–106
Infection
  bacterial pathogens and infec-
    tion sites, 228–229, 231,
    233–243
  cancer association, 189
  cardiovascular disease risk
    factor, 187
  diagnosis
    bacteremia, 231
    fungemia, 231
    pneumonia, 232
    urinary tract infection, 232
    wound infection, 233
  dosages of antimicrobials
    antibiotics, 244–245
    antifungals, 247
    antivirals, 246
  empirical antibiotic therapy,
    243
  fever, 177, 233
  fine-needle aspiration cytology
    bacterial infection, 309–310
    differential diagnosis, 309
    fungal infection, 309–310
    viral infection, 309
  foodborne infections, 405
  fungal infection, 243, 247–255
  histopathology, 303
  late posttransplantation
    period, 187–188
  management. *See specific*
    pathogens
  mixed infection management,
    241–242
  nonbacterial pathogens and
    infection sites, 228, 230

Infection (*contd.*)
  pathogenesis in kidney allo-
    graft recipients, 227–231,
    233, 238
  pediatric kidney recipient
    evaluation, 345
  pneumonitis pathogens and
    treatment, 248–249
  postoperative characteristics
    and management, 153,
    231
  pregnancy, posttransplanta-
    tion, 217
  pretransplantation screening
    in recipient and donor,
    222–227
  recognition guidelines,
    221–222
  risk factors, 222–223
  specific antibiotic therapy, 243
  time of posttransplantation
    onset, 221–222
  transmissible infections in
    transplantation, 227
  viral infection, 255–262
Influenza
  immunization in late post-
    transplantation period,
    210–211
  management, 261
Insomnia, treatment in posttransplantation period,
  375–376
Interferon-alpha, hepatitis
  treatment, 266–267, 269
Interleukin-2 (IL-2)
  antibodies in graft rejection
    prevention, 29
  expression in T cell activation,
    26
Interstitial fibrosis, calcineurin
  inhibitor nephrotoxicity,
  73–74, 301
Intravenous immunoglobulin
  (IVIG), immunosup-
  pression therapy aug-
  mentation, 99
Iron, posttransplantation
  requirements, 399–400
Ischemia-reperfusion injury,
  transplanted kidneys,
  171–172
Ischemia times
  cold ischemia time, 127
  rewarm time, 127
  warm ischemia time, 127

Itraconazole, indications for use,
  253
IVIG. *See* Intravenous
  immunoglobulin

J
JC virus, 260

K
Ketoconazole
  calcineurin inhibitor inter-
    actions, 70, 255
  indications for use, 253
Kidney–pancreas transplantation. *See* Pancreas transplantation

L
Lamivudine, hepatitis B treatment, 267
Late renal allograft failure
  acute rejection, 196
  chronic allograft nephrop-
    athy, 191–196
  death versus end-stage renal
    disease as cause, 183
  mortality causes
    cardiovascular disease,
      183–187
    infection, 187–188
    malignancy, 188–191
  noncompliance role, 198–199
  renal disease, recurrent and
    de novo, 196–198
Left ventricular hypertrophy
  (LVH), renal disease
  patients, 10
Legal issues. *See* Ethical and
  legal issues in kidney
  transplantation
Legionella, management of
  infection, 234, 240
Leukopenia, posttransplantation, 181
LFA-1. *See* Lymphocyte function-
  associated antigen-1
Linkage disequilibrium, human
  leukocyte antigens, 43
Listeria monocytogenes, management of infection,
  237–238

Liver disease. *See also* Hepatitis B; Hepatitis C
  effects on transplantation outcome, 140–141
  indications for liver–kidney transplantation, 141–142
Living kidney donation
  advantages and disadvantages, 111–112
  classification of donors, 381
  confidentiality rights of donors, 370–371
  donor criteria, 111–113
  ethical dilemmas, 381–385
  evaluation of donors
    exclusion criteria, 115
    fine-needle aspiration cytology, 305
    hereditary renal disease, 115–116
    infection screening, 222–227, 270
    for pediatric recipients, 343
    psychiatric evaluation, 367, 369–371
    psychosocial evaluation, 114–115
    radiologic evaluation, 272–274
    screening, 113–114
    selection among multiple donors, 116
    surgical evaluation, 116
  financial inducement for donation, 371, 383–384
  gifting of kidneys, 384–385
  immunosuppressive therapy, 105
  nephrectomy, 117–120
  outcomes versus cadaveric renal transplantation, 55–56
Lovastatin
  calcineurin inhibitor interactions, 71
  immunosuppression therapy inclusion, 105
  late posttransplantation period use, 205–206
LVH. *See* Left ventricular hypertrophy
Lymphocele
  diagnosis, 153, 278
  postoperative, 154
  presentation, 153, 278
  treatment, 154

Lymphocyte function-associated antigen-1 (LFA-1), allorecognition role, 25

M
Magnetic resonance imaging (MRI)
  donor evaluation, 274
  lymphocele, 278
Major histocompatibility complex (MHC). *See also* Human leukocyte antigen
  antigen presentation, 17–18
  class I antigens, 19–20
  class II antigens, 20
  genes, 17–18, 20
  minor histocompatibility antigen, 22
Malignancy. *See* Cancer
Malnutrition. *See* Nutrition
Mania, treatment in posttransplantation period, 377–378
May-Grünwald-Giemsa stain, acute cellular rejection, 308
Medicare
  End Stage Renal Disease Program prospects, 390–392
  immunosuppressive therapy coverage, 416–417
  reimbursement for transplantation, 1
Membranoproliferative glomerulonephritis (MPGN)
  histopathology, 303
  late posttransplantation period, 196–197
  recurrence effects on pediatric kidney transplantation outcome, 340–341
Membranous nephropathy, recurrence effects on pediatric kidney transplantation outcome, 342
MHC. *See* Major histocompatibility complex
Microcytotoxicity test
  antihuman globulin enhancement, 49
  panel-reactive antibody, 48–49
  T warm antibody, 48
  tissue typing, 44, 46

Minor histocompatibility antigen, 22, 43

MMF. *See* Mycophenolate mofetil

Mortality, late posttransplantation causes
- cardiovascular disease, 183–187
- infection, 187–188
- malignancy, 188–191

MPGN. *See* Membranoproliferative glomerulonephritis

MRI. *See* Magnetic resonance imaging

Mycobacterial infection, management, 241

Mycophenolate mofetil (MMF)
- cadaveric renal transplantation protocols, 104
- clinical trial design, 94–96
- drug interactions, 79
- ERL080A, 96
- mechanism of action, 77–78
- pediatric kidney transplantation, 354
- pharmacology, 78
- pregnancy, 218
- protocol design, 100–101
- safety, 78–79

N

National Organ Transplant Act, 52, 384–385

Nephrectomy
- allograft nephrectomy
  - complications, 160
  - indications, 159–160
  - technique, 160
- living kidney donors
  - approach, 119
  - complications, 119–120
  - endoscopically-assisted procedures, 117–118
  - open versus laparoscopic nephrectomy, 117, 119
  - postoperative management, 118–119
- pretransplantation native nephrectomy indications, 134

Nephropathic cystinosis, effects on pediatric kidney transplantation outcome, 342–343

Neuropathy
- diabetic kidney transplant recipients, 318
- pancreas transplantation outcomes in diabetics, 328

NIH test. *See* Microcytotoxicity test

Nitric oxide, calcineurin inhibitor nephrotoxicity effects, 72–73

Nocardiosis, management, 237–238, 240

Noncompliance. *See* Compliance

Nonsteroidal antiinflammatory drugs, calcineurin inhibitor interactions, 71

Nutrition management
- acute posttransplantation concerns
  - drug–nutrient interactions, 396–397
  - fluid and electrolyte balance, 396
  - protein catabolism, 395
- importance of exercise, 408
- long-term management concerns
  - bone loss, 403
  - diabetes, 404
  - foodborne infections, 405
  - herbal supplements, 405
  - homocysteine elevation, 402
  - hyperlipidemia, 402
  - hypertension, 403–404
  - hypoalbuminemia, 405
  - obesity, 402–403
  - renal disease progression, 404
- nutrient requirements in acute posttransplantation period
  - calories, 397
  - carbohydrates, 397–398
  - fat, 398
  - fluids, 399
  - magnesium, 398–399
  - phosphorous, 398
  - potassium, 398
  - protein, 397
  - sodium, 398
  - trace minerals, 399–400
  - vitamins, 399
- nutrient requirements in stable posttransplantation patients

calcium, 407
calories, 406
fat, 406
fish oil supplementation, 407
magnesium, 407
phosphorous, 407
potassium, 407
protein, 406
sodium, 407
trace minerals, 408
vitamins, 407–408
nutritional support in posttransplantation period
acute rejection, 401
indications for aggressive
intervention, 400
oral supplements, 400–401
pancreas–kidney recipients,
401
total parenteral nutrition,
401
tube feeding, 401
pediatric kidney transplantation, 348
pregnancy concerns, 408
pretransplantation management
assessment of nutritional
status, 395
dyslipidemia and cardio-
vascular disease, 395
malnutrition effects on
transplantation outcome,
142, 394
obesity, 142, 395

O

Obesity
effects on transplantation outcome, 142, 395
nutritional management,
402–403
OKT3
advantages and disadvantages
of antibody induction
therapy, 101
dosage and administration,
85–86
history of use, 62, 84
humanized form, 97
indications, 85
mode of action, 84–85
monitoring, 86–87

pediatric kidney transplantation, 354–356
rejection management,
106–108
side effects
cytokine release syndrome,
87
fever and chills, 87
hematologic complications,
89
infection, 88–89
nephrotoxicity, 88
neurologic complications, 88
pulmonary edema, 87–88
rejecton recurrence, 89
OKT4A, immunosuppression
therapy, 97
Oliguria, postoperative evaluation and management,
166–168, 179
Organ donor card, family veto,
386
Organ Procurement and Transplantation Network
(OPTN), 52
Osteonecrosis, late posttransplantation period,
211–212
Osteopenia
diabetic kidney transplant
recipients, 319
nutritional management, 403
prevention in late posttransplantation period,
211–212

P

Pancreas transplantation
cadaveric transplantation, 320
complications
enzyme leak, 324–325
graft pancreatitis, 325
hematuria, 326
intraabdominal abscess, 326
metabolic abnormalities, 327
overview, 323–324
urethritis, 326
urinary tract infection, 326
urine leak, 324–325
vascular thrombosis,
325–326
immunosuppressive therapy,
327
islet transplantation, 330–331

Pancreas transplantation
(*contd.*)
  kidney–pancreas trans-
    plantation
    indications, 329
    nutrition, 401
    outcomes, 321–322
    pancreas transplantation
      following kidney, 321
    preuremic pancreas trans-
      plantation, 321
    simultaneous transplanta-
      tions, 321
  options with kidney trans-
    plantation, 320–321
  quality of life, 329
  rejection diagnosis, 327
  secondary diabetic complica-
    tion outcomes
    coronary artery disease, 329
    microcirculation, 328–329
    nephropathy, 328
    neuropathy, 328
    retinopathy, 328
  surgical techniques
    bladder drainage, 323,
      326–327
    enteric drainage of exocrine
      secretions, 322
    systemic versus portal
      venous drainage, 323
  survival, 329
Pancreatitis, primary disease
  effects on transplantation
  outcome, 140
Panel-reactive antibody, 48–49,
  51, 56, 193
Paraproteinemia, primary disease effects on transplantation outcome, 137
Parathyroid hormone (PTH),
  alterations in dialysis
  patients, 10–11
Parvovirus B19, 261
Pediatric renal transplantation.
  See Child kidney transplantations
Peptic ulcer disease, primary
  disease effects on transplantation outcome, 140
Peritoneal dialysis
  comparison with hemo-
    dialysis, 7–8
  complications, 7–8
  initiation of therapy, 15–16

  modes, 7
  pediatric kidney recipient
    evaluation, 346–347
  posttransplantation dialysis,
    169
  principle, 7
  psychosocial stress, 413
  quality of life, 15
  survival of patients, 13–14
  technical advances, 9
Phenytoin, calcineurin inhibitor
  interactions, 69
Photopheresis, immuno-
  suppression therapy
  augmentation, 99
Pneumococcal pneumonia,
  immunization in late
  posttransplantation
  period, 210–211
Pneumocystosis carnii pneumonia, management, 255
Pneumonia, diagnosis, 232
Pneumonitis, pathogens and
  treatment, 248–249
Polycystic kidney disease
  infection, 224
  patients as donors, 115–116
  primary disease effects on
    transplantation outcome,
    137–138
Polyuria, postoperative evaluation and management,
  168
Portal hypertension, pediatric
  kidney recipient evaluation, 347
Posttransplantation care
  antimicrobial prophylaxis,
    242–243
  children. *See* Child kidney
    transplantations
  classification of postoperative
    time periods, 163, 182
  failure. *See* Late renal allo-
    graft failure
  first day
    anuria, 166–168
    bleeding, 168
    dialysis indications,
      168–169
    hemodynamic evaluation,
      164–165
    intravenous fluid replace-
      ment, 165–166
    oliguria, 166–168

orders, 164
polyuria, 168
recovery room assessment, 163
first two months
clinical course, 176–177
differentiation of infection, rejection, and cyclosporine toxicity, 177–179
laboratory findings, 179–181
patient education, 176
first week
acute tubular necrosis management, 170–173
delayed graft function patient management, 170–173
excellent graft function patient management, 169–170
incision care, 176
medical management, 175
nonimmunologic causes of dysfunction, 174–175
normal course, 169
rejection, 173–174
slow graft function patient management, 170
late posttransplantation period
aspirin therapy, 211
bone loss prevention, 211–212
cancer screening, 209–210
hematologic disorders, 214–215
hyperlipidemia management, 205–206
hypertension management, 206–209
immunizations, 210–211
immunosuppressive therapy reduction, 200–203
noncompliance prevention, 203–204
posttransplantation lymphoproliferative disease, 212–214
preventive medicine, 199–200
protocol biopsies, 205
renal function monitoring, 204–205

reproductive function, 215–218
smoking cessation, 209
nutrition. *See* Nutrition management
radiology in early posttransplantation period
collecting system dilation, 275–276
size of allograft, 274
Posttransplantation lymphoproliferative disease (PTLD)
clonality, 214
comparison with lymphomas, 212–213
Epstein-Barr virus and, 213
incidence, 212
treatment, 214
Prednisolone. *See* Corticosteroids
Pregnancy
antenatal care, 217
conception rates following transplantation, 216
counseling of transplant patients, 215–216
criteria for posttransplantation risk reduction, 216–217
diabetic kidney transplant recipients, 319
immunosuppressive therapy
azathioprine, 218
cyclosporine, 218
mycophenolate mofetil, 218
prednisone, 217
labor and delivery, 218
nutritional management, 408–409
Pretransplantation crossmatch, 51
Proteinuria
chronic allograft nephropathy risk factor, 195–196
late posttransplantation period monitoring, 204–205
Protocol biopsy. *See* Biopsy
Pseudoaneurysm, imaging, 288
Psychiatric aspects of kidney transplantation
biopsychosocial model framework, 365
donor evaluation, 367, 369–371

Psychiatric aspects of kidney
transplantation (*contd.*)
economic factors, 367
immunosuppressant and
psychotropic drug inter-
actions, 378–379
onset of renal failure, 366–367
recipient, pretransplant
evaluation
cognitive disorders,
372–373
compliance, 371–372
epidemiology of preexisting
disorders, 368
history, 373–374
interview, 368–369
substance abuse, 373
significance of end-stage renal
disease etiology, 365–366
treatment of posttransplantation psychiatric symptoms
anxiety, 376
delirium, 375
delusion, 378
depression, 376–377
hallucinations, 387
insomnia, 375–376
mania, 377–378
psychotropic agent with-
drawal, 374–375
Psychosocial issues, kidney
transplantation
assessment, overview,
411–412
benefits of transplantation,
411, 413–414
noncompliance, 415–417
risks of transplantation,
414–416
PTH. *See* Parathyroid hormone
PTLD. *See* Posttransplantation
lymphoproliferative
disease

Q

Quality of life
dialysis patients, 15
pancreas transplantation
patients, 329

R

Race
ABO blood group distribution,
53

effects on transplantation outcome, 58, 201
pediatric kidney transplantation outcomes, 337–338
Radionuclide imaging
abscess, 279
acute tubular necrosis, 283,
285
collecting system dilation,
275–276
coronary artery stenosis, 314
glomerular filtration rate
measurement, 289
graft dysfunction evaluation,
283
renal artery thrombosis, 285
segmental renal infarction,
286
tracers and excretion, 277
Rapamycin. *See* Sirolimus
Recipient evaluation, kidney
transplantation
cancer screening, 132–133
children. *See* Child kidney
transplantations
contraindications. *See* Contraindications, kidney transplant recipients
diabetes patients. *See* Diabetes mellitus
history, 132
infection screening, 222–227
organ system diseases as risk
factors
cardiovascular disease,
139–140
cholelithiasis, 140
chronic pulmonary disease,
141
liver disease, 140–142
metabolic bone disease, 141
pancreatitis, 140
peptic ulcer disease, 140
seizure disorders, 141
patient education, 134–135
patient risk factors
age, 141–142
double organ transplant
patients, 143–144
malnutrition, 142
obesity, 142
peritoneal dialysis patients,
142
predialysis patients,
142–143

previously transplanted
patients, 143
sensitization, 143
physical examination, 132
primary kidney disease
features and effects on
outcomes
Alport's syndrome, 136–137
amyloidosis, 137
diabetes, 135
Fabry's disease, 138
focal glomerulosclerosis, 136
Goodpasture's syndrome, 136
hyperoxaluria, 138
paraproteinemia, 137
polycystic kidney disease,
137–138
scleroderma, 138
sickle cell disease, 139
systemic lupus erythematosus, 135–136
thrombophilic disorders,
136
thrombotic thrombocy-
topenic purpura, 138–139
Wegener's granulomatosis,
139
psychiatric evaluation. *See*
Psychiatric aspects of
kidney transplantation
reevaluation of patients on
waiting list, 144
routine and elective evaluations, 133
smoking cessation, 134
urologic evaluation, 134
Rejection, renal graft
accelerated acute rejection,
32–33, 173–174
acute rejection, 33
diagnosis, 355
immunosuppressive clinical
trial end point, 93–96
incidence, 354–355
late posttransplantation
period, 196
refractory rejection, 356–357
treatment, 355–356
borderline acute rejection, 205
cell-mediated rejection, 174
chronic rejection, 33–34
cytomegalovirus in rejection,
34–35
diabetic kidney transplant
recipients and, 317

diet in acute rejection, 401
duplex ultrasonography of
acute rejection, 279–280,
283
fever, 177
fine-needle aspiration cytology
of acute cellular rejection
differential diagnosis, 309
immunochemical stains, 308
May-Grünwald-Giemsa
stain, 308
first postoperative week,
173–174
histopathology
antibody-mediated acute
rejection, 296–297
Banff 97 classification,
304–305
cell-mediated acute rejection, 294–296
differential diagnosis of
acute rejection, 297–298
hyperacute rejection, 292,
294
hyperacute rejection, 32
imaging of chronic rejection,
286–287
immunosuppressive therapy
management
first rejection, 106
late rejections, 107–108
recurrent rejections, 107
mechanisms, 31
pseudorejection, 317
subclinical rejection, 178, 297
xenogeneic grafts, 37
Renal artery
connection in transplantation
surgery, 148
late posttransplantation
period monitoring,
208–209
stenosis, 155–156, 208–209,
287–288
thrombosis imaging, 285
Renal graft rejection. *See* Rejection, renal graft
Renal osteodystrophy
pediatric kidney recipient
evaluation, 346
dialysis complications, 10–11,
13
Renal vein
connection in transplantation
surgery, 149
thrombosis imaging, 286

Reproductive function, post-transplantation. *See also* Pregnancy
family planning, 215, 216
female, 215
male, 215
pediatric kidney recipients, 360
Respiratory syncytial virus (RSV), 261
Retinopathy
diabetic kidney transplant recipients, 318
pancreas transplantation outcomes in diabetics, 328
Rewarm time, 127
Ribavirin, hepatitis B treatment, 269
Rifampin, calcineurin inhibitor interactions, 69

S

Scleroderma, primary disease effects on transplantation outcome, 138
Seizure disorder
pediatric kidney recipients, 344
primary disease effects on transplantation outcome, 141
Sensitization
effects on transplantation outcome, 56, 58
sensitized recipients and transplantation outcome, 143
Sickle cell disease
effects on pediatric kidney transplantation outcome, 343
primary disease effects on transplantation outcome, 139
Sirolimus
clinical trial design, 95–96
drug interactions, 80
immunosuppressive regimens, 79, 104
mechanism of action, 79–80, 97
pharmacology, 80
rapamycin, 79
SDZ RAD, 96
side effects, 80–81

SLE. *See* Systemic lupus erythematosus
Social Security disability income, 417–418
Social work. *See* Psychosocial issues, kidney transplantation
St. John's Wort, immunosuppression drug interactions, 379
Substance abuse, psychiatric evaluation of potential kidney recipients, 373
Surgery, kidney transplantation
allograft nephrectomy
complications, 160
indications, 159–160
technique, 160
antimicrobial prophylaxis, 242–243
child considerations, 150
complications
bleeding, 154–155
diabetic recipients. *See* Diabetes mellitus
differential diagnosis, 152–153
gastrointestinal complications, 158–159
infection, 153, 231
lymphocele, 153–154
renal artery stenosis, 155–156
thrombosis of grafts, 155
ureteral obstruction, 157–158
urine leaks, 156–157
dual kidney transplantation, 151–152
intraoperative fluid management, 150
kidney removal from donors. *See* Nephrectomy
postoperative care. *See* Post-transplantation care
precautions for non-transplantation-related surgery in patients, 160–161
preoperative preparations, 146
technique
drains, 146, 150
incision, 147
infection avoidance, 146

multiple artery connections,
148–149
renal artery connection, 148
renal vein connection, 149
ureter attachment, 149
Survival
end-stage renal disease
patients
data analysis, 13
diabetes impact, 14
treatment modality effects,
13–14
of grafts, factors affecting
donor age, 59
donor type, 55–56
HLA matching, 56
miscellaneous factors, 60
racial differences, 58
recipient age, 58–59
sensitization, 56, 58
transplantation center variability, 59–60
pancreas transplantation
patients, 329
pediatric recipients and
grafts, 336
rates for grafts, 13, 182–183
Syngenic graft, definition, 17
Systemic lupus erythematosus
(SLE)
primary disease effects on
transplantation outcome,
135–136
recurrence effects on pediatric
kidney transplantation
outcome, 342

T
T cell
activation
cell cycle, 26, 28
immunosuppressive agent
interference, 28–29, 97
signal transduction, 28
signals, 26
allorecognition
accessory molecules, 25–26
cytokine functions, 31
pathways, 22–23
T cell receptor–CD3 antigen
complex, 23–25
antigen presentation, 19–20
tolerance induction, 35–36
T warm antibody, 48

Tacrolimus
cadaveric renal transplantation protocols, 103
cardiotoxicity, 77
chronic allograft nephropathy
risk factor, 194
comparison with cyclosporine,
64, 100
concentration monitoring,
68–69, 178–179
cosmetic complications, 76
distribution, 67
drug interactions
lipid-lowering agents, 71
nephrotoxicity enhancers,
71
P450 inducers, 69–70
P450 inhibitors, 70–71
sirolimus, 80
fine-needle aspiration cytology of nephrotoxicity, 311
FK506, 63, 304
formulations, 67
gastrointestinal toxicity, 75
glucose intolerance as side
effect, 76
gout association, 77
histopathology of nephro-
toxicity
acute toxicity, 299–300
chronic toxicity, 301
differential diagnosis,
301–302
vascular effects, 300–301
history of use, 63
indolyl-ASC, 96
malignancy association, 77
mechanism of action, 28–29,
63, 65
metabolism, 67–68
nephrotoxicity
acute microvascular disease,
74
amelioration, 75
chronic interstitial fibrosis,
73–74
electrolyte abnormalities,
74–75
hypertension, 74
renal blood flow and filtration rate decrease, 72–73
neurotoxicity, 76
pediatric kidney transplantation, 351, 353–354
residual host defense, 65

Tenderness, graft on palpation, 179
Thrombocytopenia, posttransplantation, 181
Thrombosis, grafts, 155
Thrombotic microangiopathy. *See* Hemolytic-uremic syndrome
Thrombotic thrombocytopenic purpura, primary disease effects on transplantation outcome, 138–139
Thymoglobulin
  dose and administration, 90
  indications, 85
  mode of action, 89
  side effects, 90
Tissue typing. *See also* Anti-HLA antibodies
  anti-HLA antisera, 44
  cadaveric renal transplantation, 47
  chronic allograft nephropathy risk factor, 192–193
  cross-reacting group matching, 47–48
  DNA typing, 46–47
  lymphocyte isolation, 44, 46
  microcytotoxicity test, 44, 46
  outcome effects of HLA matching, 56, 201
  pediatric kidney transplantation, 338
  six antigen match program, 54–55
Tolerance, induction, 35–36
Total parenteral nutrition, 401
Transaminitis, posttransplantation, 181
Tube feeding, 401
Tuberculosis
  management, 241
  screening in transplant recipients, 133

U
Ultrasonography
  arteriovenous fistula, 288
  collecting system dilation, 275
  duplex ultrasonography of acute rejection, 279–280, 283
  pseudoaneurysm, 288
  renal artery stenosis, 287–288

renal artery thrombosis, 285
renal vein thrombosis, 286
segmental renal infarction, 285–286
Uniform Determination of Death Act, 381
United Network for Organ Sharing (UNOS)
  Department of Health and Human Services tensions and, 387
  ethics of organ allocation, 385–386
  ethics of patient selection, 388–390
  foreign nationals as organ recipients, 389–390
  point system for kidney allocation, 54
  six antigen match program, 54–55
University of Wisconsin solution, kidney storage, 128
Uremic neuropathy, dialysis complication, 11
Ureter
  attachment in transplantation surgery, 149
  postoperative obstruction diagnosis, 157–158
  etiology, 158
  treatment, 158
Urethritis, pancreas transplantation complication, 326
Urinalysis, postoperative findings, 179–180
Urinary tract infection (UTI)
  diabetic kidney transplant recipients and, 317
  diagnosis, 232
  pancreas transplantation complication, 326
  pathogenesis in kidney allograft recipients, 228
Urine leak, postoperative diagnosis, 156–157
  etiology, 156
  treatment, 157
Urinoma, features and imaging, 276, 278

V
Varicella zoster virus (VZV) management, 259–262

pediatric recipient infection, 361

Vascular access failure, dialysis complication, 12

Verapamil, calcineurin inhibitor interactions, 70

Very late activation molecules (VLA), allorecognition role, 25–26

Vitamins, posttransplantation requirements, 399, 408

Vocational rehabilitation, 419

W

Waiting list
  organ distribution by
    ABO blood groups, 53
    HLA matching, 54–55
    waiting time, 54
  transplant listing criteria, 52

Warm ischemia time, 127

Wegener's granulomatosis

primary disease effects on transplantation outcome, 139

recurrence effects on pediatric kidney transplantation outcome, 342

Wilms' tumor, pediatric kidney recipient evaluation, 347

Withdrawal
  immunosuppressive therapy, 105–106
  psychotropic agent withdrawal following transplantation, 374–375

X

Xenogeneic graft
  concordant versus discordant, 36–37
  definition, 17
  ethics, 385
  rejection mechanisms, 37